MANAGEMENT FOR NURSES

A multidisciplinary approach

MANAGEMENT FOR NURSES

A multidisciplinary approach

Edited by

MARIE STRENG BERGER, R.N., Ph.D.

Associate Professor and Chairperson, Graduate Studies Department,
University of Oregon Health Sciences Center,
School of Nursing,
Portland

DOROTHY ELHART, R.N., M.S.

Associate Professor,
University of Oregon Health Sciences Center,
School of Nursing,
Portland

SHARON CANNELL FIRSICH, R.N., M.S.

Formerly Assistant Professor,
University of Oregon Health Sciences Center,
School of Nursing,
Portland

SHELLEY BANEY JORDAN, R.N., M.N.

Director, Blood Services Nursing,
American Red Cross,
Pacific Northwest Region,
Portland

SANDRA STONE, R.N., M.S.

Associate Professor,
University of Oregon Health Sciences Center,
School of Nursing,
Portland

Second edition
with 25 illustrations

The C. V. Mosby Company

ST. LOUIS • TORONTO • LONDON   1980

SECOND EDITION

The C. V. Mosby Company
11830 Westline Industrial Drive, St. Louis, Missouri 63141

Library of Congress Cataloging in Publication Data

Main entry under title:

Management for nurses.

    Includes bibliographical references and index.
    1. Nursing service administration.
I. Berger, Marie Streng, 1929-
RT89.M37 1980   658′.91′36210425   79-19965
ISBN 0-8016-4815-7

GW/M/M 9 8 7 6 5 4 3 2 1   03/D/320

PREFACE

This edition reflects our continued belief that both students learning the concepts of leadership and management and the practitioner applying such concepts need a source of references that discuss the principles of good management and illustrate practical applications of those principles. The major units of the book remain the same and contain material relevant to organizations as a whole and the individual functioning within that organization. Many of the articles, however, have been replaced with newer material or with articles that present concepts not even considered when this book was originally published. Articles on conflict and confrontation, budgeting and affirmative action have been added as we feel that understanding these concepts are crucial to today's nurse manager.

This book provides stimulating materials of an interdisciplinary nature that supplement and/or highlight the many basic textbooks on management available today. The study guides at the end of each unit are exercises designed to assist the student to apply theoretical concepts and principles to an actual situation.

Marie Streng Berger
Dorothy Elhart
Sharon Cannell Firsich
Shelley Baney Jordan
Sandra Stone

CONTENTS

UNIT TWO

Personnel factors and their influence on efficient organizational functioning

MANAGEMENT FOR NURSES
A multidisciplinary approach

Structural factors and their influence on efficient organizational functioning

☐ This unit focuses on variables having a profound effect on the efficiency of an organization. The degree to which nurse-managers understand these variables and how they influence the organization determines to a great extent their own effectiveness within that organization. The statement of philosophy and objectives reflects an organization's primary purpose — whether that organization is a small individual clinical unit or a large multipurpose health center. Nurses who comprehend the philosophy, purpose, and objectives can more readily determine whether their own personal philosophy is in conflict with that of the institution or whether they can assist the organization in meeting its goals. Problems with the functioning of the organization can often be traced to contradictory or ambiguous statements of the philosophy or objectives.

Once nurses understand the philosophy or objectives, knowledge of other variables influencing organizational effectiveness, such as power and accountability, is essential. For example, nurses who understand sources of power in the organization and how they are mobilized are clearly in a better position to exert influence within that organization. Implicit in this understanding of power is the recognition of communication patterns within the institution.

Strongly affected by structural factors within the organization, and in turn strongly affecting the organization's efficient functioning, are delegation, decision-making, and evaluation. Nurses must be competent in these skills and must also recognize the effectiveness or ineffectiveness of others within the organization who carry these responsibilities.

Nurse-managers are responsible for helping to determine how effectively all of the factors discussed thus far contribute to organizational functioning. In addition, they must assess and evaluate their own performance in relation to each of the factors.

In Chapter 1, Cantor speaks directly to the necessity for well-defined, clearly stated, and operational purposes, philosophies, and objectives as a means of providing direction for an agency or for a program within an agency. As used in her article, *purpose* states the reason for being — the "why" of the system; *philosophy* is an explanation of the system of beliefs that determines the way one achieves the purpose; and *objectives* are statements of the criteria by which one measures the degree to which the purpose is achieved.

Chapter 2 deals with the concepts of power and accountability. Paula Johnson presents a theory of sex-role stereotyping and its effect on

1

the use of power. These ideas are particularly important in nursing, where the largest numbers of nurses are women and the largest number of administrative personnel above the level of director of nursing service are men. Luther Christman's article goes beyond the mere use of power into the area of accountability. He discusses the responsibility that rests on nursing staffs that have developed autonomy within the structure of the organization. To facilitate the leader's assessment, use, and evaluation of power within the organization, a list of principles developed by Wally Jacobson is presented at the end of this chapter. These principles include concepts about power, agents and methods that exert power, and principles relating to the power recipient.

Jackson, in Chapter 3, reviews some characteristics that create communication problems, identifies forces that determine the flow of communication in an organization, and finally considers the consequences that communication will have when various conditions exist within an organization.

Chapter 4 presents a discussion of decision-making in small groups. Van de Ven and Delbecq look at the performance of decision-making groups in terms of the quantity, quality, and variety of ideas generated; the emotional and expressive overtones of interaction; and the nature of facilitative and inhibitive influences on creative problem-solving. They review literature dealing with the relative effectiveness of interacting versus nominal group processes for problem-solving committees. Following this presentation is an outline for conducting nominal group process. In the last article of the chapter Volante argues that the question is not whether one delegates but rather how much and how effectively one delegates. The author identifies some definitive steps that the leader can use to improve delegation.

Chapter 5 presents two articles containing useful ideas for planning the evaluation of nursing care. Zimmer's article provides a theoretical model that could be used to design an evaluation process for virtually any setting in which the nurse works. She also provides clear definitions for key terms such as quality assurance, effectiveness, and efficiency.

Ramey sets up a logical plan for preparing the standards against which care is to be measured within her evaluation system. Most of the individual ideas in Ramey's article are not new to those active in nursing care administration over the past few years, but her presentation is clear and practical and provides useful guidance for putting these ideas into operation. Although the hospital is the setting in which her tool would be useful, the process of setting standards and evaluating care could be readily adapted to any agency.

Together, the two articles of this chapter provide (1) a theoretical means of examining how evaluation may be designed to assess the effectiveness and efficiency of nursing care delivered to the population served by a health care unit, and (2) a concrete example of how that evaluation might be carried out for a specific kind of institution.

Chapter 1

PHILOSOPHY, PURPOSE, AND OBJECTIVES

Philosophy, purpose, and objectives: why do we have them?

MARJORIE MOORE CANTOR, R.N., PhD.

Most nursing departments can produce documents entitled, "Philosophy, Purpose, and Objectives," designed either for the department or for special units, divisions, or programs. They usually are carefully prepared by conscientious nurses. But if examined closely, these statements frequently have no referents in the activities for which they are to provide guidance. In other words, many of these statements are written as a task which one does because it is there, and these statements have no function other than to be viewed by accreditors and other distinguished visitors.

Because of some undefined, uneasy feeling about the task, it is not uncommon for nurses developing such documents to seek help from "authorities," from whom they are likely to receive advice on *how* these statements should be written and *what* they should contain. Seldom are they told *why* these statements are written or *what one does with them* after they have been completed. For this reason, the writers of such statements tend to focus on the task of developing the wording rather than the ideas, and the statements are seldom thought of as a base for planning and implementing the operations with

which the documents are supposedly concerned.

Because of this focus on the writing, the documents tend to include concepts phrased in professional jargon, which have been accepted uncritically. The statements achieve social approval within the group, but they are difficult to translate into action. Concern with "man as a unique entity interacting with his environment," and "providing the patient with individualized care," "the democratic process as a basis for administration," or similar thoughts are frequently encountered within these papers. To the individuals who expound them, such ideas can provide satisfaction at only a verbal level because any attempts at implementation reveal that they are not clearly conceptualized by the individuals proposing them. This tendency to make use of pot-boiler statements culled from the folklore of nursing does serve a purpose of sorts: it protects nurses from looking at the realities of their jobs and evaluating their own activities. If the philosophy, purpose and objectives are stated in sufficiently nonfunctional terms, the ideas in question cannot be used as a basis for checking whether activities are in line with what one *says* she believes and is trying to achieve. This avoidance of self-examination is not restricted to nurses; we share it with the rest of humanity.

Reprinted with permission from *The Journal of Nursing Administration*, July-August, 1973.

Why bother with statements of philosophy, purpose, and objectives if they are seldom functional? Would the time be better spent in developing the operation itself? The answer to the latter question is *yes,* if such statements are developed as an end rather than as a beginning. *However, they can be very useful if they are developed to be functional;* if the philosophy, purpose, and objectives are developed as statements from which the operation of the unit, service, or program takes its direction. It is helpful to look at the development of philosophy, purpose, and objectives from the standpoint of how they can provide guidance in the operation for which they were written.

The statement of *purpose* describes the reason for being — the why of the operation. A clear understanding of purpose by all involved is primary to the total operation. The statement of *philosophy* as it is used in this context is an explanation of the system of beliefs that determines the way one achieves the purpose. The *objectives* are statements of the criteria by which one measures the degree to which the purpose is achieved.

PURPOSE

Clarification of purpose, then, has first priority for the development of any operation. For any nursing agency or program the ultimate purpose is to provide quality nursing care to patients. But a nursing department may be established to accomplish different aspects of this purpose, and programs within the department will have various goals that contribute to the major purpose. It is important, for example, that a nursing department within a teaching and research hospital recognize that the nursing department was established to provide a nursing environment which supports and encourages research and teaching. To provide such an environment, the research and teaching function must be reconciled with the ultimate goal of all nursing — the provision of quality nursing care to patients. The reconciliation of these two purposes determines the kind of operation to be established.

Any nursing department must determine how the purposes of nursing relate to the purpose for which the establishment was formed. Furthermore, when a program is developed *within* a nursing department, a realistic appraisal of its contribution to the overall purpose of quality nursing care is necessary. If the expected contribution is not stated in realistic terms, is not clearly understood, and is not used as a basis for planning, it is probable that the program initiated will be ineffective in the achievement of excellence in nursing care.

The inservice education programs of many nursing services demonstrate what is likely to happen. The purpose of an inservice education program is to educate the staff to the requirements of the job and to improve the quality of work they do. But time after time programs are selected for their interest value only, and they are evaluated in terms of the nurses' *pleasure* in the program. If the purpose of a program is to build morale, then providing programs that make the staff feel contented achieves the purpose. But if the purpose is to teach staff to perform in a way that realizes benefits to *patients,* it is likely that such an approach would garner minimal benefits in improved function.

If one is establishing a unit for the care of ambulatory patients who are either in the process of diagnosis or preparation for returning home, it is important to determine first whether the purpose is to reduce the cost of care to the patient and the hospital, or whether it is to help patients adjust to and cope with changes related to their illness. It would make a difference in the kind of staff required. It is customary in many hospitals to think of this type of unit as a minimal care unit and, if one defines minimal care as reduced services and care provided by nonprofessional personnel, one could achieve the purpose of reduced cost to the hospital and patient. However, the second purpose can not be achieved in this way. This is not to say that one purpose is superior to the other—only that knowledge and clarification of purpose are necessary for effective operation.

Almost any operation can benefit from a careful examination of its purpose and the extent to which the procedure involved is related to that purpose. Even the establishment of a policy becomes more meaningful when the purpose is thoughtfully determined. Examination of policies and practices long adhered to in nursing departments will frequently reveal that, although the policy is supported vigorously, the reason for it has long been forgotten or no longer exists.

PHILOSOPHY

A philosophy for an institution, department, committee, or program is a statement of the system of beliefs which direct the individuals in a particular group in the achievement of their purpose. It should be a statement that can be referred to as an explanation of why things are carried out in the way they are.

A collective philosophy covers those things about which the group is collectively concerned and on which decisions are required. Nurses involved in the preparation of a statement of philosophy about their nursing department may have been encouraged to develop first a statement about Man, then one about nursing generally, and then one about the department. This is a pretentious approach and one that has little usefulness in helping to establish desirable practices within the department. A nursing department does not operate as a group with respect to issues on Man, his concerns about his identity, his relations to society, or his habit patterns. The concerns of the nursing department are the patient who comes to the institution for nursing care and the nursing care that is provided for him. The more a statement of philosophy restricts itself to the actual collective concerns and a clear expression of them, the more meaningful will that statement be.

A statement of philosophy can be useful only

if it serves as a directive to those involved regarding the way the purpose is to be achieved. It should state clearly the premises which govern the operation. If one cannot look to the philosophy for this kind of direction, then it, too, becomes no more than an exercise in the manipulation of words and phrases.

Many philosophies deal with socially accepted ideas such as the "democratic ideal" and the "rights of the human being as an individual." Yet if nurses would ask themselves how the nursing department manifests this belief in a democratic system, they would be hard put to come up with an answer. If, in contrast, the nursing department asserts that it believes each patient should be treated in relation to his nursing needs rather than his economic situation or other social factors, one can show that this belief has been implemented because, in fact, the indigent patient is provided with nursing care equal to that received by the wealthiest patient, and the delinquent is cared for as assiduously as the pillar of the church. This kind of conformity of action to belief can be continually examined for the extent to which it is being observed by members of the nursing staff. A statement to the effect that one believes in the democratic process or that one believes in the inherent dignity of man is too ill-defined to have meaning and to serve as a basis for determining how one might operate. If a department cannot say that this is what we do or expect of our members in order to conform to our beliefs, the philosophy is simply a group of words set down to meet some need of those writing them. It will have little to do with the department's actual operation.

There are many values and beliefs to be examined when considering the operation of a nursing department within a hospital. How do the department's members feel about the skill level required for a minimal care as opposed to a special care unit? What do they believe about the difference in nursing care requirements for different kinds of nursing units? Are they planning to have specialists function in special care units and less prepared individuals in general or minimal care units? What do they believe about the role of educational programs in the department? Should the people responsible for developing the programs be the same individuals who provide the direct care? If not, should the former be at least as competent as the latter?

A philosophy about a nursing department or a program within the department that simply reiterates the accepted generalities of the day might better not be written at all because it not only fails to serve as a basis for clarifying the values of the group, but it also requires time and energy to prepare. Even without thoughtful expression of group values, time can be wasted on the sheer mechanics of writing and the creation of literary effect.

OBJECTIVES

If an objective is to be useful, it must be stated in terms of the results to be achieved so that it can be used as a basis for assessing the effectiveness of the process carried out. To be sure that whatever objectives are chosen can serve this purpose, one must consider them in terms of the purpose and philosophy of the operation.

For example, a nursing care objective for a hospital nursing department might state, "arrangements will be made or patient will be prepared for continuation of necessary regimen of post-hospitalization care." An objective stated in this way indicates the group believes that nursing responsibility should extend beyond the confines of the hospital and that they intend to assess the achievement of this purpose by observing results with patients.

In contrast, as an objective, "Public Health referrals are sent as needed," indicates a focus on process rather than on results. If the objectives are written in terms of the method to be used rather than the results to be gained, there is greater danger that certain nursing interventions will continue to be implemented whether they are effective or not. Objectives for most

projects are written in terms of the process rather than results. Some familiar examples: Patients will be taught about their illness. Patients will receive nursing care appropriate to the stages of their illness. The patient will be treated as an individual and his care modified according to his needs.

Although in each case the patient is mentioned, the focus tends to be on the activities of the nurse rather than on what the patient will manifest to indicate that the process *was appropriate*. Because nurses do tend to concentrate on the activities of nursing rather than on the effects to be achieved, it is necessary to emphasize the difference. The distinction may seem to be unimportant, but it must be kept in mind if objectives are to be written with thought given to why they are written and how they are to be used. If one is to use objectives as criteria for assessing the extent to which purposes have been achieved, then it is important to structure the objectives to indicate *what must be observed in the patient* to show that the nursing care in question was appropriate.

For purposes of explicitness, the general objectives that are written for the whole department must be defined in more specific terms to apply to particular groups of patients. In the case of the post-hospital regimen objective, specification of post-hospital regimen for newborn babies might include such items as the mother's demonstrating that she can bathe and feed the baby and that she understands and uses information about particular situations in infant care. For a group of patients who have had radical mastectomies, concern may be focused on the ability to perform required exercises and the ability to identify symptoms that they must look for and what they should do if those symptoms exists. Or the interest might be in a family's ability to provide care when a patient cannot or will not assume responsibility for his own care.

When evaluating the achievement of these objectives, one should not ask "Was the mother taught?" More appropriate questions are "What does the mother know and what can she do?" Instead of "Did someone teach the exercises to the patient?" ask "Can the patient do the exercises and will she be likely to do them?"

Of course, the most meaningful evaluation would come from direct observation of the patient outside of the hospital. To the extent that one could have access to such information, she could revise the objective to "carries out regimen of care prescribed." But few hospital nursing departments have access to this kind of information, and since objectives need to be stated in terms of evidence that can be evaluated *directly,* this particular goal may have to be formulated with a focus on determining what behavior can be observed *now* (prior to leaving the hospital) that is most likely to lead to desired *future* behavior.

Most of the other objectives of a nursing department can be evaluated directly. For example, nursing departments will want to see that patients do not develop such complications as post-operative pneumonia, contractures, decubiti, and infections. In the case of post-operative pneumonia, for example, what one would look for in the patient to determine that he was free of pneumonia would need to be described. This description, which might include "full, easy respirations involving excursion of the chest, rate of breathing within normal limits, and body temperature normal," would serve as the definition for "freedom from post-operative pneumonia." The patient might have been "turned, coughed, and deep breathed" as a means of achieving the goal, but the evaluation criteria of the effectiveness of nursing care, or in other words, the objectives, would be in terms of the description of the patient's condition, not the method used. If one accepts results as manifested in the patient's condition as the only criteria for quality care, then one can be sure that nursing measures will be more critically examined for their effectiveness in achieving their purpose.

In the case of programs that contribute to the total purpose, the principle objective is

the same—to evaluate the effectiveness, one must identify the objectives in terms of what is to be accomplished.

The staff development, or inservice education program, can again be used as a point of illustration. One would assume that the purpose of the staff educational program is to prepare staff members to be able to achieve the nursing care objectives. The program would presumably include a variety of activities. Of recent concern has been the training of individuals to meet the emergency care requirement for patients experiencing cardiac arrest. If one of the objectives of the inservice education program is to "provide training in the cardiopulmonary resuscitation procedure," then the presentation of the training materials will satisfy that goal. If, on the other hand, the objective is to prepare staff so that "patients receive immediate care in emergency situations (cardiac arrest)" then the educational program takes on an entirely different dimension. To make sure that individuals continue to perform adequately requires time for planned practice, review, and frequent evaluation with use of predetermined evaluation criteria. Educating a staff member to carry out procedures evaluated in terms of results with patients is quite a different matter from presenting programs and training materials—different in the material to be presented and techniques of teaching.

As is true of statements of purpose and philosophy, statements of objectives call for thoughtful examination of the reason for which they are being developed. If objectives are presented in terms of results to be achieved and defined in terms of what can be observed, they can serve as useful tools for evaluation of nursing care and personnel performance, and as a basis for planning educational programs, staffing, requisition of supplies and equipment, and other functions associated with the nursing department. If they are not written in such terms, they may serve only to obscure actual departmental purposes.

Nurses embarking on the development of

statements of purpose, philosophy, and objectives as described here, will find that it is easier to state ideas in vague generalities than to state them in terms that can be measured in the reality of everyday activities. But this more difficult task of stating what we want to accomplish in measurable terms is essential to the provision of a service that is beneficial to patients. Thoughtfully prepared statements of purpose, philosophy, and objectives based on reality, understood and used by those responsible for implementation, can promote efficiency and effectiveness in the operation of institutions, departments, and programs. Statements lacking these qualities are merely collections of words.

Chapter 2

POWER AND ACCOUNTABILITY

Women and power: toward a theory of effectiveness

PAULA JOHNSON, Ph.D.

What do the following have in common? (a) A young woman pleads teary-eyed with the detective to help find her missing brother because she just doesn't know what to do. (b) The wife wants the husband to take her to Hawaii; she doesn't tell him, but puts travel brochures all over the house—in his socks, in the refrigerator, etc. (c) Mrs. A lets Mr. A know he can sleep on the couch if he won't allow their son to go off to college. All three scenarios are stereotypical presentations of how women use power.

This paper will explore the methods by which sex-role stereotypes work in human interaction, specifically in the influence situation, and how stereotyped power use may lead to unequal positions in society. Previous research has shown that people do indeed have stereotypes of the sexes (Broverman, Vogel, Broverman, Clarkson, & Rosenkrantz, 1972) and it has shown how the stereotypes work in general (Goldberg, 1968), but there has been little research to demonstrate how stereotypes effect social relationships and social position.

Power and influence are a part of everyday life, from the requests people make of each other to the demands which governments hand down to the citizenry. The present perspective will focus on power as an aspect of social interactions. In simple terms, interpersonal power

may be defined as the ability to get another person to do or to believe something he or she would not have necessarily done or believed spontaneously. In more technical terms, power is the amount of tension toward changes which one person can bring to bear on another person's "life space" (Cartwright, 1959). If one uses power, the behavior may be called an influence attempt. We use power almost unconsciously—rules about power are built into our norms, and its use it an integral part of our daily interactions with others. To live one's own life as one wishes requires that each person be able to have some power with which to influence those around him or her.

Researchers have studied both how much power people have and the ways in which they use their power (Schopler, 1965, presents an excellent review). High power can be associated with many resources, social status, self-confidence, and expertise; one of the consequences of high power is obtaining what one wants. Researchers, however, have noted that there are many other consequences of power use in addition to a success vs. failure dichotomy. It has been hypothesized (Raven & Kruglanski, 1970) that the mode or style of influence one chooses is important not only for immediate success but for how one feels about oneself, how others feel about the influencer, and how successful one might be in future situations. In addition, these consequences of influ-

Reprinted with permission from *Journal of Social Issues*, vol. 32, no. 3, 1976.

ence attempts are not only a function of the mode, but are hypothesized also to be a result of the sex-role expectations of our society interacting with each mode.

It is proposed that men and women are expected to use power styles differently, and that, for women in particular, there are negative consequences of this differential use (Johnson, 1974). Three dimensions of power styles are posited.

Indirect vs. direct power

Indirect power, often called manipulation (Tedeschi, 1972), may be said to occur when the influencer acts as if the person on the receiving end is not aware of the influence. The influencer may try to keep the other from knowing in order to facilitate the effectiveness of the influence or to avoid personal confrontation. Since women are expected to be less direct than men and more sneaky (Broverman et al., 1972), women should be more expected to use indirect forms of power. This is not to say that men do not or are not supposed to use it, only that there are constraints against women being direct. Women can be hypothesized to use indirect power because of its short-term effectiveness and its personal and status appropriateness. That is, women may not expect a direct approach by a woman to succeed, nor are they willing to take the consequences for its use if it is perceived as out-of-role by others. If a woman does use direct power, she may risk becoming known as pushy, overbearing, unfeminine, and/or castrating. An additional reason why women may use indirect power is that they are explicitly trained to do so. For example, Stein (1971) shows that nurses are trained to present their diagnosis indirectly to doctors. The training, whether explicit or subtle, of low status persons such as women and other minorities to be indirect in their power use so as not to shake up the status quo may be quite a common phenomenon with far reaching implications.

The use of indirect (manipulative) power, though perhaps effective in the short run, may

have negative consequences for its users in the long run. Since the source of the power is concealed, use of indirect power could easily keep its user in a subordinate position. It is not surprising that people whose abilities to influence are known are seen as much more powerful in our society (Michner, Lawler, & Bacharach, 1973). Furthermore, the user of indirect influence is not likely to view her or himself as a strong person. The woman's view that she needs to use indirect power to get what she wants will be reinforced, and it is therefore unlikely that her self-concept will change.

Personal vs. concrete power

There are two types of resources one can possess: those which depend on a personal relationship, such as liking or approval; and those which are independent of relationships, the concrete resources. In this society, males control the concrete resources—money (Domhoff, 1970; Bird, 1971), knowledge, and physical strength. Millett (1970) pointed out that men are in the highest positions of our society's institutions of strength, wealth, and learning—all the military, technical, scientific, intellectual, and political institutions. Whether on an individual or institutional level, men have the opportunities to use concrete resources, and even when women do possess such resources, they are discouraged from using them directly.

There are, however, resources women can possess and which are often stereotypically ascribed to them. These are personal resources such as liking, love, affection, and approval. A woman may influence others by appealing to needs to be liked or loved. This use of personal resources is consistent with the Broverman et al. (1972) evidence that women are stereotyped as being higher in warmth and affection than men. Another resource based on a personal relationship which a woman may be able to use is sexuality. Sexual influence has been ascribed to women since the time of Aristophanes, if not before.

Unfortunately, the use of personal resources

is another power mode that is often effective only in the short run. It limits the user to those areas of influence that are affected by a personal relationship, and leaves him or her highly dependent on others. In addition, one of the requisites for the successful use of power is that one have the resources and the ability to get them for oneself (Stogdill, 1959). If one is dependent on others for resources, one's power is lessened. This theory can be extended to personal resources: To successfully use liking to influence others, one must be able to like oneself enough so that one is not entirely dependent on others for social payoffs. Consistent with this hypothesis, Wolfe (1959) found that women with a high need for affection tended to be in husband-dominant marriages rather than egalitarian or wife-dominant marriages. These women may have had needs for affection from their husbands such that the amount of personal power they could use was effectively low. To use personal power women must like themselves. Unfortunately, there are considerable (though inconsistent) data indicating that women tend to have negative self-concepts (Frieze, Parsons, Johnson, Ruble & Zellman, in press).

Helplessness vs. competence

Women often do not feel competent: They underestimate their successes (Parsons, Ruble, Hodges, & Small, 1976); they are expected to be less intelligent, logical, and wordly-wise than males (Broverman et al., 1972); they are expected to be weak and not very knowledgeable. Even women who are quite capable seem to fear others' knowing about it and may inhibit their own success (Horner, 1971).

Women often must rely on helplessness because of both their lack of concrete resources, e.g., superior knowledge, and the expectation that they lack competence. Raven and Kruglanski (1970) present the classic example of the woman standing by the side of the road with a flat tire "influencing" someone to stop. Helplessness such as this—and my opening example (a)—can be quite effective in the short run; low

power people can get others to do things for them which they can't do themselves. However, trading on one's weaknesses may make it difficult later for one to influence from a position of strength. Raven and Kruglanski (1970) also hypothesized that helplessness leads to a loss of self-esteem. Certainly the use of this type of power by females (or any group) does not establish them as strong influencers; it may be a contributing factor both to their low power status and to their low self-esteem.

SEX ROLES AND THE BASES OF POWER

Raven (1965) proposed six power bases, ways in which power is used. I will use these bases as they relate to the above dimensions to operationalize specific hypotheses about the differential use of power by males and females.

Reward and coercion

When someone has the ability to provide positive or negative sanctions to another, he or she has reward or coercive power. Promises and threats are reward and coercion, respectively. Direct use of concrete reward and coercion, such as the offering or withdrawing of money, is hypothesized to be more likely to be used by males; males possess the concrete resources and the societal approval to use them. There is initial evidence from Dunn (Note 1) that students rated reward and coercion as masculine, regardless of whether it was used by a male or a female. Coercion is predicted to be seen as the most masculine as it is aggressive and unpleasant.

On the other hand, indirect and personal reward and coercion are hypothesized as more apt to be used by females. Reward and coercion can be used in personal modes, for example, through threats of anger, through nagging, or as offers of friendship or sexual rewards. And all reward or coercion is not directly administered; it is possible to manipulate reward and punishment without letting the other persons know. One type of reward that is both personal and manipulative is ingratiation—being nice to someone and then making a request.

Thus, direct use of reward and coercion is hypothesized to be expected of males and personal and indirect reward and coercion by females. The helplessness/competence dimension does not apply clearly to reward and coercion.

Referent power

Referent power is based on the psychological process of identification: If one person sees another as similar and likeable, the person may feel a oneness and want to do and believe as the other. This is a type of power that can be appropriate to either sex. It should be open to women as it is personal, rather inactive, and therefore consistent with sex-role expectations for women.

Referent power, however, being personal, may leave its users tied to the relationships it necessitates. It is also posited to improve personal relationships (Raven & Kruglanski, 1970) and to increase similarity—if successfully used. To the extent that women are taught to be more concerned with personal relationships, though Frieze et al. (in press) find inconsistent data on this, referent power may appeal to women.

Raven, Centers, and Rodrigues (1975) found referent power to be the most common form of power used by both spouses in a marriage, and even more likely for wives to use than husbands. Thus, referent power as a personal base is appropriate for females. The competence and directness dimensions do not apply.

Expert power

Expert power is based on having superior skills or knowledge, and trustworthiness. Since men are the acknowledged experts in our society—even in areas considered "feminine" (viz., cooking, childrearing, sewing, teaching, art, and literature)—expert power should be seen as quite out of role for women. It should be attributed to men.

The Raven et al. (1975) study found that wives saw their husbands as using expert power much more than husbands saw their wives using it, though there were some areas where wives were granted expertise. This study is consistent with the hypothesis that expert power as a competent base will be more expected of males. It usually is used directly and is not very personal.

Legitimate power

Legitimate power is the most complex base, as it relies heavily on prior socialization. For people to use legitimate power, they must feel they have the right to influence and the influencer must feel obligated to comply. Common examples of legitimate power are found within hierarchical social structures—the sergeant has the right to influence the private; and the employer, the employee. It is unlikely that women find themselves in positions of authority over subordinates, with the interesting exceptions of children and "domestic servants," so power of legitimate position is to be expected of males. Even when a woman is in a position of authority, she may not be granted legitimacy, because she has a woman's status and is expected to conform to the stereotype (Epstein, 1971).

Another norm of legitimacy is the expectation of reciprocity: "If I do something for you, you are obligated to do something for me." Use of this norm would be more expected of males, if it were used directly (e.g., "you owe me"). In addition, males may be able to initiate favor-giving due to more concrete resources—as women accepting dinner dates well know. Although the last example seems indirect, the forms of legitimacy are quite competent and are hypothesized to be used by males. The norm of social responsibility, however, leads to another type of legitimacy—legitimate helplessness. Helplessness, highly stereotyped as a female form of power, was found by Gruder and Cook (1971) to be more effective for a woman than legitimacy of position, and more effective for a woman than for a man. Thus, helpless vs. position or obligation legitimacy varies on the competence dimension. Helplessness may also be less direct and more personally based.

Informational power

Informational power means the ability of one person to provide explanations for why another person should believe or behave differently. It differs from expert power in that the influencer does not just say he or she knows best but explains why. Women rarely have societal roles allowing access to the quantity and quality of information that men do. In addition, telling someone what to do and why is a direct action, out of role for women. Thus, direct information would be expected of men rather than women.

A woman might have the opportunity to use information indirectly, for example, by leaving it around the house—as in opening example (b). The sneaky, nontrustworthy stereotype also leads to the hypothesis that women may be very indirect by using false information to get their way. Thus, information may be competent and concrete, but it can also vary on the direct/indirect dimension.

AN EMPIRICAL TEST

Two "hypothetical situation" questionnaires were constructed with items operationalizing the Raven (1965) power bases and the above modifications of them. Fifteen types of power were tested for differential expectations as to the sex of the influencing agent. The situation was presented as one in which a student ("X") wanted to get another student ("Y") to change his/her opinion on a legal case (Questionnaire I) or to do something he/she would not ordinarily do (Questionnaire II). Hypothetical ways in which X could attempt to influence Y constituted the items to be rated. For example, in the first questionnaire (QI), "X tells Y that X has studied the case and knows a lot about it" represented a primarily competent form of expert power; helpless legitimacy was "X tells Y that

X really needs Y's help and support." A personal form of personal reward (form QII) was "X asks Y and indicates to Y that X will like and admire Y if Y does it"; a more concrete form of reward (from QI) was "X asks Y and tells Y that X will do Y a favor if Y does it." Direct and indirect forms of information were: "X asks Y to do it and explains the reasons why it is best to do it that way" and "X does not ask Y directly but mentions in Y's presence some reasons why it is best to do it that way."

Subjects were 60 students in a psychology class. There were 12 of each sex who on QI rated how likely it was that the influencer (X) was a male and how likely it was that X was a female. For QII, 18 students of each sex rated the influence method X used on a masculine-feminine dimension.

Results

For QI, rated likelihood of use by males was compared with rated likelihood of use by females by analysis of variance. In QII, scores on the masculinity-femininity scale for each influence method were contrasted by analysis of variance.

As is evident in Table 1, coercion, legitimate, expert, and informational power were significantly more expected of males than females. Comparing specific forms of the power dimensions on masculinity and feminity in QII, coercion was seen as more masculine than personal coercion, expert as more masculine than referent or helplessness, direct information more masculine than indirect information or deceit, and legitimate more masculine than helplessness. Direct reward was, however, not more masculine than indirect reward.

Two of the feminine power types, personal reward and sexuality, were seen as significantly more likely for females than males on QI. In QII, these types were significantly more feminine than their counterparts. No significant differences in expectations for females and males in QI were found for ingratiation, indirect information, reward, helplessness, referent, nag-

Table 1. Perceptions of types of power

Base and relevant dimensions	QI likelihood that influencer is:		QII femininity of type
	Male	Female	
Coercion (concrete)	2.54*	4.54	2.00
Legitimate (competent)	2.91*	4.29	3.83
Expert (competent, concrete)	3.00*	4.17	2.89
Information (direct, competent, concrete)	3.08*	4.21	3.06
Ingratiation (indirect, personal)	3.13*	3.83	4.67
Indirect information	3.16*	4.00	4.39
Indirect reward (indirect, concrete)	—	—	3.83
Reward (concrete)	3.54	4.08	3.94
Helpless legitimacy (helpless)	3.63	3.25	5.00
Referent (personal)	3.71	3.33	4.00
Deceit (indirect, competent)	—	—	4.10
Nagging (personal, indirect)	3.70	3.33	—
Personal coercion (personal)	3.70	3.54	4.17
Personal reward (personal)	4.25*	2.79	4.17
Sexuality (personal)	4.83*	2.25	5.83

Note. For QI, higher score = less likely; for QII, higher score = more feminine (neutral point = 4). A blank indicates that type was not included.
*$p < .001$

ging, or personal coercion—all hypothesized female power types. However, several of these were found to differ on masculinity and femininity as rated in QII (Table 1).

Discussion

It was predicted that people would view personal rewards and coercions, referent, helplessness, and indirect forms of power as stereotypic of females; and expert, legitimate, information, and direct reward and coercion as stereotypic of males. The evidence supports the hypothesized male sources as strongly expected of males. Evidence for the female sources of power was not as strong, though in the hypothesized direction; it was significant only for personal reward and sexuality. This may indicate a phenomenon similar to that reported in the Broverman et al. review (1972), namely, males are allowed to show "feminine characteristics" but females are not allowed to have "masculine traits." That is, it's acceptable (or expected) that only males will use the strong aggressive types of power; yet males are also allowed to use the other bases. Females, however, are limited in

our society's expectations to the less powerful bases. These results do differ from popular notions that men are highly restricted in sex-role behavior (e.g., the idea that it's worse for a boy to be a sissy than for a girl to be a tomboy). However, the area of power use, even on a day-to-day level, may be seen as overwhelmingly a male domain in which men may do as they please. This would be consistent with the idea that high status persons accumulate "idiosyncracy credits" (Hollander, 1964) and can engage in a wide range of behaviors.

CONCLUSION

If women's power use conforms to expectations and is limited in range to personal, helpless, and indirect power, women will be guaranteed of maintaining a powerless status in relationships with others and in society. Indirect and helpless modes of power, while useful in the short run, leave a woman as the unknown influencer or as known to be weak. Likewise, reliance on personal forms of power can leave women dependent on the relationships that are a part of the power use.

In order to change this system we need to provide women with wider access to more forms of power. This means making inroads on both the expectations our society has of women and the real opportunities they have to use other forms of power.

Shirley Chisholm (1970) provides us with two guidelines for these changes. One is the *taking* of power, for as Chisholm states, "no one is giving it away." This necessitates accruing power through increased access to concrete resources, to expertise, and to the status systems to which power is tied in our society.

The second guideline is that the point of getting power is not to act like the traditional, stereotypic male, but to support women's positive self-interests (such as welfare reform and childcare) and to promote the acceptance of such positive human values as nurturance, gentleness, and empathy by all people. These vital values are now defined as stereotypically feminine, and they are in the hands of a powerless underclass. It's time, says Chisholm, to "spread them around." So Chisholm's plan is a basic one-two—women are to accrue solid power while continuing to share the gentler forms with males, so that everyone will have the opportunity to be strong and to be humane. If women are to play society's power game, we might as well play to win; but hopefully not just to win but to change the rules as well.

Reference notes

1. Dunn, L. *A consideration of variables involved in reward and coercive influence attempts.* Unpublished manuscript, Tufts University, 1972.

References

Bird, C. The sex map of the work world. In M. H. Garskof (Ed.), *Roles women play.* Belmont, Calif.: Brooks/Cole, 1971.

Broverman, I. K., Vogel, S. R., Broverman, D. M., Clarkson, F. E., & Rosenkrantz, P. S. Sex role stereotypes: A current appraisal. *Journal of Social Issues,* 1972, 28 (2), 59-78.

Cartwright, D. Power: A neglected variable in social psychology. In D. Cartwright (Ed.), *Studies in social power.* Ann Arbor: Institute for Social Research, 1959.

Chisholm, S. Black women and politics. *Black Scholar,* 1970, *1,* 40-45.

Domhoff, G. W. *The higher circles.* New York: Random House, 1970.

Epstein, C. *Woman's place.* Berkeley: University of California Press, 1971.

Frieze, I., Parsons, J., Johnson, P., Ruble, D., & Zellman, G. *Women and sex roles: A social psychological perspective.* New York: W. W. Norton, in press.

Goldberg, P. Are women prejudiced against women. *Transaction,* April, 1968, pp. 28-33.

Gruder, C. L., & Cook, T. D. Sex, dependency, and helping. *Journal of Personality and Social Psychology,* 1971, *19,* 290-294.

Hollander, E. P. *Leaders, groups, and influence.* New York: Oxford University Press, 1964.

Horner, M. S. Femininity and successful achievement: A basic inconsistency. In M. H. Garskof (Ed.), *Roles women play.* Belmont, Calif.: Brooks/Cole, 1971.

Johnson, P. *Social power and sex role stereotyping.* Unpublished doctoral dissertation, University of California, Los Angeles, 1974.

Michner, H. A., Lawler, E. J., & Bacharach, S. B. Perception of power in conflict situations. *Journal of Personality and Social Psychology,* 1973, *28,* 155-162.

Millett, K. *Sexual politics.* Garden City, N.Y.: Doubleday, 1970.

Parsons, J. E., Ruble, D. N., Hodges, K. L., & Small, A. W. Cognitive-developmental factors in emerging sex differences in achievement-related expectancies. *Journal of Social Issues,* 1976, *32*(3).

Raven, B. H. Social influence and power. In I. D. Steiner & M. Fishbein (Eds.), *Current studies in social psychology.* New York: Holt, 1965.

Raven, B. H., Centers, R., & Rodrigues, A. The bases of conjugal power. In R. E. Cromwell & D. H. Olson (Eds.), *Power in families.* New York: Wiley, 1975.

Raven, B. H., & Kruglanski, A. W. Conflict and power. In P. Swingle (Ed.), *The structure of conflict.* New York: Academic Press, 1970.

Schopler, J. Social power. In L. Berkowitz (Ed.), *Advances in experimental social psychology* (Vol. 2). New York: Academic Press, 1965.

Stein, L. Male and female: The doctor-nurse game. In J. P. Spradley & D. W. McCurdy (Eds.), *Conformity and conflict: Readings in cultural anthropology.* Boston: Little, Brown, 1971.

Stogdill, R. M. *Individual behavior and group achievement.* New York: Oxford University Press, 1959.

Tedeschi, J. T. *The social influence processes.* Chicago: Aldine, 1972.

Wolfe, D. M. Power and authority in the family. In D. Cartwright (Ed.), *Studies in social power.* Ann Arbor, Mich.: University of Michigan Press, 1959.

Power principles

WALLY D. JACOBSON, Ph.D.

The following power principles are derived from an extensive examination of social science journals and books. They reflect 150 discrete power principles. Because some power principles overlap one another, it is useful to compress them into fewer principles characterizing the essential nature of the data from which each was derived.

In the principles, *A* represents the power holder and *B* indicates the recipient of the power attempt.

AGENT EXERTING POWER

1. Either an individual or group may exert power over others.
2. A will be able to exert power over B if A controls resources (e.g., task abilities, information, wealth) B values.
3. A may exert power over B because of the position A occupies in the status hierarchy, the communication network, or the economic structure.
4. A will be able to exert power over B if A can reward or punish B's behavior.
5. A may have fate control over B (A can influence B's behavior regardless of what B does).
6. Power is a property of the social relationship rather than an attribute of a person.
7. A will be able to exert power over B by talking more often.
8. A will incur certain costs when he exerts power over B.

9. A will make more power attempts and be more successful with them than will B.
10. A will affect the group product in cohesive groups.
11. Interpersonal attraction increases A's power over B.
12. A will enjoy using power and will be less susceptible to power attempts by B.
13. Group power over its members will be greater if they perceive that common outcomes will result for all of them.
14. Group power over members has special significance because there is a tendency for group products to be superior to individual efforts in many cases.
15. A will be able to exert power if he has a record of past success which is known to the group.

METHODS OF EXERTING POWER

16. The method of exerting power is a mediating activity, which sets up a force field on the basis of A's power base in which B must choose alternatives and respond.
17. There must be a time lag between A's power attempt and B's response.
18. A power attempt is successful if it results in behavior in B that would otherwise not occur.
19. A will be able to exert power over B by exerting physical force.
20. A will be able to exert power over B by offering him rewards or punishments for his behavior or by increasing his own (A's) alternatives.
21. A will be able to exert power over B by manipulating B's perception rather than by actually changing what is.

From *Power and Interpersonal Relations* by Wally D. Jacobson. © 1972 by Wadsworth Publishing Company, Inc., Belmont, California, 94002. Reprinted by permission of the publisher.

22. A will be able to exert power over B by using persuasive communication.
23. A will be able to exert power over B by actually reducing B's alternatives.
24. A will incur some cost to himself regardless of the method of exerting power which he chooses.
25. The power method which A chooses will reflect his own thoughts and experiences.
26. A will be able to exert power over B by increasing B's advantages or disadvantages or by using legitimate authority.
27. A will be able to exert power over B by reducing the power distance between them and displaying coordinative behavior or by participating more actively in the discussion.

POWER RECIPIENT

28. B is the crucial part of any power attempt, because power resides implicitly in his dependency.
29. Dependence of B on A is directly proportional to B's motivational investment in goals mediated by A.
30. Dependence of B on A is inversely proportional to the availability of desired goals outside the A-B relationship.
31. Power is a potential to act as well as overt behavior; a successful power attempt may result either in a readiness to act or in an act itself.
32. To complete an effective power attempt, A must cause a change in B attributable to A's power.
33. B will conform to a power attempt if it is consistent with his own beliefs and values.
34. B will conform to a power attempt if it will help him attain his own goals through attaining group goals.
35. B will conform to a power attempt if he perceives that A can observe his behav-

ior and reward or punish him for it, especially if the reward is greater group acceptance and social approval for B.
36. The more homogeneous a group is the more attractive it is to B, the more B will conform, although B may resist conformity if he has support from at least one other member.
37. Members who are less accepted and who rate others highly will conform to power attempts, but the highest and the lowest power members will be most resistant to power attempts.
38. B will attribute high power to members who give him positive responses.
39. B will conform to a power attempt if he admires A and wishes to be like him.
40. B will conform to a power attempt if he perceives that A has a legitimate right to influence him or if he feels that A has no intention of influencing him.
41. B will conform to a power attempt if he believes that A is an expert, but B may resist expert power if A attempts to use it outside his own area of expertise.
42. Personality needs and self-perceived ability will affect how readily B will conform to a power attempt.
43. If B deviates from the group, he will receive numerous power attempts until it is clear he will not conform, at which time communication to him will drop sharply.
44. B will attempt to reduce his dependence on A through cost reduction, withdrawal, status giving, extension of the power network, and coalition formation.
45. Low power members will communicate less frequently than high power members, but they will direct their communications—mostly requests for information and opinions—to high power members.
46. Status consistency within a group may

increase its productivity and will definitely increase its cooperative, social-emotional climate.

47. Each group member will reach a stable final opinion, which will be the opinion of the power subgroup, if all power subgroups have equal final opinions.

48. Conformity can be constructive or destructive to group effectiveness depending on the situation, membership, and task that compose the group setting.

The autonomous nursing staff in the hospital

LUTHER CHRISTMAN, Ph.D., R.N.

Nurses have had an equity, that is, a stake in the health care endeavor since its inception. They have not, however, enjoyed parity. Parity, which connotes equality, is vital if nurses are to exert power and influence decision-making in the care process. Symmetry and balance, on the other hand, are organizational means by which parity can be built into the structure.

By employing the concepts of symmetry and balance, the three major departments controlling the care of hospitalized patients—hospital administration, medicine and nursing—can be aligned into an organizational system which facilitates the role expression of each and eases communication between and among them. Other professional departments such as dentistry, social work, and physical therapy are needed in the care of patients but they generally provide *ad hoc* services to the patient population as demands for their specialized services arise.

ACCOUNTABILITY

Symmetry and balance are not sufficient in themselves for the emergence of parity. Each of the three major departments also must be organized in such a design that systemic accountability is assessed for each participant. The

Reprinted with permission from *Nursing Administration Quarterly*, Fall, 1976.

model for nursing care, for instance, must reflect the constancy of patient assignment, a 24-hour responsibility for the clients, scientifically ordered care plans, and a method for unerringly fixing responsibility for outcomes including the detection of errors of either omission or commission. A highly desirable concomitant of this model is the identification of excellence so that effective functioning may be rewarded. Using the notion of perfect accountability is one of the best means of placing each practitioner on his/her mettle. It is a practical form of supervision since primary accountability for patient outcomes is placed clearly on the practitioners themselves. It elicits the finest application of the knowledge that each practitioner possesses.

MODEL CONCEPT VS. PRACTICE

A brief comparison of this conceptual model with the manner generally employed by nurses to organize the nursing care patients receive might be instructive. The behavior generated by team nursing, or care by proxy, can more accurately be labeled "reflex practice" than scientific care. The mechanical similarity of care that exemplifies the behavior of nursing staff members throughout the country can be orchestrated in the ritualized way that care is given. Patients are managed by "morning routines," "afternoon routines," procedure books, policies, and rules—none of which is based firmly on scientific or experimental data. Nurses have not yet shed the heritage of the matron system which originated with the earliest form of organized nursing. Nurses must recognize the problem, but not be dismayed or distraught over its existence. The growing number of nurses with baccalaureate and graduate training has strengthened and broadened the scientific base possessed by nurses. A shift in attitude is the main requirement for changing the posture of the profession. To make critical decisions about the form and nature of new practice is an awesome, but far from impossible, task. In the face of the great uncertainty caused by ambiguous data which surface continuously in this period of rapid technological and social change, it is the only recourse of the true professional. Knowledge and the responsibility to apply it are essential to development.

DEVELOPMENT

To develop and implement an autonomous nursing staff, the concept of parity, with all its implications, must be in central focus. An autonomous nursing staff is essentially an organization designed explicitly to permit:

1. the expression of clinical self-direction among nurses;
2. the fulfillment of their responsibility to patients; and
3. the acceptance of after-the-event sanctions rather than before-the-event controls over their practice.

Instead of relying on the control of practice through such mechanisms as an appointed hierarchy of nurse supervisors and administrators, individual practitioners will have to submit to the same risks that physicians accept in the area of legal and professional malpractice. Thus, all the repressive "protective" measures such as prior administrative consultation, excessive supervision, and the rubrics of functional nursing, must be abandoned.

Autonomy is not anarchy. Nurses' autonomy will precipitate very heavy demands on practitioners for greatly increased competence and skill. Autonomy also requires the formation and maintenance of a primary nurse-patient relationship. Autonomy demands methods for determining the skills possessed by each member of the staff, for maintaining those skills, and for requiring certain preconditions for entry to any of the several departments of the staff. Autonomy means having the right to obtain consultation on request and the obligation to undergo periodic reviews of clinical consistency and results. The medical model can serve as a general prototype even though the particular techniques of the process may be different.

IMPLEMENTATION

Staff autonomy places the responsibility for adequacy and safety in nursing care directly on the nurses themselves. The nurses are collectively accountable to their patients, *and* to the governing boards of hospitals and agencies.

To implement this responsibility, nurses must use a process similar to that employed by the medical staff. They must:

1. control access to staff and practice privileges,
2. confirm background education and certification,
3. review clinical work through appropriate committees,
4. see that shortfalls (less than adequate care) in practice are determined and remedied,
5. delimit practice privileges,
6. develop quality assurance mechanisms,
7. delineate requirements for continuing education,
8. participate in the educational preparation of nursing students, and
9. engage in research to improve care.

Because specialization in nursing is increasing greatly, the departmental responsibility for peer review and quality of care is just as necessary as it is in the medical departments.

Through the committee structure and the di-

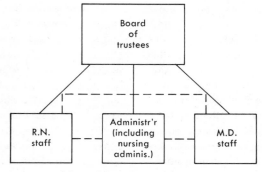

Schema for non-teaching hospitals

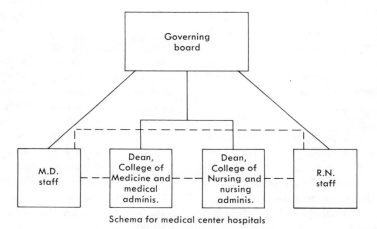

Schema for medical center hospitals

Fig. 1. Autonomous staff relationships.

recting body (usually an executive committee and an elected chief-of-staff), the autonomous staff will maintain consultative relationships:

1. with the board of trustees over qualifications for nursing staff membership and appointments and for standards of care.
2. with administration over logistical, material, and management related issues, and
3. with the medical staff and the departments of the other health professions, e.g., dietary, social work, physical therapy, occupational therapy, clinical psychology, and with whatever other departments may exist in order to share power and accountability (see Figure 1).

FUNCTION AND COORDINATION

The functions of an autonomous nursing staff would depart to a considerable degree from the principles stated in the *Accreditation Manual for Hospitals,* JCAH, as updated in 1973. The principles stated by JCAH clearly delineate the medical staff as a self-governing body responsible and accountable to the Board of Trustees for its professional practice, but the nursing staff bears its primary relationship to hospital administration. If nurses are to achieve full professional status, they must assume, with alacrity and zeal, all the obligations and accountability which accompany that privilege.

The work of all professional staff members

must be coordinated to insure the protection and amelioration of patients. The nursing and medical staff can best accomplish this objective by means of joint practice committees which examine the congruency of their role functions and interventions. A future development for hospital care process management might well be the formation of a hospital professional staff that would include the departments embraced by medicine, nursing, clinical pharmacy, psychology, dentistry, podiatry, and those other clinical departments which are organized and available for the care of patients. Hospital administration should have representation on this professional staff in order to aid the coordination effort and to allocate resources to attain the care objectives.

Administration

The functions and activities of the directors of nursing and other administrators will change in direct proportion to full autonomy. As is now evident in medical staffs, some full-time chiefs of services on salary will continue to exist, as well as other types of roles, such as educators and consultants. An autonomous staff will increase the options for career patterns rather than limit them, but the role expression of professional competence will have a different emphasis.

Patient billing

The patient-nurse relationship in the accountability model being discussed virtually demands individual patient billing for nursing services rendered. The cost will be based on actual time requirements and actual forms of service needed to assist the patient. Such a billing arrangement is quite feasible; it presently is being used in at least one hospital. Whether the patient pays directly or not is beside the point: the patient can determine from the bill precisely those services which nurses have performed. All types of permutations and combinations on this theme of direct billing are possible. Nurses

could contract with their respective hospital administrations under direct billing of nurses' service through the hospital to collect their compensation solely from such billings, knowing full well they would have the same bad debt problem that faces physicians. Another possibility is to have departmental contracts for each of the specialty departments. These contracts might vary in terms and conditions according to the desires of the participants and to the services generated, and the option to all nurses to remain on salaried reinbursement with variations according to levels of practice continues to be a possibility. At this point of conceptualization, it is unnecessary to cite a variety of types of reimbursement models. The few mentioned here are suggestive of the variations that can be implemented.

NEW LIFESTYLES

It appears that medical center hospitals and their affiliated hospitals and care networks have the nursing resources, as well as the skills and understandings of hospital administrators and physicians, to enable the creation of autonomous nursing departments as a viable model. Wholly new lifestyles for nurses must be experienced and learned before such a professional system can be transmitted to students and to colleagues working in less sophisticated settings. The full responsibility for standards of care is more than rhetoric. Standards must be empirical and based on scientific content. It will take time and energy to master the lifestyle embracing all the issues attendant to this process if the performance of an autonomous nursing staff is to have credibility with patients, governing boards, and colleagues among the other professions.

The many problems that are perceived at first as being almost unmanageable probably will disappear after the enterprise is underway. As one example, the staff may show a greater tendency to stabilize because of the intrinsic satisfaction derived from helping to control their own destiny. A system of a courtesy staff living side by side with a full active staff is one way of distinguishing between the comers and goers and the core professional staff. Status will abide in full staff membership as so much energy is devoted to becoming competent enough to earn full status. Nurses who have originally organized for collective bargaining have previously manifested this experience with beginning autonomy even though that autonomy is ordinarily limited to highly specific issues. This experience can be tempered and used by nurses in an exciting professional adventure to develop fully the service of nurses to patients and to greater satisfaction for themselves. Collective bargaining may diminish in economic importance as direct billing provides a marketplace indicator for nursing services and is a provider of income for nurses, but it may portend the rise of other self-realizations. A word of caution: it would be unwise to allow the organization of the autonomous nursing staff to develop in the manner of a fad. If this occurs, more form than substance almost surely will result. The move toward an autonomous staff should proceed with deliberate staging and orderliness until a critical mass of hospital nursing staffs have successfully adopted the model. It cannot be implemented so swiftly that nurses fail to understand the endeavor.

SOCIAL CONTRACT

Professions are social monopolies. As with all monopolies, obligations as well as rights and privileges accrue to them. How well each profession carries out its social contract to society will determine its social worth and its apportionment of social rewards, esteem and other forms of extrinsic incentives. Nurses must begin seriously to put it all together in a paradigm of scientific excellence, precise measurement, and sustained improvement of competence if they expect to have a greater image among their fellow practitioners and the public. Nurses no longer can blame "them" (meaning hospital administrators and physicians) for lack of development and for innovative change. The true professional looks to himself for the emergence of self-control and self-actualization.

OPEN DOORS

The National Joint Practice Commission had recommended the formation of autonomous nursing staffs as a basic prerequisite to effective collaboration between the nurses and physicians on the staffs of hospitals. Patients, physicians, and hospital administrators are expecting nurses to respond to new developments. The doors have been opened; it remains to be seen whether nurses will pass through and grapple with the future or remain comfortable, passive, and inert. There is risk, but the professional excitement of improving care to patients can become a marked stimulus to the growth of the profession and to the elimination of outmoded stereotypes. This air of excitement can be the catalyst that insures success — and it can be infectious.

The concept of an autonomous nursing staff is essentially a means of organizing so that the mutual expectations of nurses and physicians for each other can be met with regularity. Resultantly, the expectations of patients for both will be met with a fullness and richness never before present. To create an autonomous nursing staff requires a change of attitude, but not a new technology. It can be achieved without a large capital outlay or the use of esoteric sciences. Autonomy has, as its basic components, personal accountability and shared power and influence. This accountability and influence are outcomes of the organizational format and the style of behavior whereby nurses organize for practice. An autonomous nursing staff is feasible. It is professionally exciting. It cannot be done *for* nurses; it must be done *by* them. Will nurses aspire to this level of professional development?

Chapter 3

LINES OF COMMUNICATION

The organization and its communications problem[1]

JAY M. JACKSON, Ph.D.

Business executives, I am told, are very similar to other people: they have communication problems, too. They are concerned, of course, about better understanding among all persons. They are interested in overcoming barriers to communication between members of the public and their own particular industry. They are especially concerned, or should be, about problems of communication within an organization, since business administration by its very nature is a collective enterprise, and people in this profession must spend their days in organized groups, or organizations.

First, I want to discuss some characteristics of all organizations that create communication problems. Second, I shall present some conclusions based on recent research findings regarding the forces which determine the flow of communication in an organization. Next I shall consider the consequences of communication in a number of conditions that often exist within an organization. Finally, I shall attempt to indicate that what we call problems of communication are often merely symptomatic of other difficulties between people.

CHARACTERISTICS OF ORGANIZATIONS

What is it about organizations that seems to make communication especially difficult? An organization may be considered a system of overlapping and interdependent groups. These groups can be departments located on the same floor of a building, or they can be divisions scattered over the face of the earth. Other things being equal, people will communicate most frequently to those geographically closest to them, even within a relatively small organization. Spatial distance itself can thus be a barrier to communication.

Each one of the subgroups within an organization demands allegiance from its members. It has its own immediate goals and means for achieving them. It distributes tangible or intangible rewards to members of the group, based on their contribution to these objectives. When any particular communication is sent to a number of subgroups in an organization, each group may extract a different meaning from the message, depending upon its significance for the things the group values and is striving to accomplish.

The groups in an organization often represent different subcultures—as different, for example, as those inhabited by engineers, accountants, and salesmen. Each occupation or professional group has its own value system and idealized image, based on its traditions. These are guarded jealously, since to a considerable degree they give the members of that group their feelings of identity. Other groups in an organization, based on experience, age, sex, and marital status, have to varying degrees similar tendencies. Each develops along with its

[1]Reprinted with permission from the author.

peculiar value system a somewhat specialized system of meanings. What is required to communicate effectively to members of different groups is a system of simultaneous translation, like that employed by the United Nations. This simultaneous translation must be taking place both within the sender and the receivers of a communication.

It is also characteristic of organizations that persons are structured into different systems of relationships. A work structure exists: certain persons are expected to perform certain tasks together with other persons. An authority structure exists: some people have responsibility for directing the activities of others. The status structure determines which persons have what rights and privileges. The prestige structure permits certain persons to expect deferential behavior from others. The friendship structure is based on feelings of interpersonal trust.

These systems of relationships overlap but are not identical. Each has an important effect upon communication in an organization, by influencing the expectations people have regarding who should communicate to whom about what in what manner. Now, how often do people openly and freely discuss these matters and come to agreement? Since these areas involve ranking of persons and invidious distinctions, they are commonly avoided. Yet disagreements and distorted perceptions about questions of relationship in an organization are the source of many communication difficulties.

What intensifies these communication problems is the fact that relationships among persons in an organization are in a continual state of flux. Personnel losses, transfers, promotions and replacements are occurring. Decisions about new policies and procedures are being made, and often modify peoples' relationships. Some people are informed about changed relationships before others; some are not informed at all. Although it is common practice to communicate decisions to all the persons who are affected by them, the problem is often to determine who are the relevant persons. Unless

we are extremely sensitive to the social structure of our organization, it is likely that we shall restrict communication too narrowly. The restrictive communication of decisions about change, however, can be extremely disruptive to any consensus people have about their relationships to one another, and thus can create for them problems of communication.

THE FLOW OF COMMUNICATION

Any solution of a communication problem must be based on analysis of the particular situation in which the problem occurs, and an application of general principles about communication. It is possible on the basis of findings from research, to formulate a number of principles about the forces in an organization which direct the flow of communication.

You may have heard at one time or another that communication flows downward all right in an organization; the problem is to get communication from below. This is only partially true. In fact, any generalization that communication flows down, up, or across, is equally false. Communication is like a piece of driftwood on a sea of conflicting currents. Sometimes the shore will be littered with debris, sometimes it will be bare. The amount and direction of movement is not aimless, nor unidirectional, but a response to all the forces—winds, tides and currents—which come into play.

What forces direct communication in an organization? They are, on the whole, motivational forces. People communicate or fail to communicate in order to achieve some goal, to satisfy some personal need, or to improve their immediate situation. Let us examine briefly some of the evidence from research which supports this statement.

A study was made of the communication patterns among the personnel of a medium-sized government agency.[2] Everyone was included in

---

[2]Jay M. Jackson. Analysis of Interpersonal Relations in a Formal Organization, Ph.D. Thesis, University of Michigan, 1953.

the research, from the director to the janitor. It was found that people communicated far more to members of their own subgroups than to any other persons. They also preferred to be communicating to someone of higher status than themselves, and tried to avoid having communication with those lower in status then themselves. The only exception to this tendency was when a person had supervisory responsibilities, which removed his restraints against communicating with particular lower status persons. When people did communicate with others of the same status level in the organization, there was a strong tendency for them to select highly valued persons, and to avoid those they thought were making little contribution.

Let us see if we can find a principle which explains these results. The formal subgroupings in an organization are usually based upon joint work responsibilities. There are strong forces, therefore, to communicate with those whose work goals are the same as one's own. A supervisor can accomplish his work objectives only by having relatively frequent contact with his subordinates: and he probably would like to have more contact than he has. The people in an organization who are most valued for their ability to contribute are those who can give the best information and advice. People seek them out. These findings all seem to point to the same conclusion:

1. *In the pursuit of their work goals, people have forces acting upon them to communicate with those who will help them achieve their aims, and forces against communicating with those who will not assist, or may retard their accomplishment.*

In the midst of one study of a housing settlement,[3] a rumor swept through the community and threatened to disrupt the research. The investigators turned their attention to this rumor and were able to trace its path from person to person. They were trying to understand the forces which led people to communicate. Later on they tested their understanding by deliberately planting a rumor in an organization and again tracing its path by the use of informants.[4] They concluded that people will initiate and spread rumors in two types of situation: when they are confused and unclear about what is happening, and when they feel powerless to affect their own destinies. Passing on a rumor is a means of expressing and alleviating anxiety about the subject of the rumor.[5]

Let us consider one more fact before we draw a general conclusion from these findings. Studies in industry, in a hospital, and in a government agency all yield the same result: people want to speak to higher status rather than lower status persons.[6] Why are there these strong forces on people to direct their communication upwards? Higher status persons have the power to create for subordinates either gratifying or depriving experiences. These may take the form of tangible decisions and rewards, or perhaps merely expressions of approval and confidence. Lower status persons need reassurance about their superiors' attitudes, evaluations, and intentions towards them. We can conclude that:

2. *People have powerful forces acting upon them to direct their communication toward those who can make them feel more secure and gratify their needs, and away from those who threaten them, make them feel anxious, and generally provide unrewarding experiences.*

---

[3]Leon Festinger, Dorwin Cartwright, et al., "A Study of a Rumor: Its Origin and Spread," *Human Relations,* 1948, 1, pp. 464-486.

[4]Kurt Back, Leon Festinger, et al., "The Methodology of Studying Rumor Transmission," *Human Relations,* 1950, 3, pp. 307-312.

[5]For an illustration of this in a hospital setting, see: Jay Jackson, Gale Jensen, and Floyd Mann, "Building a Hospital Organization for Training Administrators." *Hospital Management,* September, 1956, p. 54.

[6]See Elliot Mishler and Asher Trepp. "Status and Interaction in a Psychiatric Hospital." *Human Relations,* 1956, 9, pp. 187-206; Jay Jackson, *Analysis of interpersonal Relations in a Formal Organization,* Ph.D. Thesis. Univer. of Michigan, 1953; Tom Burns, "The Directions of Activity and Communication in a Departmental Executive Group." *Human Relations,* 1954, 7, pp, 73-79.

People's needs largely determine content of their communication to others of different status. There is evidence that subordinates will often be reluctant to ask supervisors for help when they need it, because this might be seen as a threatening admission of inadequacy.[7] And superiors tend to delete from their communications to subordinates any reference to their own mistakes or errors of judgment.[8] I am sure that these findings are in accord with the experiences that many of us have had in organizations.

A third principle which helps us understand the flow of communication is this:

3. *Persons in an organization are always communicating as if they were trying to improve their position.*

They may or may not be aware of their own behavior in this respect. But the evidence indicates that they want to increase their status, to belong to a more prestigeful group, to obtain more power to influence decisions, and to expand their authority. It has been said that talking upwards is a gratifying substitute for moving upwards. Persons in an organization who are attracted to membership in a particular department or group will feel inclined to direct much more communication in that direction than will those who do not want to belong to it. If they are excluded or barred from membership and their desire to belong persists, they will increase their communication even further, as if this represented a substitute for actually moving into the desirable group.[9]

In a study of the role relationships of three types of professionals who work together in the mental health field[10]—psychiatrists, clinical psychologists, and psychiatric social workers— it was found that the direction, amount, and content of their communication to one another could be predicted largely from two factors. These were: their perception of the other professions' power relative to their own; and how satisfied they were with their own power position compared to that of the other groups. The general principle that forces act on persons to communicate so as to improve their relative position in the organization seems to be supported by all these findings.

THE CONSEQUENCES OF COMMUNICATION

Recent research also has something to tell us about the consequences that communication will have when various conditions exist within an organization. Again we find that it is not possible to state that a particular type of communication will always have the same effect, without specifying the conditions in which the generalization will hold true. At the present time, however, the evidence from research appears to warrant four general conclusions.

1. *The effect of any particular communication will depend largely upon the prior feelings and attitudes that the parties concerned have towards one another.*

Findings from a number of different studies support this statement. During World War II, hostile attitudes and negative stereotypes existed between the inhabitants of a housing project for industrial workers, and members of the surrounding community. An action research project was undertaken, to increase contact between these two groups of people.[11] It was

---

[7]Ian Ross, *Role Specialization in Supervision,* Ph.D. Thesis, Columbia University, 1957.

[8]This finding is from an unpublished study of a public utility company by Alvin Zander.

[9]Experimental evidence exists for this statement in: Jay Jackson and Herbert Saltzstein, *Group Membership and Conformity Processes,* Ann Arbor: Research Center for Group Dynamics, Univers. of Michigan, 1956, p. 89; see also: Harold Kelley, "Communication in Experimentally Created Hierarchies," *Human Relations,* 1950, 4, pp. 39-56.

[10]Zander, A., Cohen, A. R., and Stotland, E. *Role Relations in the Mental Health Professions.* Ann Arbor: Institute for Social-Research, Univer. of Michigan, 1957.

[11]Leon Festinger and Harold Kelley, *Changing Attitudes Through Social Contact.* Ann Arbor: Research Center for Group Dynamics, Univer. of Michigan, 1951.

found, however, that after increased contact the attitudes and feelings of these people had become polarized; those that were initially positive became even more positive, and those that began by being negative became even more negative. The effect of stimulating greater contact could have been predicted only from a knowledge of the pre-existing attitudes and feelings.

In another study of the communication patterns in a large organization, it was found that increased communication did make people more accurate about others' opinions, but only when they initially trusted one another and already were in considerable agreement.[12] When people are in disagreement or do not trust one another, an increase in communication will not necessarily lead to greater understanding.

It was found in another study that frequent communication among personnel made working for the organization either more or less attractive for them. The mediating factor was whether or not the persons who were in constant communication valued each other's contribution to the work of the organization.[13]

2. The effect of any particular communication will depend upon the preexisting expectations and motives of the communicating persons.

Executives of a large organization were asked to indicate on a checklist how much time they spent with each other, and the subject of their interaction.[14] In one-third of the answers they were in disagreement about the subject of their communication. For example, one reported that he had been discussing personnel matters with another; the latter thought they had been discussing questions of production. When these executives differed, each assumed that the problem with which he was personally most

concerned was what they had really been talking about.

The subjects of this study were men with an engineering background. They consistently overestimated the amount of time executives spent on production matters and underestimated the amount of time spent on personnel problems. The impressions their communication made upon them had been shaped by their own goals and motives.

From this and other studies it seems clear that the consequences of communication are limited by people's interest in achieving certain effects, and lack of concern about achieving others. They will be inclined to remember and feel committed to those decisions which are consistent with their own expectations and motives.

3. The effect of a superior's communication with a subordinate will depend upon the relationship between them, and how adequately this relationship satisfies the subordinate's needs.

Communication between superior and subordinate often has consequences which neither of them anticipates nor welcomes. It is especially difficult to avoid problems of misinterpretation or ineffectiveness in this area.

In one organization it was found that some employees who received frequent communication from their supervisor became more accurately informed about their supervisor's real attitudes; but this was not true for other employees who also had constant contact with their supervisor.[15] The difference was traced to whether or not a supervisor said he trusted his subordinates. When he did not trust them, he was more guarded in what he said to them, revealing less of his true feelings. A lack of trust between superior and subordinate can thus act as a barrier to the creation of mutual understanding.

We have discussed how people's need for security directs their communication toward

[12]Glen Mellinger, "Interpersonal Trust as a Factor in Communication." *Journal of Abnormal and Social Psychology,* 1956, 52, pp. 304-309.
[13]Jay Jackson, op. cit.
[14]Tom Burns, op. cit.
[15]Glen Mellinger, op. cit.

higher status persons in an organization. A study was conducted in a public utility company,[16] where it was possible to vary experimentally the kind of communication supervisors gave their subordinates. People became anxious and threatened in response to two different conditions: when communication from their supervisor was unclear, and when the supervisor was inconsistent in what he said from one time to another.

We have also pointed out that the persons in an organization tend to communicate as if they were constantly attempting to improve their positions. This is consistent with the finding that the experienced employees in an organization resent close supervision,[17] since it implies that their power and prestige are less than they want them to be.

The study of the senior staff members in a British engineering plant, referred to earlier, led to the discovery of a process of "status protection." When these men received instructions from their superiors, they often treated them as merely information or advice. In this manner they in effect achieved a relative improvement in their own position in the authority structure, by acting as if no one had the right to direct their activity.

Thus the findings from laboratory and field research point unequivocally to the supervisor-subordinate relationship as one of the crucial factors determining the effect of a supervisor's communication to subordinates. Another major factor is whether or not the subordinate stands alone in his relationship to the supervisor, or belongs to a group of peers in the organization.

4. *The effect of a superior's communication with a subordinate will depend upon the amount of support the subordinate receives from membership in a group of peers.*

An experimental study has demonstrated the remarkable effect of belonging to a group of equals on a subordinate confronted by a powerful and directive superior.[18] Being a member of a group decreased a person's feelings of threat and freed him to disagree with his supervisor and make counterproposals. The person who had the moral support of membership in a group reacted to his supervisor's communication with less defensive and more problem-oriented behavior.

There is a considerable body of evidence, too, that a group acts as a source of "social reality" for its members, providing them an opportunity to validate their ideas and opinions.[19] When communication from a superior is directed to a group as a whole rather than to isolated individuals, it is likely that more accurate transmission of information will be achieved.

PROBLEMS OF COMMUNICATION ARE OFTEN SYMPTOMATIC

From our discussion thus far, I think it should be clear that what we call communication problems are often only symptomatic of other difficulties which exist among persons and groups in an organization. To summarize what has been said or implied, I should like to point to four problems which people in organizations must solve in order to overcome barriers to communication.

1) *The problem of trust or lack of trust.* Communication flows along friendship channels. When trust exists, content is more freely com-

---

[16]Arthur Cohen, "Situational Structure, Self-Esteem, and Threat-Oriented Reactions to Power." A chapter in Dorwin Cartwright, et al., *Studies in Social Power.* Ann Arbor: Research Center for Group Dynamics, Univer. of Michigan, (in press).

[17]This finding is from an unpublished study by Jay Jackson, Jean Butman, and Philip Runkel of the communication patterns and attitudes of employees in two business offices.

[18]Ezra Stotland, "Peer Groups and Reaction to Power Figures." A chapter in Dorwin Cartwright, et al., *Studies in Social Power.* Ann Arbor: Research Center for Group Dynamics, Univer. of Michigan, (in press).

[19]See, for example, Jay M. Jackson, and Herbert D. Saltzstein, "The Effect of Person-Group Relationships on Conformity Processes," *The Journal of Abnormal and Social Psychology,* (in press).

municated, and the recipient is more accurate in perceiving the sender's opinion.

2) *The problem of creating interdependence among persons: common goals and agreement about means for achieving them.* When persons have different goals and value systems, then it is especially important to create mutual understanding about needs and motives.

3) *The problem of distributing rewards fairly,* so that people's needs are being met, and so that they are motivated to contribute to the overall objectives of the organization. Nothing can be so restrictive of the free flow of ideas and information, for example, as the feeling that you may not obtain credit for your contribution.

4) *The exceedingly important problem of understanding and coming to common agreement about the social structure of the organization.* I can think of nothing which would facilitate more the free and accurate flow of communication in an organization than consensus about questions of work, authority, prestige, and status relationships.

Chapter 4

DELEGATION AND DECISION MAKING

Mastering the managerial skill of delegation

ELENA M. VOLANTE, R.N., B.A.

Delegation is a key managerial function. It is a means, or process, if you will, through which a supervisor (or manager) gets the necessary work done through other personnel or sources.

The question for every R.N. who supervises others is not whether she delegates. In fact, the nature of her role requires that she assign work to those who report to her. Rather, the question is how much and how effectively does she delegate. A second question is whether she is content to delegate, as best she can, instinctively acting by trial and error as she goes along; or whether she wishes to go about improving her skill in delegating as she would any other skill, by conscious analysis of what is involved and concentrated effort to master the skill.

The ability to delegate skillfully is a major issue concerning all kinds of supervisory positions in hospitals. There was a time when what is inelegantly but accurately referred to as "seat of the pants" management was enough. But today, our organizations are becoming increasingly complex and require more sophisticated managerial techniques than ever before. These

Reprinted with permission from *The Journal of Nursing Administration*, January-February, 1974.

skills do not come easily, but many can be learned with conscious effort.

Delegation is a major skill that must be mastered by the RN in a supervisory role. Failure to delegate effectively has the potential for many negative results:

1. It results in higher management costs. If tasks that could be done ty those who report to a supervisor are, in fact, done by the supervisor herself, they are more costly. Obviously, she is paid more than those who work for her. This is one of the biggest hidden costs in management, i.e., work done at the wrong level by the wrong person.

2. If a supervisor is busy doing things that those who report to her could well do, she has little time left over to plan and do those things only she has the skill, knowledge, and authority to handle. This is a second hidden cost for all kinds of institutions; namely, professional personnel are not finding time to do the work they have been hired and paid to do. They are too busy doing work others are paid to do.

3. Still another major cost of ineffective delegation is engendered by the supervisor who cannot bring herself to delegate and thus does not enable her staff to grow.

Most developmental theorists believe that employees best develop by doing, by being given challenging opportunities to increase their skills and abilities on the job. The supervisor who is reluctant to "let go" deprives those who work for her of the opportunity to develop as individuals. And she deprives her organization of potentially higher employee contributions.

ATTITUDES THAT LEAD TO UNDERDELEGATING

There are many attitudes on the part of supervisors that lead to their not delegating as much as they should or might like. Some are valid and some are not. Time and risk factors as well as feelings about subordinates and the self underlie some of the attitudes commonly expressed by supervisors to explain or rationalize why they do not delegate more:

Time factors
1. Initially, it takes more time to explain what's needed than for me to do the job myself.

2. I'm constantly interrupted to answer questions and give guidance while the work is in progress.
3. Finally, at some point, I have to check that it's been done and done right—something I could avoid if I did it myself.
4. If the task involves other departments, I can usually get decisions and cooperation from them easier and faster than the people who work for me can.

Risk factors
1. If my people make a mistake, I'll be blamed.
2. If they make more than a couple of mistakes while they're learning, their performance may be unjustly judged.

Feelings about subordinates
1. My people are not experienced enough.
2. They are already too busy.
3. They have less knowledge than I about the total situation and are more likely to overlook something.
4. If I ask them to do more, they will expect higher salaries.
5. I can't depend on them to keep me informed about developing problems before they reach a crisis stage.

Exhibit A □ SELF-TEST

Are you an effective delegator? Here are some indicators by which you can make a rough judgment about whether you are delegating enough and well.

Are you:	Yes	No
1. Regularly working long overtime hours?	□	□
2. Unable to move key projects forward to fruition as fast as you'd like?	□	□
3. Often rushed in meeting deadlines?	□	□
4. Always busier than the poeple who work for you?	□	□
5. Doing much of the same kind of work your people are doing?	□	□
6. Doing work similar to work you performed before you were promoted?	□	□
7. So busy you haven't planned any new priorities or projects for your unit for a long time?	□	□
8. Coming back from vacation and finding a lot of things on your desk waiting for decisions and action?	□	□
9. Unable to identify a subordinate whom you've sufficiently brought along that she might replace you should you be promoted or leave your unit for other reasons?	□	□

The more yes answers you have, the more likely it is that you must work at improving your skill in delegation.

Personal feelings

1. I like doing some of this work myself.
2. I get less personal recognition for work I get done through others than for work I do myself.
3. By sharing responsibility and knowledge, I lose control, power, and prestige.
4. Delegating to others involves planning for and with them—if you're action-oriented like I am, the real satisfaction comes from doing something rather than planning for someone else to do it.

Do you see anything of yourself in these kinds of comments? If you do, you probably should take another look at the attitudes expressed and ask yourself whether in your situation and in your unit those attitudes are valid and justifiable. The Self-Test in Exhibit A will further help you judge whether you need to work at improving your skill in delegating.

STEPS TOWARD BETTER DELEGATION

Whenever you ask someone to do something in your unit, you are engaged in delegation. What are some steps to follow to insure that you delegate as wisely as possible? Some of the important ones follow:

Define the task to be done

Determine in your own mind just what it is you wish to have done. That is, define the task. So often, supervisors go to someone who works for them with a fuzzy concept of precisely what is needed. Without careful conceptualization, without a clear understanding of what you want done and why, you cannot possibly communicate effectively with someone else. If you really want to work at delegating, you should not hesitate at this stage of the game to put in writing—for your own use—a few sentences describing the task. This is a simple technique whose chief value is that it forces you to recognize whether or not your thinking has crystallized. If you cannot put the key facts down on paper, the chances are that trying to "wing it" orally will not be fully effective.

Relay your definition of the task

Tell the person you have selected to perform the task precisely *what* you want done, as you have defined it in your own mind. Go on to explain the reasons behind the task, the purpose it is to serve, etc. Ask for and take time to answer questions. If people have an understanding of why something is needed, chances are they can bring a great deal more thought of their own to the project and help both themselves and you.

Notice that we have said define "what" you want done. This means the end results you expect, including when you wish it done and what standards or yardsticks you will use to determine whether it is adequate. In delegating, whether or not you should prescribe "how" to do the task depends very much on the subordinate involved. For example, if the subordinate is an experienced, fairly knowledgeable person, it is best for that person's own self-development that the step-by-step means to achieve the results you have requested not be mapped. If you define only the "what's" and leave room for them to develop the "how's," they will have greater opportunity to relate to the task and feel a sense of responsibility. Obviously, however, you can invite such persons to come back and talk with you after they have thought through how they are going to go about it, what approaches they plan to use, etc. And you can make it clear that you are there as a resource person for support and interest.

Other employees may be relatively inexperienced, afraid of responsibility, or otherwise uncomfortable about your not indicating how to go about producing the results you have defined. In such cases, direction and guidance on step-by-step possibilities for achieving assignments will need to be greater on your part. This is a large area of judgment for the supervisor and it requires her to familiarize herself with the different skills, abilities, and personal characteristics of those who work for her.

Establish controls and checkpoints

Another important step in delegating is the establishing of controls and checkpoints to insure feedback. Since you remain accountable for work you delegate, it is essential that you follow through here. Lawrence Appley, former president of the American Management Association, once said, "Employees respect what the manager inspects." Very often supervisors delegate a task, assume it will be done, and then go on to something else. Obviously, a supervisor does not have to check every piece of work. On the other hand, she should have some means of periodically assessing the work going on. This may be done by informal meetings, by formal meetings, through written reports, or by just walking out onto the nursing floor periodically and actually observing what is going on. If employees sense that you are interested in following through, chances are they will do likewise.

Establish dialogue

Finally, open dialogue between the supervisor and each of the individuals who report to her will help. How do they feel about what is being delegated to them? What is her judgment about how they are handling delegated tasks? Can some joint goals be worked out to enable them to develop more as individuals and release time for the supervisor for tasks only she can tackle?

SUMMARY

While many management practices are open to debate due to different philosophies and styles of managing, there is substantial agreement on the need to delegate effectively. The purpose of this article has been to help the supervisor examine how well she delegates and how she might go about improving this managerial skill. The payoffs from effective delegation are important for the supervisor herself, for those she supervises, and for her institution. The supervisor wins time to plan and do important work which requires her special knowledge and skills. This is often work which could help her unit become more effective, but which she has had to put off or let slide for lack of time. Those she supervises have increased opportunities for responsibility and growth. The institution benefits from the broadened activities of both the supervisor and her people.

Profile of small group decision making

ANDRE L. DELBECQ, Ph.D., ANDREW H. VAN de VEN, Ph.D., and DAVID H. GUSTAFSON, Ph.D.

Our scientific knowledge of small group decision-making processes is incomplete. Nevertheless, a significant body of empirical knowledge exists that can provide the practitioner with general guidelines for structuring group decision-making processes for different types of problems. In particular, a number of research studies have examined the effects of alternative processes on the performance of decision-making groups in terms of (1) the quantity, quality, and variety of ideas generated; (2) the affectional (emotional and expressive) overtones of interaction; and (3) the nature of facilitative and inhibitive influences on creative problem solving. This chapter[1] will at-

[1]The material in this chapter draws heavily from Van de Ven, 1974.

tempt to summarize the research by comparing the relative effectiveness of interacting,[2] nominal, and Delphi decision-making processes.

INTERACTING VERSUS NOMINAL PROCESSES

The past fifteen years have seen a rapid growth of interest in the comparative effectiveness of individuals versus groups, and nominal versus interacting group methods in decision situations that require individuals to generate information concerning a problem. Osborn (1957), a major proponent of "brainstorming" techniques in problem solving, posited "the average person can think up twice as many ideas when working with a group than working alone." When comparing the average number of ideas produced by groups with the average number of ideas produced by individuals, brainstorming groups were found superior to an equal number of individuals brainstorming independently (Hall, Mouton, and Blake, 1963; Osborn, 1957). Further, brainstorming groups were found superior to conventional discussion groups in problem-solving situations (Bouchard, 1969; Osborn, 1957; Parnes and Meadow, 1959). Taylor, Berry, and Block (1958) found interacting groups superior to individuals in problem-solving situations when comparing the performance of individuals working alone with that of a group in which the same individuals participate at another time. They state: "Such group superiority may very well account for the widespread impression that group participation does facilitate the production of ideas."

---

[2]"Interacting" in the context of this chapter refers to a conventional discussion group format, which is generally an unstructured, free-flowing meeting, with minimal direction by the leader other than the presentation of the issue to the group. Obviously, a trained leader can create increasing degrees of structure in a discussion group, so that an interacting group can approximate a structured group process. However, one should then read "interacting" in this chapter as "unstructured discussion group."

Since the pioneering work of Osborn, various modifications have been made on the brainstorming technique. The method receiving the greatest research interest has been the *nominal group process*, where people work in the presence of each other but write ideas independently rather than talk about them. Three measures have generally been used to compare the relative effectiveness of nominal versus interacting group processes: (1) the average number of unique ideas; (2) the average total number of ideas; and (3) the quality of ideas produced.

In terms of these three measures of performance, nominal groups have been found to be significantly superior to interacting groups in generating information relevant to a problem (Bouchard, 1969; Bouchard and Hare, 1970; Campbell, 1968; Dunnette, Campbell, and Jaastad, 1963; Leader, 1963; Taylor et al., 1958; Vroom, Grant, and Cotton, 1969). Researchers have concluded that when the group task is to generate information on a problem, interacting groups inhibit creative thinking. (This is not a generic statement of superiority. For other purposes, such as attitude change, team building, and consensus generation, interacting groups are superior. The emphasis here is on *idea generation*.) Individual inhibitions and premature evaluation in interacting groups result in a decrease in quality of group ideas in terms of creativity, originality, and practicality (Collaros and Anderson, 1969). A focus effect is also characteristic of interacting groups; that is, the group tends to pursue a single train of thought for long periods (Dunnette et al., 1963; Taylor et al, 1958).

NGT VERSUS THE DELPHI TECHNIQUE

A comparison of the decision-making steps in NGT and the Delphi Technique, outlined in Chapter 1, suggests that the two techniques are strikingly similar.

First, both rely on independent individual

work for idea generation. In the Delphi process, isolated and typically anonymous respondents independently write their ideas or reactions to a questionnaire. NGT group members write their ideas on a sheet of paper in silence, in the presence of other group members seated around a table.

Second, individual judgments are pooled in both techniques. Delphi respondents mail their completed questionnaires to the design and monitoring team who, in turn, pool and collate the judgments of the respondent group in a feedback report. In NGT, the judgments of group members are pooled via the round-robin procedure, wherein the ideas of each member are presented to the group and written on a blackboard or flip chart.

Third, both allow for an idea-evaluation stage. In the Delphi process, the monitoring team mails the feedback report to the respondent group, and each respondent independently reads, evaluates, and interprets the ideas on the feedback report. In NGT, the group discusses, verbally clarifies, and evaluates each of the individual ideas of group members that were written on the blackboard or flip chart.

Finally, in both processes, mathematical voting procedures are used (e.g., rank-order or rating methods), and the group decision is arrived at by a mathematical decision rule for aggregating the individual judgments (Huber and Delbecq, 1972).

As indicated above, the major differences between the two processes appear to be:

1) Delphi respondents are typically anonymous to one another, while NGT group members become acquainted with one another.

2) NGT groups meet face to face around a table, while Delphi respondents are physically distant and never meet face to face.

3) All communications between respondents in the Delphi process occur via written questionnaires and feedback reports form

the monitoring team. In NGT groups, communications occur directly between members.

INTERACTING, NGT, AND DELPHI PROCESSES

The Delphi Technique was the product of studies of technological forecasting and transfer. The NGT technique was a synthesis of social-psychological group studies. As a result, relatively few researchers have crossed the two traditions to experimentally compare the Delphi Technique with nominal or interacting group methods; however, there are a few notable exceptions.

Gustafson and his associates (1973) tested the comparative effectiveness of independent individuals and interacting, NGT, and Delphi processes on a problem of subjective probability estimation (e. g., "What is the probability that it will rain tomorrow?"). It was found that NGT groups were superior to all other processes in terms of lowest percentage of error and variability of estimations. The Delphi process obtained the poorest outcome, while interacting groups and individuals working independently in nominal groups emerged second and third best, respectively.

Contrary to the findings of Gustafson et al., experiments carried out by Dalkey at Rand (1968, 1969) and Campbell at the University of California (1966) found the Delphi process more effective than interacting meetings. In these experiments, the problem required respondents to estimate the accuracy of a set of facts. The pooled estimates resulting from the Delphi Technique were found more accurate than the estimates resulting from the interacting meetings.

Further comparison

While the above research studies compared decision-making techniques for purposes of probability-estimation problems, one may question whether the research results would be the same if a more real-life, controversial, and emotionally involving problem were chosen. Van de Ven (1974) subjected the NGT, interacting, and Delphi techniques to a formal experimental comparison on an applied problem that was considered by participants to (1) be very difficult; (2) have no solution that would be equally acceptable to all interest groups involved; and (3) evoke highly emotional and subjective responses. Sixty heterogeneous groups (twenty NGT, twenty Delphi, and twenty interacting), each with seven members, were asked to define the job description of a university dormitory counselor. Comparisons between the NGT, Delphi, and interacting groups were based on the quality of ideas generated and the immediate perceived satisfaction of participants with the decision-making technique in which they had participated. Van de Ven (1974) found that the NGT and Delphi processes generated almost twice as many ideas as interacting groups, and that NGT groups generated slightly more ideas than Delphi groups. In terms of satisfaction, NGT group participants expressed a significantly higher level of satisfaction than did participants in the interacting and Delphi processes. Further, no significant differences were found in perceived group satisfaction between interacting and Delphi techniques.

CHARACTERISTICS OF GROUP PROCESSES

The above research studies clearly show that on problems requiring groups to generate information, differences exist among NGT, interacting, and Delphi processes. These quantitative findings, however, do not qualitatively explain why such differences exist. A number of researchers have investigated these differences. They found several key process characteristics which are structured into the NGT, Delphi, and interacting techniques which either facilitate or inhibit group performance. These key process characteristics are:

1) *Overall methodology* — the overall structure of decision-making processes.
2) *Role orientation of groups* — the tendency for groups to direct attention toward social roles (e.g., friendship acts or congeniality) or task-oriented roles (e.g., idea giving or judgment sharing).
3) *Search behavior* — the style used by a group to generate task-relevant information, and the amount of effort directed by a group to identify problems.
4) *Normative behavior* — the felt freedom to express ideas in discussions, and the level of conforming behavior in a process.
5) *Equality of participation* — the number of individuals in the group who contribute to search, evaluation, and choice of a group's product or output.
6) *Group composition and size* — the homogeneity or hetereogeneity of personnel in a group, as well as the number of individuals involved in the decision-making process.
7) *Method of conflict resolution* — the procedure used by groups to resolve disagreements and conflicts.
8) *Closure to decision process* — the extent to which the meeting arrives at a clear termination point providing an agreed-upon decision and a sense of accomplishment.
9) *Utilization of resources* — the time, cost, and effort involved for administrators and participants in each process.

In the following sections, we will comparatively analyze NGT, Delphi, and interacting processes on these key dimensions.

Role orientations of groups

When an individual works alone, as in the Delphi process, he can focus his entire attention on the problem-solving task. When he works in the presence of others, as in the interacting and NGT processes, then he must also attend to the social, interpersonal obstacles which are dictated by the need for joint task efforts and which are inevitably present when groups meet face to face. For the group member, then, a meeting implies two sets of problems: (1) those which stem directly from the task of problem solving (task-instrumental problems); and (2) those which stem directly from the need to build interpersonal relations with other group members in order to attain the greater problem-solving potential available in the face-to-face group (social-emotional problems). Further, many of the problems created by the presence of other people have no relationship to the task (Collins and Guetzkow, 1964). The greater the amount of effort a decision-making process demands of a group in maintaining social-emotional relationships, the less proportionate time and effort remain for task-instrumental problem solving (Campbell, 1968). It is appropriate, therefore, to compare NGT, Delphi, and interacting processes in terms of task-instrumental versus social-emotional role orientations.

Van de Ven (1974) utilized follow-up questionnaires and interviews with group participants and leaders in order to qualitatively interpret his research results (reported above), and to investigate more deeply the basic characteristics of NGT, Delphi, and interacting groups to account for their clear differences in performance. He reported that the interacting group participants indicated that they most enjoyed the cohesion, friendliness, and agreement among group members, while a majority expressed dislike for the lack of task accomplishment. The interacting group leaders indicated that their groups avoided controversies and heated discussions. Rather, discussions centered around those issues on which group members agreed. Group cohesion and interpersonal relationships, therefore, were developed and maintained around areas of agreement. Clearly, the results that emerged in the interacting groups indicate a predominant orientation toward stimulating and maintaining social-emotional cohesion among members.

The participants who aspired to solve the problem, however, felt the process frustrating because of "dangling conversations."

An opposite situation was found in the Delphi groups. Since group members do not meet face to face in the Delphi Technique, there is a complete absence of social-emotional behavior, and all attention focuses on task-instrumental activities. Van de Ven (1974) found, however, that the total absence of interpersonal relationships inhibits task performance because of the lack of verbal clarification or comment on ideas in the feedback report. As anonymous senders and recipients of information, Delphi respondents stated that they did not know to whom they were expressing their ideas or who their group was. Thus, they were unsure of how to express their responses in language understandable to their group. They also questioned whether their interpretations of the ideas in the feedback report were accurate. As a result, 25 percent of the Delphi groups suggested that a discussion with others would be a more interesting and stimulating way to investigate the problem.

NGT stimulates a balanced orientation among group members between task-instrumental and social-emotional concerns. The silent (nominal) period of independent thought and writing forces participants to think and work through the problem. The round-robin listing of ideas followed by a group discussion period clarifies the meaning of each participant's ideas and generates alternative interpretations of the ideas by group members. In the follow-up interviews, a majority of the NGT group leaders reported that while group members appeared to enjoy interaction during the discussion period, with intermittent intervals of laughter and humor, the group remained focused on the task.

Van de Ven (1974) concludes that neither the socially oriented nature of the interacting process, nor the task-oriented nature of the Delphi Technique, are very acceptable to participants or particularly conducive to problem solving. Rather, NGT, which provides a balanced concern for task accomplishment and interpersonal social maintenance functions, appears most acceptable to participants and facilitates problem solving. These qualitative conclusions were quantitatively supported. Van de Ven found no statistical difference between the interacting and Delphi groups concerning perceived group satisfaction, while participants' satisfaction with the NGT process was significantly greater than with either the Delphi or interacting process.

Search behavior

One of the critical process characteristics facilitating creativity is the separation of problems from solutions. Group problem-solving processes which separate ideation (problem identification) from evaluation (solution getting) are superior to group processes which combine them (Brilhart and Jochem, 1964; Maier, 1958; Maier and Hoffman, 1960; Maier and Maier, 1957). According to Maier and Hoffman (1960), ''It appears to be a human tendency to seek solutions even before the problem is understood. This tendency to be 'solution minded' seems to become stronger when there is anxiety over the nature of the decision.'' Research indicates that the success of problem-solving groups in arriving at creative decisions is related to the proportion of time spent working on the problem (Rotter and Portugal, 1969). Significantly better ideas are generated in the final third period of an individual's independent thought on a topic than in the first two-thirds of the period (Parnes, 1961; Zagona, Ellis, and MacKinnon, 1966). Thus, the quality of group performance can be increased by group processes which (1) retard speedy decisions; and (2) cause the group to perceive the task with an attitude of problem-mindedness as opposed to solution-mindedness (Maier, 1958; Maier and Solem, 1952).

Van de Ven (1974) found clear differences in the nature of search behavior in NGT, Delphi, and interacting groups. A *reactive search* process, wherein group members tended to react to the opinions of others rather than generate their own ideas, existed in interacting groups. The reactive search process was characterized by short periods of focus on the problem, frequent interruptions and drifting comments by various participants, tangential discussions, and high efforts at maintaining social relationships. Due to the lack of opportunity for group members to independently think through the problem, ideas were expressed as generalizations, and members were reluctant to become specific in their remarks. This was the case even after leaders repeatedly asked members to specifically state what they meant (Van de Ven, 1974). Other researchers have also observed a focus effect in unstructured group meetings, whereby members fall into a rut and pursue a single train of thought for extended periods of discussion (Taylor et al., 1958).

Van de Ven (1974) found that a *proactive search* process existed in the NGT and Delphi processes because each participant was required to write and/or articulate his ideas without the opportunity for other group members to react or evaluate until all ideas were presented. In the Delphi Technique, the respondent group stated that the act of writing responses forced them to think through the problem, and that the repetitive feedback and multiquestionnaire approach was a sensible way to systematically break down a complex problem into workable steps. In addition, written expression of ideas induces a greater feeling of task commitment and a greater sense of permanence than does spoken expression (Bouchard, 1969; Horowitz and Newman, 1964).

Thus, the proactive search behavior that is structured into NGT and the Delphi Technique facilitates problem-mindedness by extending the period of problem-centered focus and by requiring individuals to record their thoughts

(Dunnette, 1964; Maier and Solem, 1952; Van de Ven, 1974). The reactive search behavior characteristic of interacting groups results in short, interrupted periods of problem concentration and a tendency to reach speedy decisions before critical dimensions of the problem have been considered (Maier and Hoffman, 1960).

Finally, since NGT and the Delphi Technique structure procedures for decision making, Van de Ven (1974) found high consistency in group performance and low variability in member and leader behavior across groups. However, when interacting meetings are unstructured, high variability in member and leader behavior and in group performance occurs.

Normative behavior

A number of researchers have examined the impact of group norms on the behavior of individuals within a group. In general, research suggests that the normative pressures for conformity prevalent in conventional discussion groups (1) constrain the felt freedom and openness of members to express their ideas; and (2) inhibit creative decision making.

Tersely summarized, the prevalence of conforming behavior in interacting groups seems to relate to the following causes:

1) The fact that covert judgments are made by group members even though they are not expressed as overt criticisms in the meeting (Collaros and Anderson, 1969).
2) The inevitable presence of status incongruities in most organizational groups, wherein low-status participants may be inhibited and go along with opinions expressed by high-status participants (Torrance, 1957).
3) The implied threat of sanctions from the more knowledgeable members (Hoffman, 1965).
4) The influence of dominant personality types upon the group (Chung and Ferris, 1971).

NGT minimizes many of the conforming in-

fluences of face-to-face group meetings which act to reduce their performance (Van de Ven and Delbecq, 1971). This is due to a number of nonconformance characteristics that are structured into NGT. Because of the nominal phase (silent generation of ideas in writing), the round-robin presenting and recording of ideas on a flip chart, the serial review and clarification of all ideas on the flip chart, and the independent mathematical voting on idea priorities:

1) Hidden agendas and covert group dynamics are minimized (Fouriezos, Hatt, and Guetzkow, 1950).
2) Minority opinions and ideas are more likely to be generated and voiced (Maier and Hoffman, 1960; Shaw, 1954).
3) Conflicting and incompatible ideas are tolerated in writing (Deutsch, 1949; Guetzkow and Gyr, 1954; and Torrance, 1957).
4) All participants are equally expected and given an opportunity to produce their share of ideas and to contribute to the group product (Bales, 1953; Benne and Sheets, 1948).
5) All participants are allowed the opportunity for influencing the direction of group decision outcome (Goldman, Bolen, and Martin, 1961; Maier, 1958; Pelz, 1956).

In a similar manner, the Delphi process minimizes conforming influences because face-to-face discussion is eliminated and respondents are anonymous to one another (Dalkey and Helmer, 1963).

Researchers also suggest that individuals in a group hesitate to identify personal problems when dealing with tasks having social-emotional dimensions (Delbecq and Van de Ven, 1971). They tend to focus upon organizational, institutional, or conventionally accepted problem characteristics. When the social-emotional dimensions of a problem are important and need to be identified, a structured nominal process of separating personal (inside) from institutional or organizational (outside) categories is helpful. For example, in a group setting, elderly persons who were exploring services easily mentioned outside or organizational problems, such as cost of drugs, transportation, etc. Only when they were asked to separately list personal problems did elderly groups bring out areas such as fear of death, loneliness, preoccupation with sickness, feeling disliked by younger people, and other critical social-emotional issues.

Equality of participation

Closely related to normative behavior is the equality of participation among members when contributing to the search, evaluation, and group decision. To the extent that decision making is dominated by a few high-status, expressive, or strong individuals, there will be a lower felt freedom for open discussion and a reduction in the quality of decision making (Chung and Ferris, 1971).

When comparing the evaluations of NGT, interacting, and Delphi participants, Van de Ven (1974) found that only in the interacting process did groups indicate that not all participants felt free to participate and contribute their ideas. There was also a tendency for discussions to polarize on issues and be dominated by a few members, and for issues to be personalized with individuals.

In the NGT groups, on the other hand, there was an absence of felt pressure from dominant individuals, and an expressed freedom to ask objective questions on controversial ideas. Van de Ven (1974) reports that while dominant individuals were the most expressive during the discussion period. they did not take over the meeting because all group members had already had an opportunity to express their views. As a result, the opinions of dominant individuals were simply included in the sample of ideas already under consideration.

Because there is no face-to-face contact among respondents in the Delphi process, there is no opportunity for a few strong individuals to dominate the group's output.

Group size and composition

Numerous researchers have studied group size in terms of number of ideas generated, difficulty in reaching consensus, and patterns of interaction. They have found that, for groups involving interaction, as size increases above some limit (about size seven), restraints against participation also increase and the most active participants become increasingly differentiated. As the size of the group increases, the superiority of NGT over the conventional interacting group increases in terms of the total number of nonoverlapping ideas produced (Carter, Merrowitz, and Lanzetta, 1951; Delbecq, 1968; Gibb, 1951; Hare, 1952; Holloman and Hendrich, 1971; Leader, 1963; South, 1924).

NGT can accommodate larger numbers of participants (up to a limit of approximately nine members) without the dysfunctions of conventional interacting groups (Bouchard and Hare, 1970). There is no limit to the number of participants in a Delphi survey, and the Delphi process is frequently used as a technique to survey one or more target groups. The number of participants is generally determined by the number of respondents required to constitute a representative pooling of judgments for each target group and by the information-processing capability of the design and monitoring team.

Several studies have tested the effects of homogeneous or heterogeneous group composition on problem-solving effectiveness. Heterogeneous groups, characterized by members with widely varying personalities and substantially different perspectives on a problem, were found to produce a higher proportion of high-quality, high-acceptance solutions than homogeneous groups (Hoffman, 1959; Hoffman and Maier, 1961; Hoffman and Smith,

1960). On the other hand, homogeneous groups were found to facilitate group performance because of the reduced likelihood of interpersonal conflict and dominance of the group by one or a few (Grace, 1954; Haythorn, 1953). The mixed results found in these studies suggest that there is value in using the heterogeneous group if its detrimental effects can be controlled. Given the composition of group membership, Bouchard (1969) suggests structured group processes (such as NGT) can facilitate problem solving by (1) specifying clearly the role requirements, i.e., expectations of how participants should behave (Speisman and Moos, 1962); and (2) structuring communication networks, i.e., clarifying when sequential vs. random discussion is desired (Leavitt, 1951).

Method of conflict resolution

N.R.F. Maier (1964) and A. C. Filley (1973, 1974) suggest that disagreement among group members can lead either to hard feelings or to creative decision making, depending upon how it is controlled. Conflict can lead to hard feelings by allowing disagreements to be resolved in personalized emotional pitches, or to be smoothed over by humor or withdrawal. Conflict can lead to creative problem solving by separating persons from problems and attacking the problem rather than the person. In addition, Burke (1970) examined the effect of alternative conflict resolution methods on (1) the constructive use of disagreements; and (2) the perceived satisfaction of conflicting parties with a resolution to disagreements. It was found that withdrawing (remaining silent) and forcing (using status or aggression to dominate) methods as a means to resolve conflict were negatively related to (1) and (2) above. The smoothing-over method was inconsistently related (sometimes positive, sometimes negative). Only confrontation or problem solving always related positively to the above.

Van de Ven (1974) observed that different methods for conflict resolution were generally used in the interacting and NGT groups. In the interacting groups, cohesion and interpersonal relationships developed around areas of agreement. In efforts to maintain these social interrelationships, the interacting groups avoided or smoothed over disagreements by dwelling upon noncontroversial issues. When disagreements did openly emerge, the contending members became polarized on issues, and remarks were personalized during the discussion.

In direct contrast to the problem-solving methods followed to resolve conflicts in the interacting process, the NGT groups confronted disagreements openly and more frequently and depersonalized the problem. Since participants' ideas were recorded on a chart during the round-robin phase of the NGT meeting, during the discussion phase group participants attacked items on the chart—not individuals. Rhetorical, ideological, and emotional comments were more easily transformed into objective problem issues. As a result, groups reported that a positive, constructive attitude toward problem solving emerged among participants in the NGT meetings (Van de Ven, 1974).

Closure to decision process

When comparing the three decision-making processes, Van de Ven (1974) found in his research that in the interacting groups there was less perceived closure, lower felt accomplishment, and lower interest in future phases of problem solving than was true of either NGT or Delphi groups. (NGT and Delphi Technique, of course, are so structured that they do have a clear termination point.) Van de Ven concluded:

"The negative reactions of interacting group participants to the task also manifested itself in the severe difficulties leaders encountered in conducting their meetings. Interacting leaders reported a reluctance of groups to get into the task at hand at the beignning of the meeting.

Leaders felt much time was wasted in reacting to diversionary questions, personal statements, and ideologies regarding the task. Leaders also indicated they encountered difficulties in concluding their meetings, getting groups to set priorities on the ideas expressed during the meetings, and in arriving at a sense of closure to the meeting'' (p. 136).

In direct contrast to the difficulties encountered by interacting leaders, a majority of the NGT leaders reported their groups became sincerely concerned with and motivated by the task at hand, and expressed interest in future phases of the study (Van de Ven, 1974). In terms of closure and felt accomplishment, Delphi groups would score intermediately between interacting and NGT groups.

Utilization of resources

Thus far, attention has been directed toward making quantitative and qualitative comparisons among NGT, interacting, and Delphi processes without regard to the administration of these three procedures. From a practical standpoint, however, the choice of a decision-making procedure in the applied field must also consider the length of time and the amount of administrative cost and effort required to obtain information. This is particularly true when a practitioner needs input from a large number of groups. Suppose, for example, the practitioner is faced with a planning or problem-solving situation which requires information input from multiple reference groups (e.g., consumers, providers, suppliers, administrators, resource controllers, etc.). He or she is offered three alternative processes for obtaining this information: NGT, Delphi, or interacting group techniques. Purely from an administrative perspective of time, cost, and effort, which process should be chosen?

Table 2-1 summarizes the time, cost, and effort for administrators and participants in the 20 NGT, 20 interacting, and 20 Delphi groups conducted in the Van de Ven study. In that study, on the average, the *total administrative*

working hours required to prepare for, conduct, and follow through *for one group* was 4.4 hours, 4.2 hours, and 7.1 hours, respectively, for NGT, interacting, and Delphi processes. The *average cost per group* was $11.50 for NGT, $11.00 for interacting, and $22.00 for the Delphi process. The Delphi process required almost twice as much administrative time and cost as did the NGT and interacting groups involving a comparable number of participants.

As indicated in Table 2-1, however, from the participants' perspective the *average working hours per participant* in the Delphi Technique were far less (one-half hour) than in the NGT groups (one and one-half working hours), or in the interacting groups (one and one-quarter working hours). The Delphi process also saved participants the additional time and cost of having to attend face-to-face meetings.

In terms of the *calendar time* required to collect the same information, *on the average,* the NGT or interacting group meetings required four evenings, while a two-round Delphi required 5 months. Thus, is is clear that the Delphi process requires significantly more calendar time than the other two processes in collecting the same information.

On the basis of time and cost required for *participants,* the Delphi Technique is superior to NGT and interacting groups. If, on the other hand, participants have the time and no large travel costs are entailed in bringing people together, NGT and interacting processes require less *administrative* cost and effort, and the information can be collected in far less calendar time.

SUMMARY PROFILE

Based upon the preceding review of research findings, Table 2-2 presents a recapitulation of the qualitative differences among interacting, NGT, and Delphi groups. The research suggests that different phases of problem solving require different group-process strategies. A profile of the comparative merits of the three decision-making techniques for generating information and group ideas on a problem or issue can now be summarized.

Interacting groups

For *fact-finding problems,* interacting groups contain a number of process characteristics which inhibit decision-making performance:

1) Because interacting group meetings are unstructured, high variability in membership and leader behavior occurs from group to group.

2) Discussion tends to fall into a rut, with group members focusing on a single train of thought for extended periods, and with relatively few ideas generated.

3. The absence of an opportunity to think through independent ideas results in a tendency for ideas to be expressed as generalizations.

4) Search behavior is reactive and characterized by short periods of focus on the problem, tendencies for task avoidance, tangenital discussions, and high efforts in establishing social relationships and generating social knowledge.

5) High-status, expressive, or strong personality-type individuals tend to dominate in search, evaluation, and choice of group product.

6) Meetings tend to conclude with a high perceived lack of closure, low felt accomplishment, and low interest in future phases of problem solving.

There are, however, a number of techniques that can be adopted during conventional discussion group meetings to improve their performance. When there is a need to obtain the ideas of all group members on a problem or issue to be discussed, the round-robin technique can be very helpful. This technique facilities the self-disclosure of ideas even by less secure members who may hesitate to bring some problem dimensions before the group in the conventional interacting situation (Culbert, 1968). Further, the round-robin procedure of writing problem dimensions and issues on a blackboard of flip chart reduces arguments over semantics, increases retention of ideas presented, and decreases redundancy of discussions (Delbecq and Van de Ven, 1971). Finally, evaluation and synthesis of issues can be improved in discussion groups by having the total set of ideas or issues placed in writing before the group prior to spontaneous discussion of each idea.

It should be noted, however, that interacting groups can play a very positive role with respect to: (1) increasing group motivation and cohesion; (2) increasing a sense of group consensus; and (3) increasing the feeling that each alternative solution possibility has been carefully reviewed. Thus, for certain motivational purposes, the problems associated with the interacting group may not cancel out its benefits.

NGT

NGT is a structured group meeting which follows a prescribed sequence of problem-solving steps. The NGT process includes a number of characteristics which facilitate decision-making performance:

1) Low variability among groups in member and leader behavior leads to consistency in decision making.

2) A balanced concern for social-emotional group maintenance roles and performance of task-instrumental roles offers both social reinforcement and task accomplishment reward to group members.

3) The silent independent generation of ideas, followed by further thought and listening during the round-robin procedure, results in a high quality of ideas.

4) Search behavior is proactive, characterized by extended periods in generating and clarifying alternative dimensions of the problem, tendencies for high task-centered group effort, and the generation of new social and task-related knowledge.

5) The structured process forces equality of participation among members in generating information on the problem.

6) NGT meetings tend to conclude with a perceived sense of closure, accomplishment, and interest in future phases of problem solving.

Associated with the positive characteristics of NGT are difficulties that are frequently encountered in conducting NGT meetings. While these difficulties and possible solutions will be discussed in detail in Chapter 3, the include:

1) Extended preparation for NGT meetings is necessary to clearly identify the information desired from a group, and to provide the necessary supplies. NGT, therefore, is not a spontaneous group meeting technique.

2) Inflexibility of the structured NGT format makes it difficult to make adjustments or to change topics in the middle of a meeting. NGT is generally limited, therefore, to a single-purpose, single-topic meeting.

3) Conforming behavior to a structured format is required on the part of all participants, a condition which is not immediately comfortable to inexperienced participants.

The Delphi technique

The Delphi process is a survey technique for decision making among isolated anonymous respondents. The characteristics of the Delphi process which facilitate decision-making performance are:

1) The isolated generation of ideas in writing produces a high quality of ideas.

2) The process of writing responses to the questions forces respondents to think through the complexity of the problem, and to submit specific, high-quality ideas.

3) Search behavior is proactive since respondents cannot react to the ideas of others.

4) The anonymity and isolation of respondents provides freedom from conformity pressures.

5) Simple pooling of independent ideas and judgments facilitates equality of participants.

6) The Delphi process tends to conclude with a moderate perceived sense of closure and accomplishment.

7) The technique is valuable for obtaining judgments from experts geographically isolated.

The major characteristics of the Delphi process which inhibit decision-making performance are:

1) The lack of opportunity for social-emotional rewards in problem solving leads to a feeling of detachment from the problem-solving effort.

2) The lack of opportunity for verbal clarification or comment on the feedback report creates communication and interpretation difficulties among respondents.

3) Conflicting or incompatible ideas on the feedback report are handled by simply pooling and adding the votes of group respondents. Thus, while this majority rule procedure identifies group priorities, conflicts are not resolved.

This chapter has summarized research on NGT, Delphi, and interacting groups concerned with judgmental problem solving. The present burden of evidence favors NGT and Delphi approaches to idea or estimate generation, interaction for purposes of clarification, and mathematical voting in the form of rank-ordering or rating for aggregating group judgments. Chapters 3 and 4 will detail NGT and Delphi formats which combine these group processes at different stages of analysis. Both techniques should greatly enhance the quality of group effort for judgmental tasks.

References

Bales, R. F. "The Equilibrium Problem in Small Groups." In *Working Papers in the Theory of Action*. T. Parsons, R. F. Bales, and E. A. Shils. Free Press, 1953.

Benne, K. A., and P. Sheets. "Functional Roles of Group Numbers." *Journal of Social Issues*, 2 (1948): 42-47.

Bouchard, T. J., Jr. "Personality, Problem-Solving

Procedure, and Performance in Small Groups," *Journal of Applied Psychology,* 53, 1, Part 2 (February 1969): 1-29.

Bouchard, T. J., Jr., and M. Hare. "Size, Performance, and Potential in Brainstorming Groups." *Journal of Applied Psychology,* 54, 1 (February 1970): 51-55.

Brillhart, J. K., and L. M. Jochem. "The Effects of Different Patterns on Outcomes of Problem-Solving Discussions." *Journal of Applied Psychology,* 48 (1964): 175-79.

Burke, R. J. "Methods of Resolving Superior-Subordinate Conflict: The Constructive Use of Subordinate Differences and Disagreements." *Organization Behavior and Human Performance,* 5 (1970): 393-411.

Campbell, J. P. "Individual versus Group Problem Solving in an Industrial Sample." *Journal of Applied Psychology,* 52, 3 (1968): 205-10.

Campbell, R. M. "A methodological Study of the Utilization of Experts in Business Forecasting." Doctoral dissertation, University of California, Los Angeles, 1966.

Carter, L. F., A. Haythorn, B. Merrowitz, and J. Lanzetta. "The Relation of Categorizations and Ratings in the Observation of Group Behavior." *Human Relations,* 4 (1951).

Chung, K. H., and M. J. Ferris. "An Inquiry of the Nominal Group Process." *Academy of Management Journal,* 14, 4 (1971): 520-24.

Collaros, P. A., and L. R. Anderson. "The Effect of Perceived expertness upon Creativity of Members of Brainstorming Groups." *Journal of Applied Psychology,* 53, 2 (April 1969): 159-63.

Collins, B., and H. Guetzkow. *A Social Psychology of Group Processes for Decision Making.* Wiley, 1964.

Culbert, S. A. "Trainer Self-Disclosure and Member Growth in Two T-Groups." *Journal of Applied Behavioral Sciences,* 4, 1, (1968): 47-74.

Dalkey, N. C. *Experiment in Group Prediction.* Rand Corporation, 1968.

Dalkey, N. C. *The Delphi Method: An Experimental Study of Group Opinion.* Rand Corporation, June 1969.

Dalkey, N. C., and O. Helmer. "An Experimental Application of the Delphi Method to the Use of Experts." *Management Science* (1963).

Delbecq, A. L. "The World Within the 'Span of Control': Managerial Behavior in Groups of Varied Size." *Business Horizons* (August 1968).

Delbecq, A. L., and A. H. Van de Ven. "A Group Process Model for Problem Identification and Program Planning." *Journal of Applied Behavioral Sciences,* 7, 4 (July-August 1971).

Deutsch, M. "An Experimental study of the Effects of Cooperation and Competition on Group Process." *Human Relations,* 2 (1949): 199-231.

Dunnette, M. "Are Meetings Any Good for Problem Solving?" *Personnel Administration* (March-April 1964): 12-29.

Dunnette, M., J. Campbell, and K. Jaastad. "The Effect of Group Participation on Brainstorming Effectiveness for Two Industrial Samples." *Journal of Applied Psychology,* 47, 1 (1963): 30-37.

Filley, A. C. *Organization Invention: A Study of Utopian Organizations.* Bureau of Business Research and Service, University of Wisconsin, Madison, Graduate School of Business, 1973.

Filley, A. C. *Interpersonal Conflict Resolution.* Scott, Foresman and Company, 1974.

Fouiezos, N. T., M. L. Hatt, and H. Geutzkow. "Measurement of Self-Oriented Needs in Discussion Groups." *Journal of Abnormal and Social Psychology,* 45 (1950): 682-90.

Gibb, J. R. "The Effects of Size and of Threat Reduction upon Creativity in Problem-Solving Situations." *American Psychologist,* 6 (1951).

Goldman, M., M. Bolen, and R. Martin. "Some Conditions Under Which Groups Operate and How This Affects Their Performance." *Journal of Social Psychology,* 54 (1961): 47-56.

Grace, H. A. "Conformance and Performance." *Journal of Social Psychology,* 40 (1954): 333-35.

Guetzkow, H., and J. Gyr. "An Analysis of Conflict in Decision-Making Groups." *Human Relations,* 7 (1954): 367-82.

Gustafson, D. H., R. M. Shukla, A. L. Delbecq, and G. W. Walster. "A Comparative Study of Differences in Subjective Likelihood Estimates Made by Individuals, Interacting Groups, Delphi Groups, and Nominal Groups." *Organizational Behavior and Human Performance,* 9 (1973): 280-91.

Hall, E. J., J. Mouton, and R. R. Blake. "Group Problem-Solving Effectiveness Under Conditions of Pooling versus Interaction." *Journal of Social Psychology,* 59 (1963): 147-57.

Hare, A. P. "A Study of Interaction and Consensus in Different-Sized Groups."*American Sociological Review,* 17 (1952): 261-67.

Haythorn, A. "The Influence of Individual Members on the Characteristics of Small Groups." *Journal of Abnormal and Social Psychology,* 48 (1953): 276-84.

Hoffman, L. R. "Homogeneity of Member Presonality and Its Effect on Group Problem Solving." *Journal of Abnormal and Social Psychology,* 58 (1959): 27-32.

Hoffman, L. R. "Group Problem Solving." In *Advances in Experimental Social Psychology,* Part II. L. Berkowitz, ed. Academic Press, 1965.

Hoffman, L. R., and N. R. F. Maier. "Quality and Acceptance of Problem Solutions by Members of Homogeneous and Heterogeneous Groups." *Journal of Abnormal and Social Psychology,* 62 (1961): 401-407.

Hoffman, L. R., and G. G. Smith. "Some Factors Affecting the Behavior of Members of Problem-Solving Groups." *Sociometry,* 23 (1960): 273-91.

Holloman, C. R., and H. W. Hendrich. "Problem Solving

in Different-Sized Groups.'' *Personnel Psychology, 24* (1971): 489-500.

Horowitz, M. W., and J. B. Newman. ''Spoken and Wirtten Expression: An Experimental Analysis.'' *Journal of Abnormal and Social Psychology, 68* (1964): 640-47.

Huber, G., and A. L. Delbecq. ''Guidelines for Combining the Judgment of Individual Members in Decision Conferences.'' *Academy of Management Journal,* 51, 1 (June 1972): 161-74.

Leader, A. ''Patterns in Judgmental Decision Making: Individual and Group Performance Across Tasks.'' Unpublished doctoral dissertation, Indiana University Graduate School of Business, 1963.

Leavitt, H. J. ''Some Effects of Certain Communication Patterns on Group Performance.'' *Journal of Abnormal and Social Psychology,* 46 (1951): 38-50.

Maier, N. R. F. *The Appraisal Interview: Objectives, Methods, and Skills.* Wiley, 1958.

Maier, N. R. F., and L. R. Hoffman. ''Quality of First and Second Solution in Group Problem Solving.'' *Journal of Applied Psychology,* 44, 4 (1960): 278-83.

Maier, N. R. F., and A. R. A. Maier. ''An Experimental Test of the Effects of 'Developmental' Group Decisions.'' *Journal of Applied Psychology,* 41 (1957): 320-23.

Maier, N. R. F., and A. R. Solem. ''The Contribution of the Discussion Leader to the Quality of Group Thinking.'' *Human Relations,* 3 (1952): 155-74.

Osborn, A. F. *Applied Imagination.* Scribners, 1957.

Parnes, S. J. ''Effects of Extended Effort in Creative Problem Solving.'' *Journal of Educational Psychology,* 52 (1961): 117-22.

Parnes, S. J., and A. Meadow. ''Effects of Brainstorming Instructions on Creative Problem Solving by Trained and Untrained Subjects.'' *Journal of Educational Psychology,* 50 (1959): 171-76.

Pelz, D. C. ''Some Social Factors Related to Performance in a Research Organization.'' *Administrative Science Quarterly,* 1 (1956): 310-25.

Rotter, G. S., and S. M. Portugal. ''Group and Individual Effects in Problem Solving.'' *Journal of Applied Psychology,* 53, 4 (August 1969): 338-41.

Shaw, M. E. ''Some Effects of Problem Solution Efficiency in Different Communication Nets.'' *Journal of Experimental Psychology,* 48 (1954):211-17.

South, E. B. ''Some Psychological Aspects of Committee Work.'' *Journal of Applied Psychology,* 2 (1924).

Speisman, J. C., and R. H. Moos. ''Group Compatibility and Production.'' *Journal of Abnormal and Social Psychology,* 54 (1962): 190-96.

Taylor, D. W., P. L. Berry, and C. H. Block. ''Does Group Participation When Using Brainstorming Facilitate or Inhibit Creative Thinking?'' *Administrative Science Quarterly,* 3 (1958): 23-47.

Torrance, E. P. ''Group Decision Making and Disagreement.'' *Social Forces,* 35 (1957): 314-18.

Van de Ven, A. H. *Group Decision-Making Effectiveness.* Kent State University Center for Business and Economic Research Press, 1974.

Van de Ven, A. H., and A. L. Delbecq. ''Nominal versus Interacting Group Processes for Committee Decision-Making Effectiveness.'' *Academy of Management Journal,* 14, 2 (June 1971): 203-12.

Vroom, V. H., L. D. Grant, and T. J. Cotton. ''The Consequences of Social Interaction in Group Problem Solving.'' *Journal of Applied Psychology,* 53, 4 (August 1969): 338-41.

Zogona, S. V., J. E. Ellis, and W. J. MacKinnon. ''Group Effectiveness in Creative Problem-Solving Tasks: An Examination of Relevant Variables.'' *Journal of Psychology,* 62 (1966): 111-37.

Chapter 5

EVALUATION OF CARE

A model for evaluating nursing care

MARIE J. ZIMMER, R.N., M.S.

Despite some nursing profession action to ready its members to implement mechanisms to ensure the quality of the health and sickness care delivered by nurses and despite at least one legislative reference to the responsibility of all health care practitioners for the quality of their services, nursing has not quite "made the connection." First, the impact of nursing's separate and interdependent contributions to the delivery of health and illness care has not generally been recognized by nursing's inclusion in required quality monitoring and control mechanisms. Second, nurses currently do not have a single, well-defined, and well-understood focus and a well-developed and widely communicated method for quality assurance. In an attempt to remedy that lack, this article presents and recommends a model and method for quality assurance for nursing.

One of the difficulties in the development of quality assurance is the lack of a consistent and understood language. A good place to start to remedy this difficulty is with the questions, "What is quality assurance?" and "What are the components?"

Reprinted with permission from *Hospitals, Journal of the American Hospital Association,* March 1, 1974, and the American Nurses' Association. Condensed from the keynote speech presented at an institute on "Quality Assurance for Nursing Care," sponsored jointly by the American Hospital Association and the American Nurses' Association, Kansas City, Mo., Oct. 29-31, 1973.

A QUALITY ASSURANCE GLOSSARY

Quality assurance involves both evaluation and improvement actions. In the delivery of health and illness care, quality assurance is estimation of the degree of excellence in patient health outcomes and in activity and other resource cost outcomes. Quality assurance includes the use of the results of estimation to secure improvements in order to fulfill the public trust that professionals continually search for means to secure more advantageous consumer health and resource cost outcomes. To narrow and sharpen its focus, my discussion will be limited to assessment of the effectiveness and the efficiency of the health care delivered to the population who receives care through a specific institution, agency, or organization.

Effectiveness is the extent to which preestablished objectives, that is, outcomes, are attained as a result of activity. *Efficiency* is the cost of the activities and other resources that are used to achieve the outcomes.* Because efficiency cannot be calculated without an effectiveness factor to place in the mathematical formula, determination of effectiveness must precede determination of efficiency; my discussion, therefore, will concentrate on effectiveness.

*Deniston, O. L., Rosenstock, I. M., and Getting, U. A. Evaluation of program effectiveness. *Public Health Rep.* **83:**323, April 1968.

Outcome means the end result, that is, the alteration in the health status of the patient caused by goal-directed nursing care activities. The degree to which the desired outcomes are attainable is influenced by the characteristics of the served population. If patient health outcomes are assessed for a population of patients with a diagnosis of diabetes mellitus, the degree of positive health will be different for a population of 10- to 25-year-olds than for a population of 65- to 80-year-olds. The degree of positive health will influence the degree to which some desired health outcomes can be realistically attained. Thus, in reviewing the quality of attained patient health outcomes, it is essential to view them in the context of the population characteristics.

Activity is a goal-directed transaction between the nurse and the patient. Some persons refer to transactions as encounters. ''Goal-directed'' means that the activity is aimed at achieving a specific objective, that is, a desired health outcome. Sometimes a single activity is used. At other times, a cluster of several different activities is needed to achieve the single health outcome. An activity is the cause for the effect or outcome.

The degree to which desired patient health outcomes are attained and the degree to which activities are maintained in a consistent and clear relationship with an objective are influenced by the *continuity* among members of the interdependent team. Objectives and activities of various team members should enhance rather than cancel or confuse those of other members.

The degree to which outcomes are attained also is influenced by continuity in health care objectives and activities as the patient receives sequential care in various segments of the health care system. In a single episode of sickness, the patient may receive preadmission care in a physician's office, inpatient care in a hospital, and posthospital ambulatory care in a hospital-based clinic, along with home care by a community health nurse. Frequently, full progress to the desired outcome is not achieved while the patient receives care in a single segment of the system, and there is a need for continuation of objectives and activities by persons in the next segment. When each new participating professional develops his or her own objectives and activities, the possibility of the patient's realizing his full potential for health is in jeopardy.

Resources are the manpower, building, equipment, supply, and financial means and their organization. Traditional methods for evaluation focus primarily on resources. In nursing, more recent efforts single out one of these—manpower—and focus on the nurse and/or the nurse's activities. Supporters of this approach believe that excellence in resources results in excellence in patient health outcomes. There is little research either to support or to refute this assumption; furthermore, such research will not be productive until we can name and evaluate outcomes and can connect activities with the outcomes.

THREE STEPS TO QUALITY ASSURANCE

Given this three-part model (outcome, activity, and resource) with two influencing variables (population characteristics and continuity), where do we start? I am convinced that in quality assurance efforts nurses first must start with determination of desired patient health outcomes and of the degree to which these are attained. When outcomes are identified and assessed, nurses must proceed to the second step, identification of the most powerful and cost-effective activities that cause these outcomes. When activities are identified and their relationship with specific outcomes is clear, nurses must proceed to the third step, determination of the cost of the activities (that is, goal-directed patient-nurse transactions or encounters) and the cost of the related resources used to achieve specific outcomes. If nurses name and quantify activities before they clearly identify the full span of patient health objectives, they will not answer the questions, "How effective was nursing of these patients?" or "How cost-effective, that is, efficient, was nursing of these patients?"

Many nurses are reluctant to take a position that establishes patient health outcomes as a priority first step. Their reluctance stems partially from their awareness that nurses are not always able to assist patients in all dimensions of need. Nurses ought to be freed of this obstacle, because nursing *does* make a difference in patient health outcomes. Even though some desired health outcomes seem not to be achievable with our current armamentarium of activities, nurses should never be reluctant to present the best they can do, given the current state of the nursing art.

QA: MORE THAN EVALUATION

Quality assurance involves evaluation, but it also involves a second action, the use of evaluation to secure improvement. Evaluation is the determination of the results attained by an activity designed to accomplish a valued goal or objective. In important respects, quality assurance in an ongoing health delivery service is different from project evaluation or evaluative research and from traditional employee performance evaluation.

First, the primary function of quality assurance evaluation is to assess the results of an *ongoing program* for delivery of health and illness care to a specific population. The assessment is done in the context of the patient population of the institution, agency, or organization and of a mutually agreed-upon prior definition of objectives. As the notion of public accountability becomes widespread, it will be increasingly important in defining objectives to consider citizens' definitions of expected results and citizens' rights to an equivalent standard of care regardless of geographic location and resources.

Second, quality assurance is accomplished by assessment. "Assess" means to estimate or judge the value, rank, or degree of excellence. I emphasize both estimate and judge. Quality assurance methods involve the use of judgment. The goal is accuracy, and the closer the estimation is to scientific measurement, the more accurate or valid the judgment. Evaluation as applied in quality assurance, however, is not research, for it may not always require the rigorous measurement and control required of research.

Third, methods and systems for quality assurance must be practical in terms of both the required quantity of resources and the significance of the findings for providers' decisions. This need for practicality accounts for an emphasis on monitoring of critical events in performance. One or two per cent of the total manpower effort has been mentioned as the amount of institutional or agency manpower and other resources that should be dedicated to quality assurance. Even one per cent of the total manpower effort is substantial. For a nursing unit with eight RNs and eight nursing aides, one per cent of annual time is equivalent to eight weeks of one RN's time.

Fourth, the results of the quality assurance assessment are used to make decisions that will be immediately implemented in the institution or agency. Thus, quality assurance requires a method that will enable nurses to move from findings to action that will result in improvement. In the literature, continuing education is the predominantly mentioned method. Findings also may indicate a need for other kinds of decisions, such as a different allocation of manpower, a change in activities or procedures, or a need for further research.

Fifth, there must be a method for reporting the results of quality assurance assessment to successively higher levels in the organization.

Persons at all levels, including members of the board of trustees, are accountable and need to develop acceptable and useful methods to monitor and evaluate data and to provide support for needed improvement actions. Also, judicious consideration must be given to release data to outside bodies and to the use of released data.

Finally, quality assurance assessment is not traditional employee performance evaluation. In quality assurance, the patient, not the employee, is the person being assessed. The questions asked are, "What were the alterations in the patient's health status that were caused by patient-provider encounters or transactions?" and "What were the costs in resources to achieve these outcomes?" The primary function of quality assurance assessment is improvement in *patient* health and resource cost outcomes. The primary function should not be discipline of individual professionals or weeding out of the incompetent. Similarly, the primary function should not be recognition of exceptionally effective practitioners. The patient is the focus, although there can be spinoffs, that is, secondary uses, from the process.

PEER REVIEW AND ACCOUNTABILITY

Peer review and *accountability* are two other terms in the quality assurance glossary. Some persons appear to use them as synonyms for quality assurance. In the delivery of health and illness care, *peer review* is a formal, concurrent or retrospective, critical examination with a view toward future improvement of the activities and outcomes of care for a very specific patient population. The review is made and reported by the experts who are involved in the giving of care to the particular patient population. The staff nurse, the head nurse, and the clinical nurse specialist who together deliver care to a very specific patient population are a peer group. This peer group has first-level responsibility for giving care and for assuring and reporting the quality of the delivered care. In

this instance, the inservice instructor, the director of nursing service, and the consultant for continuity are not their peers, because they are not involved as members of the group in the direct delivery of nursing care.

THE ROLE OF NURSE PEERS

Expert nurse peers or peer panels are a very important component of quality assurance, because nurse peers who are involved together in the delivery of care are the only persons who have the needed knowledge and can make the needed judgments about desired patient health outcomes, how patients should progress toward attainment of those outcomes, and activities that cause the changes. Quality assurance requires the ability to identify qualities that are imperceptible to those who are not experts. Numerous variables must be noted and the degree of their influence on outcomes and activities assessed. There is another compelling reason to involve nurse peers in quality assurance efforts. In the end, the nurse peers who are involved together in the delivery of care are the persons who will take most of the improvement actions. Change requires their acceptance that what is recommended reflects an important problem and their recognition that the problem is *their* problem.

It is important that nursing's quality assurance method include peer review by registered nurses who together are involved in the direct delivery of care to a very specific patient population. In quality assurance, peer review answers the question, "Who develops and applies patient health outcome criteria?" The term is not a synonym for quality assurance.

When a nurse peer group compares actual patient health outcomes and activities for care with a set of criteria or standards, identifies and takes improvement actions, and reports results to the board of trustees through successively higher levels of line management, the nurse peer group is fulfilling one dimension of accountability. *Accountability* is the condition of being responsible for provision of a reckoning to the persons who gave the authority to act. Such an accounting might be made to the employer; to a representative of a patient population, such as the fiscal intermediary; or to a review committee of peers. "Accountability" is a broad term, and it should not be substituted for the phrase, "quality assurance of patient health outcomes and of activity and other resource cost outcomes." The latter is a very specific component of the total area for which health care providers might be asked to make an accounting.

DEVELOPING HEALTH OUTCOME CRITERIA

How do expert nurse peers or panels fulfill their responsibility for determining patient health outcome effectiveness and for making an accounting? When the task is to develop a method for nursing quality assurance, the first step is for expert peer groups within health care delivery institutions, agencies, and organizations to develop patient health outcome criteria for use in comparisons with actual patient health results. They are equal to the task. Practicing nurses who have had good experience in the care of very specific patient populations know the desired and relevant patient outcomes. They also know the observable data that indicate steps in patient progress toward achievement of those outcomes. Furthermore, they usually find the experience of stating and scaling health outcome criteria to be both stimulating and rewarding.

What framework or protocol results in productive efforts? The following are some assumptions about sets of outcome criteria that have been developed by members of my staff at the University of Wisconsin Hospitals:

• A criterion for assessment of the quality of nursing care must be relevant to the selected frame of reference, for example, outcomes ac-

tivities, or resources. One frame of reference should be selected and stayed with; frames of reference should not be mixed. When a frame of reference is selected, the nurse should be clear about the product that will result from assessment with that type of criterion.

• Criteria stated in terms of outcome, that is, alteration in the health status of the consumer, are the frame of reference that is used in these guidelines. This frame of reference will result in conclusions about effectiveness.

• A set of criteria should include positive indexes of patient health. Examples of positive indexes include the degree of the person's increase in relevant health knowledge, the degree he applies his health knowledge, and the degree of responsibility he assumes for his health behavior. Assessment should not be limited to negative indexes, such as mortality, complications, disease, disability, discomfort, and dissatisfaction.

• A criterion that is relevant to results of nursing practice usually relates to a patient health outcome that is subject to change by an activity or group of activities carried out by the nursing staff. There may be some overlap with outcome criteria of other health professionals.

• A criterion should be stated to yield a range of scores or values. One way to achieve a range is to provide scales that depict time sequence, psychological or behavioral change, or classifications used in recognized frameworks such as crisis theory. A range of scores is needed to determine a patient's progress, to adjust for individual differences between patients, and to determine the degree of attained outcomes at the time of discharge to another health care setting or at another point in the care process.

• Data that will be used to assess the degree to which a criterion is met should be observable. Also, the criterion measure that is organized to provide a range of scores will refer to observable data.

• Criteria should be written for a population

of patients with commonalities that can be identified. A number of frameworks may be used to classify populations, for example, disease (e.g., myocardial infarction), development (e.g., adolescent), conceptual (e.g., rehabilitation), or syndrome (e.g., pain).

• In initial work, populations usually should be selected that are common in the health care institution, agency, or organization and that are responsible for a significant volume of the patients who receive care and treatment. At times and for reasons associated with significant program decisions, a low-volume population may be selected.

• In selecting from among the total possible number of criteria that could be developed for a particular patient population, priority should be given to the outcomes that make the most difference in the total result. For the ambulatory ophthalmology patient receiving photocoagulation, condition of the skin is usually not a critical factor in health outcome, and priority would not be given to a criterion for skin care.

• Each criterion measure should be free from bias. Each patient to whom the criterion is applied should have an equal opportunity to obtain a good score. Assessment of the skin condition of an aged person and of a youth might require two different criterion measures.

• Consumers provide input to professionals about what is important in health outcomes. Their input is used either to augment the range of criteria in a set or to scale criteria. Consumers also provide data about results for use in comparison of actual outcomes with criteria.

• In sets of criteria, criteria may be organized into sections according to stage of illness, for example, prevention, crisis, preconvalescent, convalescent, restoration, and health maintenance.

• The patient record is the source of data for comparison of actual outcomes with sets of criteria.

• The nursing audit is the usual method for comparing actual patient health outcomes with the set of criteria applicable to the specific patient population.

• Data about patient characteristics are used to determine the percentage of the specific patient population that will reach the most positive point on each criterion measure. Patient characteristics also are used for determining comparability of populations.

• Deductions about appropriate utilization of hospital, clinic, office, home care, nursing home, and other facilities can be made from criterion measures. From a set of criteria, judgments can be made about the point in a scale of progress at which the patient is ready for another health care setting.

• The development of a set of criteria that represents outcomes of *patient care* (as contrasted with medical or nursing care) is desirable and should be accomplished by representatives of all disciplines active in care of the very specific population, including nursing, medicine, social work, and the allied health professions. Nurse participation in interdisciplinary assessment usually will follow development of competence in naming and assessing outcomes influenced by nursing activities.

From this point, there is need for a process for abstracting data to allow comparisons of actual results with desired results, for judging results of the comparison, for making decisions about and implementing improvement actions, for making reassessments to determine patterns as they develop, and for making needed accountings for results.

CONCLUSIONS

If there is to be meaningful quality assurance for nursing, nursing must start by defining desired patient health outcomes and determining the degree to which they are attained. This is both the essential first step and the key to meaningful results. Then nurses must proceed to the second and third steps, which are (1) identification of the most powerful and cost-effective means to achieve the named patient health outcomes and (2) determination of the cost of the activities and other resources used to achieve specific patient health outcomes.

Members of the nursing profession will be able to take their place among the disciplines that function in patient health review when and only when they can identify the specific alterations in patient health status secured through nursing activities. The development and the use of nurses' capability to function in quality assurance thus deserve the highest priority in the nursing profession.

Setting nursing standards and evaluating care

IRENE G. RAMEY, R.N., Ph.D.

The "in" word in management circles these days is *productivity*. The efficiency of employees is being measured by the number of units of work they process or produce and by the degree of "zero defect" they reach. The number of units measurement deals with the speed of performance, whereas the degree of zero-defect considers the quality of performance. In the health care area, where the product consists in rendering professional services to human beings, the task of measuring productivity becomes difficult.

Professional productivity cannot be measured by tallying the tasks performed in a day and determining whether they add up to a full eight hours of "work." Nursing, for example, involves not only technical and manual tasks but also intellectual and interpersonal activities which are difficult to define and measure, both as to speed and quality. Other dimensions, such as the needs and responses of individual patients, must be taken into account even though they make it difficult to evaluate the quality of performance. Since a number of persons are involved in giving a patient nursing care, it becomes necessary to distinguish between the speed and quality of performance of an employee, which is probably best done on a daily basis by his immediate supervisor, and the qual-ity of services rendered by the nursing staff in a patient unit and by the department as a whole.

A sequence of steps is suggested to a nursing service department that wishes to evaluate the quality of nursing service provided in the patient units. The first step is to establish its philosophy, its standards of care, and its objectives so that there can be no doubt about the kinds of services to be provided to patients, the frequency with which they are to be provided, and who is to provide them. Having done this, it is then possible to develop an evaluation tool which will measure progress toward the objectives and standards.

PHILOSOPHY, STANDARDS, AND OBJECTIVES

There is a close relation between philosophies, standards, and objectives. A *philosophy* is a system of motivating beliefs, concepts, and principles; it reflects the values and beliefs held by its adherents. In her excellent article, "Philosophy, Purpose, and Objectives: Why Do We Have Them?" Moore says that a philosophy is ". . . a statement of the system of beliefs which direct the individuals in a particular group in the achievement of their purpose. It should be a statement that can be referred to as explanation of why things are carried out the way they are." She makes a strong plea for specific statements rather than broad, general, nonspecific ones.[1]

Reprinted with permission from Journal of Nursing Administration, May-June, 1973.

A *standard* may be defined as a model or example established by authority, custom, or general consent, e.g., a criterion and a level or degree of quality considered proper and adequate for a specific purpose. In nursing, we combine these two definitions when we use the word *standard*.

An *objective* is a goal toward which effort is directed—an aim or end of action. Objectives may be related to personnel, patient care services, education, and research. Nurses, in defining their objectives, may, all too often, state them so broadly that they are meaningless as a guide to evaluation, or they may state them so specifically that they are task oriented and rule out opportunities for professional judgment.

To recapitulate: A standard states what should be done; an objective describes a goal and implies an intention to accomplish it; and a philosophy states why.

Examples of professional nursing standards

The American Nurses' Association and the National League for Nursing have laid the groundwork in developing standards of nursing care. The NLN has developed and made available the following publications in this area: *Criteria for Evaluating a Hospital Department of Nursing Service, Criteria for Evaluating the Administration of a Public Health Nursing Service* and *A Guide for Assessing Nursing Services in Long Term Care Facilities.*[2-4] In addition, when the Joint Commission for Accreditation of Hospitals revised the *Accreditation Manual for Hospitals, 1970,* nursing consultants were used to assist in the revision of the section on nursing.[5] These nursing consultants drew heavily from the materials produced by the ANA and the NLN.[6] Some governmental agencies also publish standards for health care. An excellent example is the *New York City Health Code;* and there are other official and nonofficial agencies which evaluate nursing services, although they may not have written standards which are used as guidelines.[7] Examples are state boards of nurse examiners and state health departments.

The publications referred to contain standards on the various aspects of nursing, including philosophy, objectives, organization, authority, responsibilities, personnel policies, staff development, agreements with educational institutions, research, budget, supplies, equipment, participating in planning and evaluation, and patient care. This paper will focus only on standards and objectives for a nursing unit rather than for a whole department.

The ANA *Standards for Organized Nursing Services* contains the following standard on patient care: "The Nursing Department promotes safe and therapeutically effective nursing care through implementation of established standards of nursing practice."[8] The nine assessment factors then listed indicate the responsibilities of the registered nurse in planning, administering, recording, and evaluating nursing care, and in supervising others who participate in giving care. These standards are now being revised.

The NLN's *Criteria for Evaluating a Hospital Department of Nursing Service* contains this standard: "The Department of Nursing Service develops and implements the program for providing nursing care."[9] The four assessment factors then listed cite the professional nurse's responsibilities for planning, implementing, recording, and evaluating nursing care which supports the medical care plans, and her responsibilities for the supervision of others who assist in giving nursing care.

The JCAH publication, *Accreditation Manual for Hospitals, 1970,* contains the following standard with several interpretative paragraphs listing factors subsumed under the standard: "There shall be evidence established that the Nursing Service provides safe, efficient and therapeutically effective nursing care through the planning of each patient's care and the effective implementation of the plans."[10]

These three examples of standards are broadly stated. Even the assessment factors or explanatory statements accompanying them are broadly stated. They are, therefore, of limited use to a nursing service department unless an additional number of more specific statements are developed.

It immediately becomes obvious that although there are legally and professionally determined standards for minimum levels of practice, some institutions aim for higher levels. The degree of expertise of the professionals in the institution, the expectations of the community, and the financial resources available to the nursing service department all have serious implications for the standards of care which prevail in an institution. These factors also affect the philosophy and objectives, both of the institution and of the nursing service department.

In her article, "Predicting Change in Nursing Values," Thomas includes a statement of standards for nursing practice.[11] This statement, which was developed in 1968 by the California Nurses Association, contains three standards which specify the functions and responsibilities of registered nurses in providing patient care. One of the functions is the determination of the acuity of each patient's need for nursing care. Descriptive examples are provided for classifying patients into four groups: those requiring intensive, moderate, minimal, or no nursing care. Directions for the implementation of the standards indicate which levels of nurses shall provide care to the different classifications of patients, and the job descriptions for the different levels of nurses delineate differences in the level of their functioning.

McGuire, in her article "Bedside Nursing Audit," provides an example of how standards may be used to evaluate nursing care.[12] A declarative statement such as "Nursing measures are taken to prevent foot drop," is converted into a question, "Have nursing measures been taken to prevent foot drop?" This question is then included in the nursing audit.

In actuality then, a question, which is part of an evaluation tool, points to an expected level of care, a standard. Conversely, a standard points to the type of question to include in the audit or evaluation tool.

Evaluation of nursing service in a university hospital

For three years, the department of nursing service at a university hospital used the NLN's self-evaluation guide to try to measure progress during the year.[13] In the spring of each year, each head nurse was given a copy of the guide, with instructions to complete it. The guide contains seventy-five pages of questions; it took days for the nurses to answer them. The job of tabulating the answers was even more formidable. Analyzing the results was impossible. Furthermore, by doing such an evaluation only once a year, close observation of changes and developments over time could not be made. Part II of the guide, "Patient Appraisal," was based on an analysis of one patient's care; this was obviously an inadequate sample of year-round activities. Furthermore, although the guide did contain questions regarding assessment, planning, intervention, and evaluation, these questions were so scattered throughout the guide that it was impossible to discern whether the nursing process was being utilized in a logical step-by-step manner.

What was needed was an evaluation tool specifically designed to measure the quality of nursing service in the patient units. It had to be comprehensive, but reasonably short, so that it could be used frequently during the year. It was also desirable to have a tool in which the answers could be easily tabulated by clerical personnel.

Some of the head nurses had developed objectives for their units. These were synthesized by the author, who added a few others. These new objectives concern the nursing care of patients, the nursing administration of the unit, and inservice education on the unit. They are stated as follows:

1. Four steps in the nursing process are to be utilized in the care of each patient.
   a. A nursing assessment is to be done on each patient on admission with subsequent in-depth assessment by the staff nurse, team leader, head nurse, and clinical specialist.
   b. A nursing care plan is to be developed for each patient, based on information obtained on assessment. Such a plan will include short-term and long-term goals.
   c. Nursing intervention is to be skillfully administered with appropriate attention to the patient's safety and to his psychosocial, physiological, and teaching needs. Concise, accurate records are to be kept of the patient's condition, of the nursing care administered, and of the patient's response to the therapeutic measures.
   d. Frequent evaluations are to be made of the patient's responses to the nursing measures utilized.
2. Each nursing unit is to develop additional objectives for the specific care of patients admitted to that unit.
3. Each nursing unit is to develop an orientation program for new nursing personnel which is specific to the care of the patients in that unit.
4. Each nursing unit is to utilize the concept of team nursing to ensure that each patient receives attention from appropriate personnel, depending on his needs, and to ensure that nursing personnel are utilized appropriately according to their capabilities.
5. All nursing personnel are to assume responsibility, as appropriate to their position, for ensuring a therapeutic environment for the patients in their care (including visitors, noise, safety factors).
6. All nursing personnel are to strive continually to improve their knowledge and skills by utilizing reference materials and resource persons.
7. Inservice educational programs are to be designed to implement the objectives stated above.
8. The nursing personnel and the care they provide patients are to serve as models of excellence for students receiving clinical instruction in this institution.

These objectives reflect the considerable amount of inservice education that has been devoted during the past three years to the topics of team nursing and to the assessment and planning steps in the nursing process.

A format was developed for a tool to measure and evaluate progress toward the objectives enumerated (see accompanying Evaluation Form). The tool has three major sections. Section I, *Nursing Process,* is the longest, and has four headings: Assessment, Planning, Intervention, and Evaluation. The third heading, *Intervention,* has six subheadings: Interpersonal, Technical Skills, Environmental Control, Collaboration With Other Professionals, Referrals, and Record-keeping. The questions in Section I are designed for an evaluation of the care of one patient during his hospital stay. Section II, *Administration,* and Section III, *Inservice Education,* are designed to evaluate activities pertaining to the total patient unit.

A committee consisting of staff nurses, head nurses, and inservice and administrative personnel developed questions for each of the headings and subheadings enumerated. The questions were stated in such a way that a "yes" answer is the desired answer, and therefore reflects a standard of care. Columns were provided for yes or no answers with a check to be placed in the appropriate column. If the question cannot be answered, a check is placed in the column headed by a question mark. If the question is not applicable to the particular patient whose care is being evaluated, a check is

Text continued on p. 62.

NURSING SERVICE DEPARTMENT

EVALUATION OF NURSING SERVICES ON A PATIENT UNIT

Unit _____ Date _____ (Name of patient _____)

I. NURSING PROCESS

A. Assessment

	Yes	No	?	NA*
1. Was an initial assessment done on the patient?	☐	☐	☐	☐
2. Was the initial assessment done immediately after admission?	☐	☐	☐	☐
3. Was the assessment done by a Registered Nurse?	☐	☐	☐	☐
4. Did the initial assessment include:	☐	☐	☐	☐
Chief complaint	☐	☐	☐	☐
Level of consciousness	☐	☐	☐	☐
Ambulatory aids	☐	☐	☐	☐
Sensory needs	☐	☐	☐	☐
Vital signs	☐	☐	☐	☐
Skin condition	☐	☐	☐	☐
Emotional state	☐	☐	☐	☐
Nutritional habits	☐	☐	☐	☐
Sleeping patterns	☐	☐	☐	☐
Elimination patterns	☐	☐	☐	☐
5. Was a subsequent in-depth assessment done within 24-36 hours after admission?	☐	☐	☐	☐
6. Did the assessment reflect a consideration of the patient as a human being rather than as a stereotyped pathological problem?	☐	☐	☐	☐
7. Did the in-depth assessment include:	☐	☐	☐	☐
The patient's present condition	☐	☐	☐	☐
His ways of interacting with his environment	☐	☐	☐	☐
His coping mechanisms	☐	☐	☐	☐
His rhythmic life patterns	☐	☐	☐	☐
8. Were all of the patient's problems adequately identified:	☐	☐	☐	☐
Physiological	☐	☐	☐	☐
Safety	☐	☐	☐	☐
Belonging or affection needs	☐	☐	☐	☐
Self-esteem	☐	☐	☐	☐
Self-actualization	☐	☐	☐	☐
9. Did the in-depth assessment include the patient's home situation and his socioeconomic aspects as a prerequisite to discharge planning?	☐	☐	☐	☐
10. Were other resources used in the assessment:	☐	☐	☐	☐
Physician (chart, verbal)	☐	☐	☐	☐
Family	☐	☐	☐	☐
Other (e.g., assessments previously done)	☐	☐	☐	☐
11. Was the assessment written into the patient's record?	☐	☐	☐	☐

B. Planning

	Yes	No	?	NA*
1. Was the nursing care plan developed from the patient assessment?	☐	☐	☐	☐
2. Was the initial care plan developed immediately after the admission assessment?	☐	☐	☐	☐

*NA = Not applicable.

Continued.

EVALUATION OF NURSING SERVICES ON A PATIENT UNIT—cont'd

I. NURSING PROCESS—cont'd

B. Planning—cont'd

	Yes	No	?	Na*
3. Was the initial care plan developed by the nurse who did the assessment?	☐	☐	☐	☐
4. Were realistic goals and nursing actions defined in the plan:	☐	☐	☐	☐
Short-term	☐	☐	☐	☐
Long-term	☐	☐	☐	☐
Discharge planning	☐	☐	☐	☐
5. Was the patient involved in developing his/her care plan?	☐	☐	☐	☐
6. Was the family or a significant person involved in developing the care plan?	☐	☐	☐	☐
7. Did the nursing personnel caring for the patient read the care plan before giving direct care?	☐	☐	☐	☐
8. Was the care plan written so that it could be accurately understood by all levels of nursing personnel?	☐	☐	☐	☐
9. Were other members of the health team (social worker, physical therapist, etc.) utilized in planning the care?	☐	☐	☐	☐

C. Intervention

  1. *Interpersonal*

	Yes	No	?	Na*
a. Was there one particular nurse to whom the patient related?	☐	☐	☐	☐
b. Did the nursing personnel relate to the patient as a unique individual?	☐	☐	☐	☐
c. Did the nursing staff provide therapeutic intervention when necessary and appropriate?	☐	☐	☐	☐
d. Did the nursing staff provide psychological support to the patient's family?	☐	☐	☐	☐
e. Did the nursing personnel sustain an acceptable, helpful attitude toward the patient?	☐	☐	☐	☐
f. Did the patient understand the roles and functions of the various team members?	☐	☐	☐	☐
g. Were personality conflicts between patient and nursing personnel overcome?	☐	☐	☐	☐
h. Was there open communication between the nursing personnel and the physician?	☐	☐	☐	☐
i. Was a teaching plan considered and initiated in preparation for discharge?	☐	☐	☐	☐
j. Was the family or a significant person included in the teaching?	☐	☐	☐	☐
k. Did the nursing staff promote a comfortable relationship between roommates?	☐	☐	☐	☐

  2. *Technical skills*

	Yes	No	?	Na*
a. Was the patient informed of what was being done, and the reason for the activity or test?	☐	☐	☐	☐
b. Was the patient properly prepared for the procedure?	☐	☐	☐	☐
c. Did nursing personnel understand the functioning of special equipment being used in caring for the patient?	☐	☐	☐	☐
d. Did the nursing personnel use good technique when performing procedures?	☐	☐	☐	☐
e. Did the nursing personnel accurately observe and record the patient's response to the procedures?	☐	☐	☐	☐

EVALUATION OF NURSING SERVICES ON A PATIENT UNIT—cont'd

I. **NURSING PROCESS**—cont'd
  C. **Intervention**—cont'd

	Yes	No	?	NA*
3. *Environmental control*				
a. Did the patient appear comfortable?	☐	☐	☐	☐
b. Were provisions made to provide privacy to the patient?	☐	☐	☐	☐
c. Were proper precautions taken to protect the patient from infection?	☐	☐	☐	☐
d. Was the patient wearing an identification band?	☐	☐	☐	☐
e. Did nursing personnel use it to identify the patient?	☐	☐	☐	☐
f. Were precautions taken and adjustments made in placing room furniture to accommodate the patient's physical or psychological needs?	☐	☐	☐	☐
g. Did the bed function properly and have the necessary equipment?	☐	☐	☐	☐
Side rails	☐	☐	☐	☐
IV pole	☐	☐	☐	☐
h. Was the operation of the bed controls explained to the patient?	☐	☐	☐	☐
i. Was the method for contacting nursing personnel explained to the patient and made readily available to him?	☐	☐	☐	☐
j. Was the patient's room cleaned daily?	☐	☐	☐	☐
k. Was the lighting in the room adequate?	☐	☐	☐	☐
l. Was the patient satisfied with the accommodations?	☐	☐	☐	☐
4. *Collaboration with other professionals*				
a. Were needs for other services identified:	☐	☐	☐	☐
Social service	☐	☐	☐	☐
Physical therapy	☐	☐	☐	☐
Inhalation therapy	☐	☐	☐	☐
Diet therapy	☐	☐	☐	☐
Religion	☐	☐	☐	☐
b. Were the other services obtained or consulted?	☐	☐	☐	☐
c. Was there an efficient method of communication between the nursing personnel and the other services?	☐	☐	☐	☐
d. Did the nursing personnel communicate effectively with the other services?	☐	☐	☐	☐
5. *Referrals*				
a. Did the nursing personnel utilize community resources available to the patient:	☐	☐	☐	☐
Visiting nurse association	☐	☐	☐	☐
Bureau of vocational rehabilitation	☐	☐	☐	☐
Nursing homes	☐	☐	☐	☐
Extended care facilities	☐	☐	☐	☐
Community fund agencies	☐	☐	☐	☐
Private philanthropic agencies	☐	☐	☐	☐
Groups with similar physical/psycho/social problems	☐	☐	☐	☐
b. Did the nursing personnel provide the patient and his/her family with information about community resources?	☐	☐	☐	☐
c. Was a method established for two-way communication between nursing personnel and agencies or groups in the community? munity?	☐	☐	☐	☐

Continued.

EVALUATION OF NURSING SERVICES ON A PATIENT UNIT—cont'd

I. **NURSING PROCESS**—cont'd

C. **Intervention**—cont'd

5. *Referrals*—cont'd

	Yes	No	?	NA*
d. Were referrals identified and initiated early enough to facilitate the patient's discharge?	☐	☐	☐	☐
e. Did the nurses make referrals without a physician's order?	☐	☐	☐	☐

6. *Record-keeping*

	Yes	No	?	NA*
a. Was the patient's chart clearly identified?	☐	☐	☐	☐
b. Was the chart readily available to nursing personnel?	☐	☐	☐	☐
c. Did the nurses' notes reflect the patient's condition and his progress relative to the goals established in the care plan?	☐	☐	☐	☐
d. Was the "Weed System" of record-keeping properly utilized? lized?	☐	☐	☐	☐
e. Were other forms containing nursing entries carefully maintained?	☐	☐	☐	☐
f. Did nursing personnel read the chart for necessary information before caring for the patient?	☐	☐	☐	☐
g. Was the patient's previous medical record obtained?	☐	☐	☐	☐
h. Did nursing personnel have ready access to parts of the chart which had been removed for filing during a long hospitalization?	☐	☐	☐	☐
i. Were all physicians' orders noted and signed off?	☐	☐	☐	☐
j. Did consent forms contain the necessary factual information, and were they properly signed?	☐	☐	☐	☐

D. **Evaluation**

	Yes	No	?	NA*
1. Were conferences held to evaluate the patient's responses to nursing intervention?	☐	☐	☐	☐
2. Were modifications or adaptations in the care plan made as a result of the evaluation?	☐	☐	☐	☐
3. Was the evaluation of the patient's care done in an accurate and objective manner?	☐	☐	☐	☐
4. Was the patient and his/her family included in the evaluation of the patient's progress?	☐	☐	☐	☐
5. Were the goals which had been established for the patient realized?	☐	☐	☐	☐
6. Did the patient make maximal recovery?	☐	☐	☐	☐

II. **ADMINISTRATION**

A. **Objectives for the unit**

	Yes	No	?	NA*
1. Were there written objectives for the unit?	☐	☐	☐	☐
2. Were the unit objectives reviewed periodically?	☐	☐	☐	☐
3. Were the unit objectives realistic and inclusive?	☐	☐	☐	☐
4. Were the unit objectives available to nursing personnel?	☐	☐	☐	☐
5. Did the unit objectives correlate with the objectives of the Nursing Service Department?	☐	☐	☐	☐
6. Did the nursing personnel attempt to fulfill the unit objectives?	☐	☐	☐	☐

B. **Team nursing**

	Yes	No	?	NA*
1. Were the patients' physical and psychosocial needs considered when assignments were made?	☐	☐	☐	☐
2. Was continuity of patient care provided in assigning team members?	☐	☐	☐	☐

EVALUATION OF NURSING SERVICES ON A PATIENT UNIT—cont'd

II. **ADMINISTRATION**—cont'd
   B. **Team nursing**—cont'd

   3. Were assignments made according to the competencies of the nursing personnel? ☐ ☐ ☐ ☐
   4. Was the physical design of the unit considered when assignments were made? ☐ ☐ ☐ ☐
   5. Did the teams work effectively as groups: ☐ ☐ ☐ ☐
      Was an assessment done on each patient on the unit? ☐ ☐ ☐ ☐
      Was a nursing care plan developed and maintained on each patient on the unit? ☐ ☐ ☐ ☐
   6. Did the team leader have a planning conference after the shift report? ☐ ☐ ☐ ☐
   7. Was the evaluation and updating of the nursing care plan a team effort? ☐ ☐ ☐ ☐
   8. Were conferences held to help the team ventilate frustrations which they may have been experiencing? ☐ ☐ ☐ ☐
   9. Was counseling regarding job performance provided to individual staff members? ☐ ☐ ☐ ☐

   C. **Environmental control**

   1. Were appropriate measures taken when patients were diagnosed as having suicidal tendencies? ☐ ☐ ☐ ☐
   2. Did the nursing personnel help keep noise to a minimum? ☐ ☐ ☐ ☐
   3. Did the nursing personnel regulate the ventilation system to control temperature and odors? ☐ ☐ ☐ ☐
   4. Was the emergency equipment checked daily? ☐ ☐ ☐ ☐
   5. Did the nursing personnel know and understand their role: ☐ ☐ ☐ ☐
      Fire plan ☐ ☐ ☐ ☐
      Disaster plan ☐ ☐ ☐ ☐
   6. Was equipment (wheelchairs, stretchers, etc.) available and functional when needed? ☐ ☐ ☐ ☐

III. **INSERVICE EDUCATION**
   A. **Programs based on objectives**

   1. Were the objectives for inservice education shared with nursing personnel? ☐ ☐ ☐ ☐
      Written ☐ ☐ ☐ ☐
      Verbal ☐ ☐ ☐ ☐
   2. Were the personnel made aware of what was expected of them? ☐ ☐ ☐ ☐
   3. Did nursing employees participate in the programs? ☐ ☐ ☐ ☐
   4. Did the program fulfill the objectives? ☐ ☐ ☐ ☐

   B. **Orientation plan for the unit**

   1. Was there an established orientation program for the unit? ☐ ☐ ☐ ☐
   2. Were nursing personnel aware of their roles in the orientation program for the unit? ☐ ☐ ☐ ☐
   3. Was the orientation program for the unit reviewed and revised periodically? ☐ ☐ ☐ ☐
   4. Were nursing personnel on the unit given an opportunity to evaluate the orientation program? ☐ ☐ ☐ ☐

Continued.

EVALUATION OF NURSING SERVICES ON A PATIENT UNIT—cont'd

III. INSERVICE EDUCATION
  C. Utilization of reference material and resource programs
    1. Was current literature dealing with subject matter pertinent to the unit readily available to the staff? ☐ ☐ ☐ ☐
    2. Were conferences held with physicians, social workers, dietitians, and nursing personnel to discuss subject matter pertinent to the unit? ☐ ☐ ☐ ☐
    3. Were nursing personnel encouraged to attend lectures, seminars, and workshops? ☐ ☐ ☐ ☐
    4. Were nursing personnel aware of where they might obtain information and training for new skills needed in caring for the patients? ☐ ☐ ☐ ☐
    5. Was there opportunity for nursing personnel to be supervised and evaluated when performing a new procedure? ☐ ☐ ☐ ☐

---

placed in the column headed "NA" (not applicable).

Two factors that are always of concern in evaluating or measuring are reliability and validity. An attempt has been made to phrase the questions carefully, so that the terminology used is not ambiguous nor value-laden. Meetings are being held with the staff who will use the evaluation tool in order to clarify its use, to reach a common understanding regarding the concepts utilized, and to reduce errors of severity, leniency, and central tendency.

After preliminary testing, and revisions made by the author, it is planned to use the evaluation tool frequently enough during the year so that trends can be noted and generalizations can be made regarding the quality of nursing services.

The results obtained from the evaluation tool may be analyzed in a number of ways:

1. The answers to one question, or to questions under one heading, may be analyzed.
2. The total number of yes, no, ?, and NA answers on one form are compared to the total number of questions.
3. Data from one unit may be analyzed to show progress over time.
4. Data from one unit may be compared with that from other units.
5. Data from all units may be summarized for a generalization about the whole department.

Either simple or complex statistical analyses may be performed, depending upon the sophistication of the answers desired and the availability of computer resources.

It is envisioned that frequent utilization of this evaluation tool in each of the nursing units will not only assist the department in evaluating the quality and amount of care being rendered but will also serve as an educational tool in pointing out to the nursing staff the factors that comprise good nursing care.

SUMMARY

With the present-day focus on productivity, it is necessary to emphasize that although appropriate and full utilization of personnel is important, it is equally important that a high quality of nursing care be provided to patients in our hospitals. The first can be assured by diligent supervision. In order to provide a high quality of care, however, it is necessary that nurses develop standards of patient care and appropriate evaluation tools so that the professional aspects of nursing involving intellectual and interpersonal activities will be ensured, and attention will be given to the individual needs and responses of patients.

References

1. Moore, M. A. Philosophy, Purpose and Objectives: Why Do We Need Them? *J. Nurs. Admin.* **1**(3):9-14, 1971.
2. *Criteria for Evaluating a Hospital Department of Nursing Service.* New York: National League for Nursing, 1965.
3. *Criteria for Evaluating the Administration of a Public Health Nursing Service.* New York: National League for Nursing, 1968.
4. *A Guide for Assessing Nursing Services in Long Term Care Facilities.* New York: National League for Nursing, 1968.
5. *Accreditation Manual for Hospitals, 1970.* Chicago: Joint Commission on Accreditation of Hospitals, 1970.
6. *Standards for Organized Nursing Services.* New York: American Nurses Association, 1965.
7. *New York City Health Code.* New York: The City Record Office, 1964.
8. *Standards for Organized Nursing Services, op. cit.,* p. 10.
9. *Criteria for Evaluating a Hospital Department of Nursing Services, op. cit.,* p. 6.
10. *Accreditation Manual for Hospitals, 1970, op. cit.,* p. 51.
11. Thomas, L. A. Predicting Change in Nursing Values, *J. Nurs. Admin.* **1**(3):50-58, 1971.
12. McGuire, R. L. Bedside Nursing Audit, *Am. J. Nurs.* **68**(10):2146-2148, 1968.
13. *Quest for Quality: A Self-Evaluation Guide to Patient Care.* New York: National League for Nursing, 1966.

Three instruments for measuring the quality of nursing care

MABEL A. WANDELT, R.N., Ph.D., and MARIA C. PHANEUF, R.N., M.A.

Concern for measurement of quality of care provided patients is not new, but acknowledgment that quantitative measurement of quality is possible is relatively recent. Widespread demand for such measurements is a very recent development, and for a variety of reasons, it is rapidly intensifying.

This paper briefly describes three instruments that have been demonstrated effective for providing quantitative measurements of quality of nursing care and suggests some purposes for which they might be useful. The instruments are:

(1) *Slater Nursing Competencies Rating Scale,* for measuring competencies displayed by a nurse.

(2) *Quality Patient Care Scale,* for measuring the quality of nursing care received by a patient, while care is ongoing.

(3) *Nursing Audit,* for measuring the quality of nursing care received by patient, after a cycle of care has been completed and the patient is discharged.

The three instruments have varied and extensive usefulness within education and research programs. Discussion here, however, will be directed to persons whose primary responsibilities are providing nursing care for patients. The purpose is to inform readers:

• That the three instruments have been developed.

Reprinted by permission from *Hospital Topics,* August 1972, and the authors.

• That each has been extensively tested for its value as a measuring instrument and for best technics of application.

• That each has been used in studies beyond those used for testing and in agencies with various types of care programs.

• That each is available from the developers, with anticipated availability from usual publishing channels.

The measurements obtained with the three tools will serve purposes of persons with varied aspects of responsibility for providing nursing care.

For nursing administrators, the measurements:

• Provide evaluations of particular programs, such as orientation of personnel or establishment of a patient teaching program.

• Support requests for accreditation or for financing for a particular program.

• Serve as bases for planning new programs or program changes.

• Serve to identify areas of strength and weakness in the total nursing program, in specific areas of the program, and in various settings in which a program exists.

• Determine the influence of varied staffing patterns.

• May be used as data in cost effectiveness studies—for example, studies comparing the quality of care received by patients in varied situations in which costs of staffing vary.

For supervisors and head nurses, the measurements:

• Identify areas of needed patient-care improvement.

• Provide bases for planning inservice education programs.

• Identify teaching/supervision needs of staff members who give direct care to patients.

For head nurses and staff nurses, the measurements:

• Provide a "self" examination of care in their specific nursing unit or setting.

• Identify particular types of care in which

practice may be improved merely by increased attention and conscientiousness.

• Identify types of care in which improvement will depend on the staff's acquiring additional knowledge and skill.

Regardless of the particular responsibilities, concern, or interests of persons using the measurements, the process for using the tools is the same. Depending on the purpose for which evaluation is done, one, two, or all three of the tools may be used. A brief description of each tool, the process of its use, and identification of the specific measurements each is designed to make, suggest purposes each may be expected to serve.

SLATER SCALE

The Slater Nursing Competencies Rating Scale is an 84-item scale designed to measure the competencies displayed by a nurse in providing care to patients. The scale may be used in any setting in which nurses intervene in behalf of patients, either in direct nurse-patient interactions or in other interventions. Scale items identifying nurse-patient interactions include:

"Gives explanation and verbal assurance when needed."

"Encourages patient to take adequate diet."

"Encourages patient to accept dependence/independence as appropriate to his condition."

Items identifying interventions in behalf of the patient include:

"Establishes a well-developed nursing-care plan."

"Attends to patient needs through use of referrals, both to departments in the hospital and to other community agencies."

"Contributes as nurse member of medical team in planning and evaluating care."

The scale is used, in retrospect, to rate nurse performance that has occurred over a period that may be any length from two weeks to one year, as well as for on-the-spot ratings. For ratings of performance occurring over a specific period, the rater (usually the head nurse or supervisor) is a nurse who has observed the subject to be rated as she provided direct nursing care during the rating period. The rater ascribes ratings to the items on the scale on the basis of retrospective analysis of the many observations of episodes of care during the rating period.

For some purposes, the scale may be used for ratings during a one-time observation period. The nurse observer shadows the nurse to be rated as she provides care during a 2½-hour period. She ascribes rating to one or more germane items for each episode of the nurse's interactions with or interventions on behalf of patients.

The standard against which the nurse's action is compared for measurement is "Care expected of a first-level staff nurse," with a 5-point range from "Best Nurse" through "Average Nurse" to "Poorest Nurse." The ratings are given numerical values ranging from 5 for Best Nurse to 1 for Poorest Nurse. The numerical values are identified after the total ratings on the scale have been completed. This may be done by a clerk.

The 84 items are arranged into six subsections, according to the primary science and cultural bases for the nursing-care actions to be rated:

Area	Number of items
I *Psycho-social: individual* — Actions directed toward meeting psycho-social needs of individual patients	18
II *Psycho-social: group* — Actions directed toward meeting psycho-social needs of patients as members of a group	13
III *Physical* — Actions directed toward meeting physical needs of patients	13
IV *General* — Actions that may be directed toward meeting either psycho-social or physical needs of patient or both at once	16
V *Communication* — Communication on behalf of patient	7
VI *Professional implications* — Care given to patients reflects initiative and responsibility indicative of professional expectations.	17
TOTAL ITEMS	84

The items are identified in terms descriptive of observable nurse actions, which enables them to be readily matched with criteria for stated objectives for behavior of a nursing service or education program.

Among purposes for which measurements from the Slater scale may serve are:

• Periodic personnel evaluations of individual nurses, where retention, promotion, and merit salary increases are among the considerations.

• Examination of relationships between competencies displayed by nurses and the quality of care received by patients.

• Identification of areas of needed instruction for inservice-education programs, or particular learning needs of individual staff members.

Essentially, where there is interest in knowing the level of competency displayed by a nurse, for whatever reason, the Slater scale will provide discriminating measurement for each individual or group of individuals measured. The scale has been repeatedly demonstrated to be so sensitive that it will measure changes that occur (learning) in as brief a period as two weeks.

QUALPACS

The Quality Patient Care Scale (QualPaCS) is a 68-item scale designed to measure the quality of care received by patients in any setting in which nurses intervene to provide care for patients, either in direct nurse-patient interactions or in interventions in behalf of the patient.

QualPaCS derived from the Slater scale; many of the items from that scale were fitted into QualPaCS by merely structuring the wording to describe the nurse action as it was received by the patient, rather than as it was performed by the nurse. For example, "Gives full attention to patients" becomes "Patient receives nurse's full attention''; ''Allows for slow or unskilled performance without showing annoyance or impatience'' becomes ''Patient with slow or unskilled performance is accepted and encouraged.''

The standard for measurement is the same: ''Care expected of a first-level staff nurse.'' The items are arranged into the same six subsections, and are identified in terms descriptive of observable nurse actions.

Ratings of care for a patient are done by a nurse who spends two hours in direct observation of the care provided the patient. On the basis of observed interactions and of information from the patient's record and from members of the staff, the observer ascribes ratings to all applicable items on the scale. As for the Slater, the numerical values for the items are ascribed when the total rating for care has been completed.

NURSING AUDIT

The Nursing Audit is a 50-item instrument designed to measure quality of care received by a patient during a particular cycle of care, such as a period of active care from a home health-care agency or a period of one hospital or nursing-home stay. The audit is useful in evaluating the quality of the care provided in any program and setting in which a record is an integral part of providing comprehensive and continuing nursing care. In other words, it may be used wherever there is an organized program for providing nursing care.

After the patient has been discharged from the hospital or nursing home, or placed in an inactive status of a home health agency's case load, the complete, closed record is audited. The audit consists of ratings ascribed to each of the 50 items. The items identify components of the one dependent and six independent functions of nursing as they are identified in statutes of licensure for nurses. These functions are:

- Application and execution of physician's legal orders

- Observation of symptoms
- Supervision of the patient
- Supervision of those participating in care
- Reporting and recording
- Application of nursing procedures and technics
- Promotion of health by direction and teaching

There are varying numbers of items appropriate to the various functions. For example, for the dependent function, ''Application and execution of physician's legal orders,'' there are six items to be rated. Among them are: ''Order current,'' ''Orders promptly executed,'' and ''Evidence that the nurse understood cause and effect.'' For one independent function, ''Supervision of the patient,'' there are seven items to be rated. Among them are: ''Continuing assessment of patient's condition and capacity'' and ''Nursing plans changed in accordance with assessment.''

Numerical values have been ascribed to items according to a reasonableness established during the developmental testing of the audit. The evaluation for each nursing function is determined by totaling the scores for the items composing it. The audit of a record yields an overall numerical score and, in addition, scores for each of the seven subsections.

Several features of the nursing audit make it an outstanding teaching device for ongiong inservice programs, as well as one useful for evaluation:

- Each item is defined, briefly, but in a manner in which the total instrument identifies essential components of adequate nursing care.

- Ranges of the numerical scores have been established for the total score and for each of the nursing functions. These ranges have been translated into terms descriptive of quality: excellent, good, incomplete (care is good as far as it goes, but it does not go far enough), poor, and unsafe.

- The auditing is to be done by a committee composed of nurses with varied expertise, with representation for administration, supervision, and staff nursing. Representation for a hospital, a nursing home, and a home health agency is recommended for all adult committees.

• Auditing is an ongoing process, with monthly auditing of all or a sample of records of patients discharged in the previous month.

• The auditing is done by a committee composed of nurses from the staff of the agency (supplemented by representatives from other types of care agencies) — internal audit, or by a committee composed of nurses from outside the agency — external audit. Committee membership should be rotated among the staff, with half the members being replaced each year.

Each of the features has its own contribution, and combinations of various ones further enhance the audit's usefulness for teaching/learning and for planning improved nursing care at all administrative levels.

COMMONALITIES AMONG TOOLS

There are commonalities among the three instruments and between any two of them. Those between the Slater and QualPaCS scales have already been mentioned. Commonalities shared by all three include:

• The ratings are descriptive and ascribed on the basis of directly observable entities. In the audit, a rating is ascribed in one of three columns:

Yes (there is evidence in the record)

No (there is no evidence in the record)

Uncertain (some evidence toward the affirmative)

In the Slater and QualPaCS, a rating is ascribed in one of five columns:

Best Nurse/Care

Between

Average Nurse/Care

Between

Poorest Nurse/Care

The numerical values for items are identified after the total rating is completed. This may be done by a clerk.

• Items are arranged in sections so that subscores for pertinent concerns may be readily determined. These arrangements allow for not only a total over-all evaluative score, but also scores for the subsections.

• The over-all score permits comparison of quality of care received by various groups of patients, or by patients receiving care from various personnel groupings or in various settings. The scores for individual functions pinpoint areas needing attention and identify areas of adequate or better care, thus providing bases for planning immediate and long-term actions or for improvement of patient care and care programs.

The over-all score allows evaluative generalizations about a program; it serves little or not at all as a basis for improvement. Improvement and logical change can stem only from information about specific facets of a program. Improvement accrues from changes in definitive portions of a program, whether changes are made in several aspects simultaneously or in sequence.

Effects of changes can be revelaed by the over-all score, but the subsection scores are needed to identify the areas of needed change and changes that have or have not been effective. There are analogous advantages for the total and subsection scores of measurements from the Slater scale.

• The items themselves, in the Slater and QualPaCS, and the definitions of items, in the audit, identify directly observable actions of nurses as they provide care. This means that they can be matched with stated objectives of behavior that have been established for a nursing program, so that composites of items from any one of the instruments may be established to provide measurements of the degree of attainment of each program objective.

• The ratings for each of the instruments must be done by a nurse competent to judge the appropriateness of nursing-care actions to meeting the needs of the patients receiving the care.

Testing has demonstrated that the area of clinical specialization of the rater does not influence the ratings. In other words, a nurse who knows nursing care will ascribe reliable ratings to items on the instruments, regardless of the medical-care category of the patient or the setting in which the care is provided.

• The instruments may be used repeatedly to measure quality of care in the same setting and of the same subjects, and as frequently as measurements are desired. Because the rating of the items is done by an observer, there is no problem that those being rated will learn to act in a certain way merely through repeated exposure to the instrument being used to measure their nursing-care actions.

Commonalities between the audit and QualPaCS include:

• These instruments lend themselves well to evaluation without the connotation of blame-fixing or punitiveness. The detailed definitions of items for the audit and the concreteness of the items on the QualPaCS can serve all nurses as reminders of the composition of comprehensive nursing care.

The audit and QualPaCS evaluate the care received by a patient, without identification of individuals who provide the care. This aspect of their use mitigates against their being used to place blame or to punish individuals. The audit prescribes the use of a committee, with representatives from all administrative levels, and the QualPaCS recommends the use of two or more raters.

These aspects of the instruments enhance the likelihood of their being viewed by the staff as teaching/learning instruments, as well as for use to obtain numerical scores of quality of care.

• The audit and QualPaCS were developed to provide measurements of care received by individual patients, with the view not to planning change in the care of any one patient but rather to permitting evaluative generalizations about the nursing care being provided to groups of patients. The aim was to establish measurements of the quality of care provided by nursing staffs to groups of patients for whom they were responsible; to evaluate the quality of a program or nursing care with the view to identifying strengths and weaknesses, which, in turn, will serve as bases for planning a continued and future program.

SUMMARY

The measurement of an entity as complex as nursing care of patients to determine the magnitude of an attribute as complex as quality may not be expected ever to be simple. In the present state of the art, when valid and reliable measuring instruments are just beginning to be developed, there are many questions about any instrument that purports to provide measurements of quality of care. For the nursing audit, there are questions about what constitutes ''evidence'' and ''some evidence toward affirmative,'' and about the numerical values ascribed to various items. For the QualPaCS and Slater Scales, there are questions about the standard of measurement and the length of the instrument.

About all three, there are questions about validity and about subjectivity of the rater.

The presence of subjectivity is acknowledged for each instrument. For measuring attributes of the complexity of the quality of nursing care, there are two alternatives. Either some subjectivity will be accepted, or there will be no attempt to measure. The developers of the audit and scales have chosen to provide measuring devices that have some acknowledged limitations, rather than to do nothing.

The negative connotations ascribed to subjectivity are overriden by the practical connotations of professional judgment. Professional judgment is the basis for the rater's ascribing levels of quality to specific components of care identified by each item of the audit and the scales. All nurse actions that are not purely technical practive evolve from judgments made by the nurse performing the actions. The basis of such judgments is observed facts; its essence is subjectivity. A rater is an individual competent to plan and provide nursing care for patients — competent to make professional judgments about the quality of the actions composing the nursing care being rated.

Data from thousands of evaluations with each tool have been analyzed to test the usefulness of the three instruments. The report of the testing and the guides for using each instrument delineate rationale for the many facets of the instrument and its use. Tests show each to be a reliable, valid, stable, discriminating instrument for providing quantitative measurements of the quality of nursing care.

Obviously, each instrument may be used alone or by a nursing service seeking information about some particular aspect of its program. Maximum information for continued program improvement will be obtained through use of all three instruments. The purposes served by the information derived from use of the instruments will be as extensive, varied, or limited as the imagination and application of the entire nursing staff.

Unit one □ STUDY GUIDE

1. Obtain a copy of the objectives for your clinical unit. Evaluate them according to the criteria of clarity, specificity, and practicality. If possible, investigate the process by which they were developed. Compare your findings with the guidelines presented in Cantor's article.

2. Develop a statement of philosophy and objectives for a real or hypothetical patient unit. Outline a plan for putting the philosophy and objectives into practice.

3. Given that groups have more impact in affecting quality of patient care than individuals, identify actual or potential power groups in your clinical situation. Discuss how you might gain entry into these groups and the purpose for doing so.

4. Examine the written job descriptions in an agency and determine whether the responsibility and accountability are spelled out for these positions.

5. Obtain a copy of the organizational chart for your agency. How does this formal structure relate to the informal communication that occurs? Might the formal chart be made more reflective of the real situation?

6. Select a situation in which a group needs to make a decision. Speculate about the decision-making process for this group, contrasting the interactional and the nominal group processes as they might be used. Consider the possible consequences of each.

7. Choose a situation in which nominal group process might be a useful tool for decision-making and employ the steps to do so. Evaluate the results.

8. Select a decision made by you or another leader in a clinical situation. Outline how the responsibility for operationalizing that decision would be delegated. How can you ensure that authority and accountability are delegated along with responsibility?

9. When your clinical unit was last reviewed for accreditation, what process did the institution use to obtain and present information evaluating the care being provided?

10. Gather all the necessary data regarding an agency's quality assurance program: (a) examine the program objectives and the process of program implementation; (b) examine the feedback system and its relationship to both consumer and agency productivity.

Personnel factors and their influence on efficient organizational functioning

□ It is crucial that nurse-managers faced with the growing complexity of health care delivery systems and the concomitant complexity of personnel management be skilled in human relations and knowledgeable about behavior in organizations. Ultimately the effectiveness of the organization depends upon the performance of the staff and their leader.

Factors that promote staff efficiency and effectiveness are directly related to leadership behavior. Leadership can be defined as the effort "to influence or change the behavior of others in order to accomplish organizational, individual, or personal goals" (Huse and Bowditch, 1973, p. 145). A flexible and innovative leader who supports and practices open and honest communication, who understands the functional and dysfunctional aspects of conflict, and who uses confrontation appropriately provides a climate conducive to effectiveness and staff growth.

In an attempt to understand how a leader can learn to cope with and understand a variety of personnel and their behavior, it might be helpful to first examine the components of leadership. The meaning of leadership has changed over the years. It was not until shortly after World War II that the whole area of leadership became an important topic for re-

search. Since then several different theories of leadership have emerged. In order to provide a framework for these theories, a brief historical overview will be presented. The theorists who will be discussed have been selected to reflect current thinking about leadership styles and concepts of managerial behavior.

Douglas McGregor, one of the most influential management theorists, has classified managers according to two leadership styles: (1) an authoritarian style, which he labels "Theory X" and (2) an egalitarian style, which he calls "Theory Y."

The typical Theory X manager believes that people are inherently lazy, dislike work, and will therefore avoid it whenever possible. As a result, the Theory X manager exercises strong control over employees, typically by close supervision or coercion and threat of punishment. These measures are necessitated, the Theory X manager believes, because most workers are incapable of self-direction and control and because they do not care to assume any responsibility for themselves. Implicit in this view is the notion that there are two kinds of people, those who want to lead and those who want to be led.

In contrast, the Theory Y leader assumes that work is enjoyable, that people will work hard, and that people will assume responsibility. In addition, this leader believes that workers are not only capable of self-direction but welcome the opportunity for personal growth. Given the proper conditions, individuals really do want to do a good job, their performance being based on internal rather than external controls. There is no sharp division between leaders and followers in this orientation, but a tendency toward collaborative and participative decision-making.

Another theorist, Rensis Likert, feels that a manager's most important task is managing the human component of the organization because it is people who accomplish the goals of the organization. Focusing on the group and the organization within which the manager works, Likert organizes leadership styles into four categories that range from a purely exploitative, authoritarian, hierarchical approach (System 1), to one which is less exploitative, but still authoritarian (System 2), to a more consultative approach (System 3), and finally to a participative approach (System 4).

Like the Theory X manager, the System 1 manager has little confidence in subordinates, makes most of the decisions, and uses fear, threats, and punishment to force subordinates to work. Control is authoritarian and supervision is close.

At the other end of the continuum, management has almost complete trust and confidence in the abilities of subordinates. Decision-making is carried out at all levels of the organization. There is free-flowing communication and involvement between supervisors and workers.

A third approach to leadership is that described by the "Managerial Grid" developed by Robert Blake and Jane Mouton. In their model, there are two basic dimensions of leadership: the extent and degree of a manager's concern about people and the concern with production. Utilizing a standardized questionnaire, a manager's orientation can be plotted numerically on the managerial grid. Concern for peo-

ple on the vertical axis and concern for production on the horizontal axis can range from very low (1) to very high (9) — it is possible for a manager to have a high degree of concern for production (9) while showing little concern for people (1); conversely, a manager may have very low concern for both people and production (1,1). The most desirable placement, according to Blake and Mouton is the (9,9) manager, one who has a high concern for both people and production.

The fourth major theorist is Fiedler, who has developed a contingency ("it depends") theory. In sharp contrast to the three "one best approach to management" theorists discussed already, Fiedler maintains that appropriate leadership style depends on the subordinates, the set of conditions within which the leader is operating, and the particular situation. Once again, leadership style can vary from permissive, passive, and considerate to controlling, active, and structured. The appropriateness and effectiveness of each style vary with the situation.

Leadership literature has continued to identify behaviors that will promote quality output as well as individual satisfaction. Undoubtedly, ideas about what leadership is and what the functions of a leader should be will continue to change in the 1980's. It has become increasingly accepted that leadership is a significant social process and that the new leader will be one who is highly skilled in interpersonal relationships. In addition, a leader must be able to adapt the style of leadership to the situation and to the individuals being supervised.

Unit two includes articles dealing with leadership and various influences on leadership style. Each of the four theories presented earlier, that is McGregor, Likert, Blake and Mouton, and Fiedler, postulates a continuum of leadership pattern from highly leader-centered to highly employee-centered. A composite of these four theories developed by Tannenbaum and Schmidt is presented in Chapter 6. They propose a contingency or situational approach to leadership and suggest a method for selecting a leadership style appropriate to the circumstance.

Merton proposes that because leadership must necessarily take place between people, it is a social transaction and social role. He maintains that a leader assists others in achieving personal and social goals. In addition, he outlines four identifiable social processes that produce the respect that is essential for effective leadership and the four conditions that must be met before compliance with administrative requests can even take place.

Taking a different and more philosophical approach to the subject, Zaleznick compares and contrasts the work of leaders and managers. He raises questions about whether our society can have the luxury of both and traces the markedly different lines of development of a manager and a leader.

The necessity for skill in interpersonal communication is emphasized in Chapter 7. Morton maintains that the effective leader not only must communicate concrete facts but must develop skill in the technique of ''leveling'' with others on the job. Guidelines for learning and using leveling are presented and factors that determine the effectiveness of leveling are discussed.

Assessing communication in the work group is continued in the Bradford, Stock, and Horwitz article. The authors present a framework for diagnosing causes for ineffective, nonproductive groups. They describe signs one can observe to diagnose and treat group problems.

Charrier proposes a model of group growth which a leader can use in designing group meetings. The author states that while group sessions should be flexible, leaders should chart sessions up Cog's ladder to facilitate effectiveness.

Another look at diagnosing communication blocks in a group is presented in Smith's article. She outlines four major barriers to communication, including language, anxiety, tendency to evaluate, and preconceptions and stereotypes. The subtleties of interracial communications are discussed in the article by DeLo and Green. They introduce a new approach that focuses on the problem of black-white communication. Promotion of facilitative and authentic relations between blacks and whites is the issue presented in the ''Blocking and Facilitating Assumptions and Behavior Sheet.'' Assumptions and behaviors that block and facilitate interracial relations are listed.

In Chapter 8, Osterhaus discusses the way in which motivation, along with participatory management, influences greater productivity and leads to more effective performance evaluation. By analyzing three components — individual needs and desires, physical conditions, and social conditions of the job — the leader has a way of looking at factors that might be influencing employees' motivation.

Chopra's article on motivation in task-oriented groups has important implications for health care workers. The author points out the importance of the interaction between the person in authority and the group and identifies specific behaviors that promote successful interaction and high work output.

Conflict, often seen as negative, is examined in Chapter 9. Filley discusses the values of conflict, the conflict process, and the resolution of conflict. Confrontation, also typically viewed as negative, is seen by Egan as an invitation to explore attitudes and behavior in a group. After explaining five types of confrontation, Egan proposes a facilitative approach to confrontation. Chapter 10 presents McGregor's classic article on performance evaluation. Conventional evaluation procedures, in which the manager assumes the responsibility for judging employees, is contrasted with one in which the employee sets the criteria against which performance will be evaluated.

Benson, Schmeling, and Bruins, utilizing Maslow's hierarchy of needs, outline a system's approach to evaluation. They discuss the implementation of the proposed system and evaluate the outcomes.

Gerold examines the use of the position description as a basis for staff evaluation outlining the pros and the cons of the technique. He suggests many categories that encompass the mutually determined goals of employee and employer.

In Chapter 11 Rodgers reviews some of the basic issues involved in the process of change. She looks at the focus of change, some models of change, the change process itself, and the resistance it creates. She also considers some of the elements necessary for change.

Chapter 6

LEADERSHIP

How to choose a leadership pattern

ROBERT TANNENBAUM and WARREN H. SCHMIDT

FOREWORD

Since its publication in HBR's March-April 1958 issue, this article has had such impact and popularity as to warrant its choice as an "HBR Classic." Mr. Tannenbaum and Mr. Schmidt succeeded in capturing in a few succinct pages the main ideas involved in the question of how a manager should lead his organization. For this publication, the authors have written a commentary, in which they look at their article from a 15-year perspective.

Mr. Tannenbaum is Professor of the Development of Human Systems at the Graduate School of Management, University of California, Los Angeles. He is also a Consulting Editor of the *Journal of Applied Behavioral Science* and coauthor (with Irving Weschler and Fred Massarik) of *Leadership and Organization: A Behavioral Science Approach* (New York, McGraw-Hill, 1961). Mr. Schmidt is also affiliated with the UCLA Graduate School of Management, where he is Senior Lecturer in Behavioral Science. Besides writing extensively in the fields of human relations and leadership and conference planning, Mr. Schmidt wrote the screenplay for a film, "Is It Always Right to Be Right?" which won an Academy Award in 1970.

- "I put most problems into my group's hands and leave it to them to carry the ball from there. I serve merely as a catalyst, mirroring

back the people's thoughts and feelings so that they can better understand them."

- "It's foolish to make decisions oneself on matters that affect people. I always talk things over with my subordinates, but I make it clear to them that I'm the one who has to have the final say."

- "Once I have decided on a course of action, I do my best to sell my ideas to my employees."

- "I'm being paid to lead. If I let a lot of other people make the decisions I should be making, then I'm not worth my salt."

- "I believe in getting things done. I can't waste time calling meetings. Someone has to call the shots around here, and I think it should be me."

Each of these statements represents a point of view about "good leadership." Considerable experience, factual data, and theoretical principles could be cited to support each statement, even though they seem to be inconsistent when placed together. Such contradictions point up the dilemma in which the modern manager frequently finds himself.

NEW PROBLEM

The problem of how the modern manager can be "democratic" in his relations with subordinates and at the same time maintain the necessary authority and control in the organization for which he is responsible has come into focus increasingly in recent years.

Earlier in the century this problem was not so acutely felt. The successful executive was generally pictured as possessing intelligence, imagination, initiative, the capacity to make rapid (and generally wise) decisions, and the ability to inspire subordinates. People tended to think of the world as being divided into "leaders" and "followers."

New focus. Gradually, however, from the social sciences emerged the concept of "group dynamics" with its focus on *members* of the group rather than solely on the leader. Research efforts of social scientists underscored the importance of employee involvement and participation in decision making. Evidence began to challenge the efficiency of highly directive leadership, and increasing attention was paid to problems of motivation and human relations.

Through training laboratories in group development that sprang up across the country, many of the newer notions of leadership began to exert an impact. These training laboratories were carefully designed to give people a first-hand experience in full participation and decision making. The designated "leaders" deliberately attempted to reduce their own power and to make group members as responsible as possible for setting their own goals and methods within the laboratory experience.

It was perhaps inevitable that some of the people who attended the training laboratories regarded this kind of leadership as being truly "democratic" and went home with the determination to build fully participative decision making into their own organizations. Whenever their bosses made a decision without convening a staff meeting, they tended to perceive this as authoritarian behavior. The true symbol of democratic leadership to some was the meeting—and the less directed from the top, the more democratic it was.

Some of the more enthusiastic alumni of these training laboratories began to get the habit of categorizing leader behavior as "democratic" or "authoritarian." The boss who made too many decisions himself was thought of as an authoritarian, and his directive behavior was often attributed solely to his personality.

New need. The net result of the research findings and of the human relations training based upon them has been to call into question the stereotype of an effective leader. Consequently, the modern manager often finds himself in an uncomfortable state of mind.

Often he is not quite sure how to behave; there are times when he is torn between exerting "strong" leadership and "permissive" leadership. Sometimes new knowledge pushes him in one direction ("I should really get the group to help make this decision"), but at the same time his experience pushes him in another direction ("I really understand the problem better than the group and therefore I should make the decision"). He is not sure when a group decision is really appropriate or when holding a staff meeting serves merely as a device for avoiding his own decision-making responsibility.

The purpose of our article is to suggest a framework which managers may find useful in grappling with this dilemma. First, we shall look at the different patterns of leadership behavior that the manager can choose from in relating himself to his subordinates. Then, we shall turn to some of the questions suggested by this range of patterns. For instance, how important is it for a manager's subordinates to know what type of leadership he is using in a situation? What factors should he consider in deciding on a leadership pattern? What difference do his long-run objectives make as compared to his immediate objectives?

RANGE OF BEHAVIOR

Exhibit I presents the continuum or range of possible leadership behavior available to a manager. Each type of action is related to the degree of authority used by the boss and to the amount

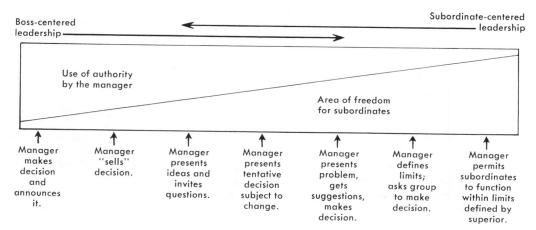

Boss-centered
leadership

Subordinate-centered
leadership

Use of authority
by the manager

Area of freedom
for subordinates

| Manager makes decision and announces it. | Manager "sells" decision. | Manager presents ideas and invites questions. | Manager presents tentative decision subject to change. | Manager presents problem, gets suggestions, makes decision. | Manager defines limits; asks group to make decision. | Manager permits subordinates to function within limits defined by superior. |

Exhibit I. Continuum of leadership behavior.

of freedom available to his subordinates in reaching decisions. The actions seen on the extreme left characterize the manager who maintains a high degree of control while those seen on the extreme right characterize the manager who releases a high degree of control. Neither extreme is absolute; authority and freedom are never without their limitations.

Now let us look more closely at each of the behavior points occurring along this continuum.

The manager makes the decision and announces it

In this case the boss identifies a problem, considers alternative solutions, chooses one of them, and then reports this decision to his subordinates for implementation. He may or may not give consideration to what he believes his subordinates will think or feel about his decision; in any case, he provides no opportunity for them to participate directly in the decision-making process. Coercion may or may not be used or implied.

The manager "sells" his decision

Here the manager, as before, takes responsibility for identifying the problem and arriving at

a decision. However, rather than simply announcing it, he takes the additional step of persuading his subordinates to accept it. In doing so, he recognizes the possibility of some resistance among those who will be faced with the decision, and seeks to reduce this resistance by indicating, for example, what the employees have to gain from his decision.

The manager presents his ideas, invites questions

Here the boss who has arrived at a decision and who seeks acceptance of his ideas provides an opportunity for his subordinates to get a fuller explanation of his thinking and his intentions. After presenting the ideas, he invites questions so that his associates can better understand what he is trying to accomplish. This "give and take" also enables the manager and the subordinates to explore more fully the implications of the decision.

The manager presents a tentative decision subject to change

This kind of behavior permits the subordinates to exert some influence on the decision. The initiative for identifying and diagnosing the problem remains with the boss. Before meeting with his staff, he has thought the problem through and arrived at a decision—but only a tentative one. Before finalizing it, he presents his proposed solution for the reaction of those who will be affected by it. He says in effect, "I'd like to hear what you have to say about this plan that I have developed. I'll appreciate your frank reactions, but will reserve for myself the final decision."

The manager presents the problem, gets suggestions, and then makes his decision

Up to this point the boss has come before the group with a solution of his own. Not so in this case. The subordinates now get the first chance to suggest solutions. The manager's initial role involves identifying the problem. He might, for example, say something of this sort: "We are faced with a number of complaints from newspapers and the general public on our service policy. What is wrong here? What ideas do you have for coming to grips with this problem?"

RETROSPECTIVE COMMENTARY

Since this HBR Classic was first published in 1958, there have been many changes in organizations and in the world that have affected leadership patterns. While the article's continued popularity attests to its essential validity, we believe it can be reconsidered and updated to reflect subsequent societal changes and new management concepts.

The reasons for the article's continued relevance can be summarized briefly:

• The article contains insights and perspectives which mesh well with, and help clarify, the experiences of managers, other leaders, and students of leadership. Thus it is useful to individuals in a wide variety of organizations—industrial, governmental, educational, religious, and community.

• The concept of leadership the article defines is reflected in a continuum of leadership behavior (see *Exhibit I* in original article). Rather than offering a choice between two styles of leadership, democratic or authoritarian, it sanctions a range of behavior.

• The concept does not dictate to managers but helps them to analyze their own behavior within a context of other alternatives, without any style being labeled right or wrong.

(We have sometimes wondered if we have, perhaps, made it too easy for anyone to justify his or her style of leadership. It may be a small step between being nonjudgmental and giving the impression that all behavior is equally valid and useful. The latter was not our intention. Indeed, the thrust of our endorsement was for the manager who is insightful in assessing relevant forces within himself, others, and the situation, and who can be flexible in responding to these forces.)

In recognizing that our article can be updated, we are acknowledging that organizations do not exist in a vacuum but are affected by changes that occur in society. Consider, for example, the implications for organizations of these recent social developments:

• The youth revolution that expresses distrust and even contempt for organizations identified with the establishment.

• The civil rights movement that demands all minority groups be given a greater opportunity for participation and influence in the organizational processes.

• The ecology and consumer movements that challenge the right of managers to make decisions without considering the interest of people outside the organization.

• The increasing national concern with the quality of working life and its relationship to worker productivity, participation, and satisfaction.

These and other societal changes make effective leadership in this decade a more challenging task, requiring even greater sensitivity and flexibility than was needed in the 1950's. Today's manager is more likely to deal with employees who resent being treated as subordinates, who may be highly critical of any organizational system, who expect to be consulted and to exert influence, and who often stand on the edge of alienation from the institution that needs their loyalty and commitment. In addition, he is frequently confronted by a highly turbulent, unpredictable environment.

In response to these social pressures, new concepts of management have emerged in organizations. Open-system theory, with its emphasis on subsystems' interdependency *and* on the interaction of an organization with its environment, has made a powerful impact on managers' approach to problems. Organization development has emerged as a new behavioral science approach to the improvement of individual, group, organizational, and interorganizational performance. New research has added to our understanding of motivation in the work situation. More and more executives have become concerned with social responsibility and have explored the feasibility of social audits. And a growing number of organizations, in Europe and in the United States, have conducted experiments in industrial democracy.

In light of these developments, we submit the following thoughts on how we would rewrite certain points in our original article.

The article described forces in the manager, subordinates, and the situation as givens, with the leadership pattern a resultant of these forces. We would now give more attention to the *interdependency* of these forces. For example, such interdependency occurs in: (a) the interplay between the manager's confidence in his subordinates, their readiness to assume responsibility, and the level of group effectiveness; and (b) the impact of the behavior of the manager on that of his subordinates, and vice versa.

In discussing the forces in the situation, we primarily identified organizational phenomena. We would now include forces lying outside the organization, and would explore the relevant interdependencies between the organization and its environment.

In the original article, we presented the size of the rectangle in *Exhibit I* as a given, with its boundaries already determined by external forces—in effect, a closed system. We would now recognize the possibility of the manager and/or his subordinates taking the initiative to change those boundaries through interaction with relevant external forces—both within their own organization and in the larger society.

The article portrayed the manager as the principal and almost unilateral actor. He initiated and determined group functions, assumed responsibility, and exercised control. Subordinates made inputs and assumed power only at the will of the manager. Although the manager might have taken into account forces outside himself, it was *he* who decided where to operate on the continuum—that is, whether to

announce a decision instead of trying to sell his idea to his subordinates, whether to invite questions, to let subordinates decide an issue, and so on. While the manager has retained this clear prerogative in many organizations, it has been challenged in others. Even in situations where he has retained it, however, the balance in the relationship between manager and subordinates at any given time is arrived at by interaction—direct or indirect—between the two parties.

Although power and its use by the manager played a role in our article, we now realize that our concern with cooperation and collaboration, common goals, commitment, trust, and mutual caring limited our vision with respect to the realities of power. We did not attempt to deal with unions, other forms of joint worker action, or with individual workers' expressions of resistance. Today, we would recognize much more clearly the power available to *all* parties, and the factors that underlie the interrelated decisions on whether to use it.

In the original article, we used the terms "manager" and "subordinate." We are now uncomfortable with "subordinate" because of its demeaning, dependency-laden connotations and prefer "nonmanager." The titles "manager" and "nonmanager" make the terminological difference functional rather than hierarchical.

We assumed fairly traditional organizational structures in our original article. Now we would alter our formulation to reflect newer organizational modes which are slowly emerging, such as industrial democracy, intentional communities, and "phenomenarchy."* These new modes are based on observations such as the following:

• Both manager and nonmanagers may be governing forces in their group's environment, contributing to the definition of the total area of freedom.

• A group can function without a manager, with managerial functions being shared by group members.

• A group, as a unit, can be delegated authority and can assume responsibility within a larger organizational context.

Our thoughts on the question of leadership have prompted us to design a new behavior continuum

*For a description of phenomenarchy, see Will McWhinney, "Phenomenarchy: A Suggestion for Social Redesign," *Journal of Applied Behavioral Science*, May 1973.

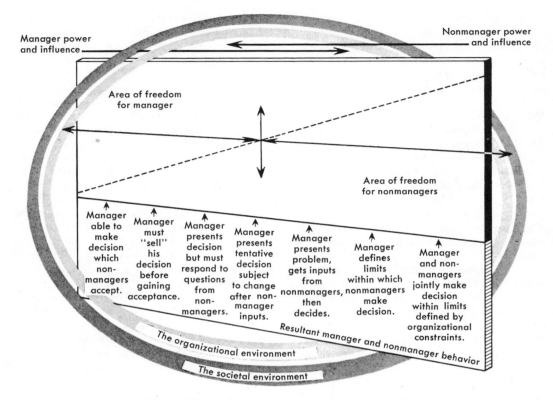

Exhibit II. Continuum of manager-nonmanager behavior.

(see *Exhibit II*) in which the total area of freedom shared by manager and nonmanagers is constantly redefined by interactions between them and the forces in the environment.

The arrows in the exhibit indicate the continual flow of interdependent influence among systems and people. The points on the continuum designate the types of manager and nonmanager behavior that become possible with any given amount of freedom available to each. The new continuum is both more complex and more dynamic than the 1958 version, reflecting the organizational and societal realities of 1973.

The function of the group becomes one of increasing the manager's repertory of possible solutions to the problem. The purpose is to capitalize on the knowledge and experience of those who are on the "firing line." From the expanded list of alternatives developed by the manager and his subordinates, the manager then selects the solution that he regards as most promising.[1]

The manager defines the limits and requests the group to make a decision

At this point the manager passes to the group (possibly including himself as a member) the right to make decisions. Before doing so, however, he defines the problem to be solved and the boundaries within which the decision must be made.

An example might be the handling of a parking problem at a plant. The boss decides that

1. For a fuller explanation of this approach, see Leo Moore, "Too Much Management, Too Little Change," HBR January-February 1956, p. 41.

this is something that should be worked on by the people involved, so he calls them together and points up the existence of the problem. Then he tells them:

"There is the open field just north of the main plant which has been designated for additional employee parking. We can build underground or surface multilevel facilities as long as the cost does not exceed $100,000. Within these limits we are free to work out whatever solution makes sense to us. After we decide on a specific plan, the company will spend the available money in whatever way we indicate."

The manager permits the group to make decisions within prescribed limits

This represents an extreme degree of group freedom only occasionally encountered in formal organizations, as, for instance, in many research groups. Here the team of managers or engineers undertakes the identification and diagnosis of the problem, develops alternative procedures for solving it, and decides on one or more of these alternative solutions. The only limits directly imposed on the group by the organization are those specified by the superior of the team's boss. If the boss participates in the decision-making process, he attempts to do so with no more authority than any other member of the group. He commits himself in advance to assist in implementing whatever decision the group makes.

Key questions

As the continuum in *Exhibit I* demonstrates, there are a number of alternative ways in which a manager can relate himself to the group or individuals he is supervising. At the extreme left of the range, the emphasis is on the manager—on what *he* is interested in, how *he* sees things, how *he* feels about them. As we move toward the subordinate-centered end of the continuum, however, the focus is increasingly on the subordinates—on what *they* are interested in, how *they* look at things, how *they* feel about them.

When business leadership is regarded in this way, a number of questions arise. Let us take four of especial importance:

Can a boss ever relinquish his responsibility by delegating it to someone else?

Our view is that the manager must expect to be held responsible by his superior for the quality of the decisions made, even though operationally these decisions may have been made on a group basis. He should, therefore, be ready to accept whatever risk is involved whenever he delegates decision-making power to his subordinates. Delegation is not a way of "passing the buck." Also, it should be emphasized that the amount of freedom the boss gives to his subordinates cannot be greater than the freedom which he himself has been given by his own superior.

Should the manager participate with his subordinates once he has delegated responsibility to them?

The manager should carefully think over this question and decide on his role prior to involving the subordinate group. He should ask if his presence will inhibit or facilitate the problem-solving process. There may be some instances when he should leave the group to let it solve the problem for itself. Typically, however, the boss has useful ideas to contribute, and should function as an additional member of the group. In the latter instance, it is important that he indicate clearly to the group that he sees himself in a *member* role rather than in an authority role.

How important is it for the group to recognize what kind of leadership behavior the boss is using?

It makes a great deal of difference. Many relationship problems between boss and subordinate occur because the boss fails to make clear how he plans to use his authority. If, for example, he actually intends to make a certain decision himself, but the subordinate group gets the impression that he has delegated this authority, considerable confusion and resentment are likely to follow. Problems may also occur when the boss uses a "democratic" façade to conceal the fact that he has already made a decision which he hopes the group will accept as its own. The attempt to "make them think it was their idea in the first place" is a risky one. We believe that it is highly important for the manager to be honest and clear in describing what authority he is keeping and what role he is asking his subordinates to assume in solving a particular problem.

Can you tell how "democratic" a manager is by the number of decisions his subordinates make?

The sheer *number* of decisions is not an accurate index of the amount of freedom that a subordinate group enjoys. More important is the *significance* of the decisions which the boss entrusts to his subordinates. Obviously a decision on how to arrange desks is of an entirely different order from a decision involving the introduction of new electronic data-processing equipment. Even though the widest possible limits are given in dealing with the first issue, the group will sense no particular degree of responsibility. For a boss to permit the group to decide equipment policy, even within rather narrow limits, would reflect a greater degree of confidence in them on his part.

Deciding how to lead

Now let us turn from the types of leadership which are possible in a company situation to the question of what types are *practical* and *desirable*. What factors or forces should a manager consider in deciding how to manage? Three are of particular importance:

- Forces in the manager.
- Forces in the subordinates.
- Forces in the situation.

We should like briefly to describe these elements and indicate how they might influence a manager's action in a decision-making situation.[2] The strength of each of them will, of course, vary from instance to instance, but the manager who is sensitive to them can better assess the problems which face him and determine which mode of leadership behavior is most appropriate for him.

Forces in the manager. The manager's behavior in any given instance will be influenced greatly by the many forces operating within his own personality. He will, of course, perceive his leadership problems in a unique way on the basis of his background, knowledge, and experience. Among the important internal forces affecting him will be the following:

1. *His value system.* How strongly does he feel that individuals should have a share in making the decisions which affect them? Or, how convinced is he that the official who is paid to assume responsibility should personally carry the burden of decision making? The strength of his convictions on questions like these will tend to move the manager to one end or the other of the continuum shown in *Exhibit I*. His behavior will also be influenced by the relative importance that he attaches to organizational efficiency, personal growth of subordinates, and company profits.[3]

2. *His confidence in his subordinates.* Managers differ greatly in the amount of trust they have in other people generally, and this carries over to the particular employees they supervise at a given time. In viewing his particular group of subordinates, the manager is likely to consider their knowledge and competence with respect to the problem. A central question he might ask himself is: "Who is best qualified to

2. See also Robert Tannenbaum and Fred Massarik, "Participation by Subordinates in the Managerial Decision-Making Process," *Canadian Journal of Economics and Political Science,* August 1950, p. 413.

3. See Chris Argyris, "Top Management Dilemma: Company Needs vs. Individual Development," *Personnel,* September 1955, pp. 123-134.

deal with this problem?'' Often he may, justifiably or not, have more confidence in his own capabilities than in those of his subordinates.

3. *His own leadership inclinations*. There are some managers who seem to function more comfortably and naturally as highly directive leaders. Resolving problems and issuing orders come easily to them. Other managers seem to operate more comfortably in a team role, where they are continually sharing many of their functions with their subordinates.

4. *His feelings of security in an uncertain situation*. The manager who releases control over the decision-making process thereby reduces the predictability of the outcome. Some managers have a greater need than others for predictability and stability in their environment. This ''tolerance for ambiguity'' is being viewed increasingly by psychologists as a key variable in a person's manner of dealing with problems.

The manager brings these and other highly personal variables to each situation he faces. If he can see them as forces which, consciously or unconsciously, influence his behavior, he can better understand what makes him prefer to act in a given way. And understanding this, he can often make himself more effective.

Forces in the subordinate. Before deciding how to lead a certain group, the manager will also want to consider a number of forces affecting his subordinates' behavior. He will want to remember that each employee, like himself, is influenced by many personality variables. In addition, each subordinate has a set of expectations about how the boss should act in relation to him (the phrase ''expected behavior'' is one we hear more and more often these days at discussions of leadership and teaching). The better the manager understands these factors, the more accurately he can determine what kind of behavior on his part will enable his subordinates to act most effectively.

Generally speaking, the manager can permit his subordinates greater freedom if the following essential conditions exist:

• If the subordinates have relatively high needs for independence. (As we all know, people differ greatly in the amount of direction they desire.)

• If the subordinates have a readiness to assume responsibility for decision making. (Some see additional responsibility as a tribute to their ability; others see it as ''passing the buck.'')

• If they have a relatively high tolerance for ambiguity. (Some employees prefer to have clear-cut directives given to them; others prefer a wider area of freedom.)

• If they are interested in the problem and feel that it is important.

• If they understand and identify with the goals of the organization.

• If they have the necessary knowledge and experience to deal with the problem.

• If they have learned to expect to share in decision making. (Persons who have come to expect strong leadership and are then suddenly confronted with the request to share more fully in decision making are often upset by this new experience. On the other hand, persons who have enjoyed a considerable amount of freedom resent the boss who begins to make all the decisions himself.)

The manager will probably tend to make fuller use of his own authority if the above conditions do *not* exist; at times there may be no realistic alternative to running a ''one-man show.''

The restrictive of many of the forces will, of course, be greatly modified by the general feeling of confidence which subordinates have in the boss. Where they have learned to respect and trust him, he is free to vary his behavior. He will feel certain that he will not be perceived as an authoritarian boss on those occasions when he makes decisions by himself. Similarly, he will not be seen as using staff meetings to avoid his decision-making responsibility. In a climate of mutual confidence and respect, people tend to feel less threatened by deviations from normal practice, which in turn makes possible a higher degree of flexibility in the whole relationship.

Forces in the situation: In addition to the forces which exist in the manager himself and in his subordinates, certain characteristics of the general situation will also affect the manager's behavior. Among the more critical environmental pressures that surround him are those which stem from the organization, the work group, the nature of the problem, and the pressures of time. Let us look briefly at each of these:

Type of organization. Like individuals, organizations have values and traditions which inevitably influence the behavior of the people who work in them. The manager who is a newcomer to a company quickly discovers that certain kinds of behavior are approved while others are not. He also discovers that to deviate radically from what is generally accepted is likely to create problems for him.

These values and traditions are communicated in numerous ways—through job descriptions, policy pronouncements, and public statements by top executives. Some organizations, for example, hold to the notion that the desirable executive is one who is dynamic, imaginative, decisive, and persuasive. Other organizations put more emphasis upon the importance of the executive's ability to work effectively with people—his human relations skills. The fact that his superiors have a defined concept of what the good executive should be will very likely push the manager toward one end or the other of the behavioral range.

In addition to the above, the amount of employee participation is influenced by such variables as the size of the working units, their geographical distribution, and the degree of inter- and intra-organizational security required to attain company goals. For example, the wide geographical dispersion of an organization may preclude a practical system of participative decision making, even though this would otherwise be desirable. Similarly, the size of the working units or the need for keeping plans confidential may make it necessary for the boss to exercise more control than would otherwise be the case. Factors like these may limit considerably the manager's ability to function flexibly on the continuum.

Group effectiveness. Before turning decision-making responsibility over to a subordinate group, the boss should consider how effectively its members work together as a unit.

One of the relevant factors here is the experience the group has had in working together. It can generally be expected that a group which has functioned for some time will have developed habits of cooperation and thus be able to tackle a problem more effectively than a new group. It can also be expected that a group of people with similar backgrounds and interests will work more quickly and easily than people with dissimilar backgrounds, because the communication problems are likely to be less complex.

The degree of confidence that the members have in their ability to solve problems as a group is also a key consideration. Finally, such group variables as cohesiveness, permissiveness, mutual acceptance, and commonality of purpose will exert subtle but powerful influence on the group's functioning.

The problem itself. The nature of the problem may determine what degree of authority should be delegated by the manager to his subordinates. Obviously he will ask himself whether they have the kind of knowledge which is needed. It is possible to do them a real disservice by assigning a problem that their experience does not equip them to handle.

Since the problems faced in large or growing industries increasingly require knowledge of specialists from many different fields, it might be inferred that the more complex a problem, the more anxious a manager will be to get some assistance in solving it. However, this is not always the case. There will be times when the very complexity of the problem calls for one person to work it out. For example, if the manager has most of the background and factual data relevant to a given issue, it may be easier for him to think it through himself than to take the time to fill in his staff on all the pertinent background information.

The key question to ask, of course, is: "Have I heard the ideas of everyone who has the necessary knowledge to make a significant contribution to the solution of this problem?"

The pressure of time—This is perhaps the most clearly felt pressure on the manager (in spite of the fact that it may sometimes be imagined). The more that he feels the need for an immediate decision, the more difficult it is to involve other people. In organizations which are in a constant state of "crisis" and "crash programming" one is likely to find managers personally using a high degree of authority with relatively little delegation to subordinates. When the time pressure is less intense, however, it becomes much more possible to bring subordinates in on the decision-making process.

These, then, are the principal forces that impinge on the manager in any given instance and that tend to determine his tactical behavior in relation to his subordinates. In each case his behavior ideally will be that which makes possible the most effective attainment of his immediate goal within the limits facing him.

Long-run strategy

As the manager works with his organization on the problems that come up day by day, his choice of a leadership pattern is usually limited. He must take account of the forces just described and, within the restrictions they impose on him, do the best that he can. But as he looks ahead months or even years, he can shift his thinking from tactics to large-scale strategy. No longer need he be fettered by all of the forces mentioned, for he can view many of them as variables over which he has some control. He can, for example, gain new insights or skills for himself, supply training for individ-

ual subordinates, and provide participative experiences for his employee group.

In trying to bring about a change in these variables, however, he is faced with a challenging question: At which point along the continuum *should* he act?

Attaining objectives. The answer depends largely on what he wants to accomplish. Let us suppose that he is interested in the same objectives that most modern managers seek to attain when they can shift their attention from the pressure of immediate assignments:

1. To raise the level of employee motivation.
2. To increase the readiness of subordinates to accept change.
3. To improve the quality of all managerial decisions.
4. To develop teamwork and morale.
5. To further the individual development of employees.

In recent years the manager has been deluged with a flow of advice on how best to achieve these longer-run objectives. It is little wonder that he is often both bewildered and annoyed. However, there are some guidelines which he can usefully follow in making a decision.

Most research and much of the experience of recent years give a strong factual basis to the theory that a fairly high degree of subordinate-centered behavior is associated with the accomplishment of the five purposes mentioned.[4] This does not mean that a manager should always leave all decisions to his assistants. To provide the individual or the group with greater freedom than they are ready for at any given time may very well tend to generate anxieties and therefore inhibit rather than facilitate the attainment of desired objectives. But this should not keep the manager from making a continuing effort

---

4. For example, see Warren H. Schmidt and Paul C. Buchanan, *Techniques that Produce Teamwork* (New London, Arthur C. Croft Publications, 1954); and Morris S. Viteles, *Motivation and Morale in Industry* (New York, W. W. Norton & Company, Inc., 1953).

to confront his subordinates with the challenge of freedom.

CONCLUSION

In summary, there are two implications in the basic thesis that we have been developing. The first is that the successful leader is one who is keenly aware of those forces which are most relevant to his behavior at any given time. He accurately understands himself, the individuals and group he is dealing with, and the company and broader social environment in which he operates. And certainly he is able to assess the present readiness for growth of his subordinates.

But this sensitivity or understanding is not enough, which brings us to the second implication. The successful leader is one who is able to behave appropriately in the light of these perceptions. If direction is in order, he is able to direct; if considerable participative freedom is called for, he is able to provide such freedom.

Thus, the successful manager of men can be primarily characterized neither as a strong leader nor as a permissive one. Rather, he is one who maintains a high batting average in accurately assessing the forces that determine what his most appropriate behavior at any given time should be and in actually being able to behave accordingly. Being both insightful and flexible, he is less likely to see the problems of leadership as a dilemma.

The social nature of leadership

ROBERT K. MERTON, Ph.D.

From the obscure time of ancient Byzantium to our own day, the practice and theory of leadership have engaged man's interest. Treading his way to the Lyceum, Aristotle was persuaded that some men were endowed by nature with the capacity for leadership, and there are still people who hold with him that "from the hour of their birth, some are marked out for subjection, others for rule."[1] Almost two millennia later, Machiavelli, in his handbook for princes, encompassed courage, conviction, pride, and strength among the qualities of leaders. And as we approach our own time, it still seems to many that the question most worth asking about leadership is this: What personal traits distinguish leaders from the rest of us? Answers to this question take us to a bottomless pit of

virtue. According to the mystique, leaders distinctively possess such traits as intelligence, emotional maturity, perseverance, tact, faith, dominance, courage, insight, and so on and on.

More recently, social science has greatly restricted the search for the personality traits distinctive to leaders. The reasons for this shift are varied. It was found that the same people proved to be leaders in one type of group and not in others. Correlatively, leaders in the same groups were of quite different kinds at different times. Few traits were found to be uniformly linked with leadership. R. D. Mann, for example, examined 125 studies of leadership which had generated 750 findings about the personality traits of leaders.[2] He could discover none which yielded a significant relation with leadership in as many as half of these studies. And to make matters worse, of the scores of traits tentatively identified in one study or another, many were diametrically opposed; in some groups, effective leaders were aggressive, in others, mild and restrained; in some, decisive, in others, diplomatic. We have come to recognize that the apparently sensible question about distinctive traits of leaders was largely misdirected, that answers to it could yield little understanding of the nature of leadership.

What we now know about leadership derives from quite another perspective. This one holds that leadership does not, indeed cannot, result merely from the individual traits of leaders; it must also involve attributes of the transactions between those who lead and those who follow. Otherwise put, we start from the assumption that the leader is only one component in that complex phenomenon we call leadership. Like other discoveries about human behavior, it may seem odd that this one was so long coming. For once announced, it appears self-evident. After all, Robinson Crusoe might have been brave, bright, innovative, courageous, adaptive, and so on, though it is plain that until his man Friday came along he could not possibly have exercised leadership. And since leadership involves directive influence upon others, since it involves collective action, we will do better to seek its workings in the system of roles and interactions between people rather than simply in the characteristics of individuals.

Leadership is, then, some sort of social transaction. Its outward and visible signs are as evident as they are familiar. Leaders exert an unusual degree of influence upon their fellows. They more often initiate ideas for the group and these ideas are apt to make good sense to their associates. When leaders are not engaged in initiating group action, they are responding to others who turn to them for counsel. As these others find that the performance of their own roles is facilitated by what leaders say and do, they tend to express deference to them. Altogether, in the useful words of Stogdill, leadership is the process of "influencing the activities of an organized group toward goal-setting and goal-achievement."[3]

LEADERSHIP versus AUTHORITY

So it is that this transactional perspective puts in question the ancient notion that leadership is only an expression of the individual qualities of leadership. This perspective does more. It requires us to recognize that leadership, as a mode of social influence, is not the same as authority, which is an attribute of a social position. The organizational executive, the judge, the foreman, the head nurse have *authority* by virtue of the positions they hold. They may or may not also exert leadership. Authority involves the legitimated rights of a position that require others to obey; leadership is an interpersonal relation in which others comply because they want to, not because they have to. This distinction between authority and leadership is more than an academic exercise. It is fundamental to our understanding the major fact that *leadership can be found at every level of an organization*. The leaders, the influentials, sometimes hold formal offices of authority; sometimes, they do not. At times, they are unofficially acknowledged leaders, recognized as such in the behavior of their associates though not in the organization blueprint.

Once we keep in mind the basic distinction between authority and leadership, all manner of problems come into focus. We can begin to understand how it is that some people who occupy positions of authority are effective in their jobs while others in such positions do poorly. The first type combine authority *and* leadership; the second have authority without leadership. In the first case, the organization thrives, in the second, it deteriorates. Sooner or later, something gives. The people in positions of authority are displaced or the organization becomes less and less effective.

One way of coaxing sociological truths about leadership out of their dark hiding places, then, is to center on cases in which people occupy varying positions of authority and to consider what is necessary for them to exercise that authority effectively. This is only another way of saying that we want to deal primarily with the question of what makes for the joint exercise of authority *and* leadership.

It was the distinctive genius of Chester Barnard to recognize, some 30 years ago, that authority, at its most effective, achieves willing rather than forced compliance. In the relation between leader and follower, there is a "zone of acceptability": that range of behavior "within which the subordinate is ready to accept the decisions made for him by his superior."*

Effective leadership operates principally within that zone of acceptability. And to do this, as Barnard pointed out, four primitive conditions must be satisfied. Evident as they are, these conditions are nevertheless often neglected in practice. First, the recipient of the communication—suggestion, advice or order, as the case may be—must be able to understand it. Experience shows that much seeming noncompliance with a directive is in fact only a case of its not having been understood. Second, the person must be able to comply with the directive; he must have the resources to do what he is being asked to do. Many an apparent failure in leadership occurs because this condition is unmet. Leaders have not seen to it that people are equipped with both the inner and outer resources, with the skills and knowledge and time and energy and tools needed to do what is being called for. Third, to comply with what is being asked of them, people must believe that the action is in some degree consistent with their personal interests and values. They may be ready to act against these interests for a time but asked to do so continually, they will develop profoundly original ways of evading orders

or suggestions. Fourth and finally, they must perceive the directive as consistent with the purposes and values of the organization.

Effective leaders intuitively or explicitly provide for meeting these four primitive requirements; ineffective leaders neglect one or more of them and are puzzled by deteriorating organizational performance. Analysis shows that the leader who is losing his grip has been violating one or more of these requirements: his communications calling for action are unclear to recipients, they are directed to people not equipped to do what they are being asked to do, they violate the personal interests or values of recipients or they are at odds with group purposes, values, and norms.

These observations bring out once again the central idea that leadership is less an attribute of individuals than of a social exchange, a transaction between leader and led. And again, though some leaders sense this intuitively, the rest of us must learn it more laboriously. Leaders assist their associates in achieving personal and social goals. In exchange, they receive the basic coin of effective leadership: trust and respect. You need not be loved to be an effective leader, but you must be respected.

Identifiable social processes produce the respect that makes for effective leadership. First, respect expressed *by* the leader breeds respect *for* the leader. As he exhibits respect for members of the group and for their shared values and norms he finds it reciprocated.

Second, he demonstrates competence in performing his own roles, whatever these may be. No one is better situated than subordinates to distinguish between a superior's authentic competence and its mere appearance.

Third, the leader is in continuing touch with what is going on within the group. For this, it helps to be located at strategic nodes in the network of communication. Located there, he provides for two-way communication. He not only lets the other fellow get an occasional word in edgewise, he lets him get a good number of words in straightaway. And the leader

---

*The concept was called the "zone of difference" by Chester Barnard, *The Functions of the Executive,* Cambridge, Mass., Harvard University Press, 1938, pp. 168-169. It was then extended and called the "area of acceptance" by Herbert A. Simon, *Administrative Behavior,* New York, Macmillan Co., 1947, p. 133 (whose language is quoted here). The term "zone of acceptability" is intended to capture the intent of both Barnard and Simon.

listens: both to what is said and to what is not said but implied. He allows for both negative and positive feedback. Negative feedback, as a cue to the possibility that he has moved far beyond the zone of acceptibility; positive feedback as a cue for support of his initiating actions.

Fourth, though the leader in positions of authority has access to the power that coerces, he seldom makes use of it. Once he has gained the respect of associates, it is they, not the leader, who tend to ensure compliance among their peers. Leaders deplete their authority by frequent exercise of power. For such action shrinks the zone of acceptibility. Group experiments have found that the more often group leaders used the coercive power granted them, the more apt were they to be displaced. These experiments confirm what has long been thought; leadership is sustained by *noblesse oblige,* the obligation for generosity of behavior among those enjoying rank and power. Force is an ultimate resource that maintains itself by being seldom employed.

Having noted this in a general way, we must note also that styles of leadership vary. The repertoire of styles is large and few leaders acquire the versatility to shift from one to another style as changing circumstances require. There is the authoritarian style in which the leader is firm, insistent, self-assured, dominating. With or without intent, he creates fear and then meets the regressive needs of his followers that that fear has created. He keeps himself at the center of attention and manages to keep communication between others in the group to a minimum. Ready to use coercion, the authoritarian may be effective in times of crisis when the social system is in a state of disorder. But extreme and enforced dependence on the leader means that the system is especially liable to instability.

The democratic style of leadership, in contrast, is responsive. It provides for extended participation of others, with policies emerging out of interaction between leader and led. The democratic leader initiates more than the rank and file but the authoritarian does so to a far greater degree. Other familiar styles of leadership can here only find mention: the bureaucratic leader, for example, who holds fast to the rule book at all costs, and the paternalistic leader, who converts direction of even the most impersonal task into inflexible but to him benevolent control. The styles of leadership emerging in particular cases are, to an unknown degree, an expansion of the personality structure and earlier socialization of the leader. Leaders lead as they have been led. But to perhaps a greater extent, styles of leadership are a function of the situation and the character of the organization; it is through the incessant process of self-selection and organizational selection that particular personality types find themselves cast in leadership roles.

WHAT DO LEADERS DO?

But whatever the styles of leadership, what are its functions? All apart from the flamboyant rhetoric in which we ordinarily talk of leaders, what in fact do they do? So many and diverse are these functions that we sometimes wonder that leaders, like self-conscious centipedes, can navigate at all. The saving grace seems to be that social systems, once established, have enough stability to limp along even though some of those many functions are served ineptly. Here, then, in swift review, are some of the chief functions of leadership.

• Leaders facilitate the adaptive capacity of social systems. They initiate change that is responsive to both the internal and external environments of the system.

• Leaders are distinctively alert to the unanticipated consequences of previous collective action. They capitalize upon the consequences that advance the group purpose and counteract those consequences that were both unforeseen and unwanted.

• Leaders are future oriented as well as present oriented. They search out currently hidden but impending problems. These anticipatory adaptations assist the group to prepare for impending problems, to curtail their impact when they do emerge and, in the ideal case, keep them from developing at all.

•Whether assigned this task or not, leaders represent the group to its environment. Central to the internal organization of the group, they are also at its boundary where interchange between the group and its environment takes place.

• Leaders evaluate resources for the system and cope with the problem of their allocation. This they do in terms of priorities of achieving group objectives and in terms of optimum technical allocations hedged in by group-defined criteria of social justice.

• Leaders express aspirations that evoke resonance among members of the group. This is often phrased as saying that leaders have vision. But vision that is remote from the values and wants of the group becomes self-defeating fantasy.

• Leaders mobilize, guide, coordinate, and control the efforts of group members. When effective, they deepen motivation and enlarge output beyond that which could be achieved without them.

• Leaders symbolize, extend and deepen collective unity among members of the system. They dramatize what would otherwise be prosy, and in doing so, tap new energies that enable people to work together.

• Leaders enunciate the values and ideals of the group, and give people pride in their group identity.

• Leaders arbitrate and mediate the inevitable conflicts that emerge in social interaction in such fashion that most members of the group feel most of the time that justice has been done.

• Not least, leaders serve as scapegoats. They must be prepared to have the sins of their followers and of the entire group symbolically laid upon them.

Having assembled these leadership functions, we should pause for a moment to take stock. We first touched upon the concept of leadership as social transaction and social role, rather than as merely a quality of individuals. We noted that leadership need not coincide with appointed office, that it is found, as potential and as actuality, on every level of organizational hierarchy. We glimpsed some of the social process engaging leaders with rank and file and noted how legitimacy and respect—prime characteristics of leadership—are generated by certain kinds of interaction within the group. We glanced at styles of leadership and noted that, to be effective, these must be geared into the character of the organization and the conditions it confronts. And we took partial inventory of the functions of leaders.

There are other aspects of this complex social phenomenon called leadership. Consider for a moment how the operation of leadership differs for relatively stationary social systems and for rapidly expanding ones. In the stationary society, where total resources are not being greatly enlarged, growth in the power, wealth, and authority of some typically means decline for the rest. This is the zero-sum situation in which what is good for one is bad for the other. But in the expanding social system, all this can change. Leaders can expand the scope of their influence without this being at the expense of others. The gap between them *can* widen. But, as Boulding has shown, there is nevertheless a basic difference between stationary and expanding systems: in the second, unlike the first, one need not rise only by pushing others down.[4]

In the same overly condensed fashion, we must take note that types of leadership required by groups change under changing circumstances. As Fiedler has found experimentally, effective group performance is contingent upon differing styles of leadership under differing conditions.[5] Again without benefit of sociological theory or experimentation, many of us sense this intuitively. Bad times and good call for different emphases in leadership. In time of crisis and gloom, when previous procedures and values are being widely questioned, groups turn to leaders who can affirm or reaffirm newly emerging values. They are concerned more with achieving a new state of the social system than with the task-performance of that system. In time of relative stability, the basic demand is not so much for this kind of leadership as for enlarging the productivity of the system.

GENERIC FUNCTIONS

All this takes us directly to one of those great simplifications about the behavior of social systems that can provide much understanding if it is not distorted into an oversimplification. The over-riding functions of leadership can be instructively reduced to two, with all the specific functions being of one or the other kind. The first is the integrative function providing for that socio-emotional support to members of a group which stabilizes systems of social relations between them. The second is the instrumental function providing for effective mobilization and coordination of activity to enlarge the amount and improve the quality of task-performance. Both generic functions are of course essential to the operation of social systems. But phases in systems vary, sometimes requiring more of the first function, sometimes more of the second. Paragons among leaders manage the difficult feat of directing their efforts chiefly toward integrative or toward instrumental functions as they diagnose the changing needs of the system. But leaders of this adaptable and comprehensive type are rare. More often, social systems evolve a division of labor, with or without plan, in which certain people serve primarily as system-maintainers and others primarily as task performers. But whether encompassed in the same people or allocated to different people these functions are basic to the effective working of social systems.

Touching upon the character, styles, conditions, functions, processes, and contexts of effective leadership might convey the monstrous idea that all leadership is a good thing, in and of itself. We all know better. Like every other instrumentality, social or technological, leadership lends itself indifferently to good or evil. After all, Stalin and Hitler were for a time effective leaders. What, then, are some of the principal dangers of leadership within small social systems as well as large?

To begin with, there is what Robert Michels excessively described as "the iron law of oligarchy."[6] He examined the paradoxical case of leaders initially committed to democratic values who abandoned these values as their attention turned increasingly to maintaining the organization and especially their own place within it. The danger is plain: leaders long established are often the last to perceive their own transition toward oligarchy, toward a form of control in which power is confined to the same few persons. And leaders long established are apt to confuse the legitimacy of their rule with themselves. It was not only Louis XIV who announced "*L'état, c'est moi!*" As the more recent story goes, De Gaulle periodically intoned to himself: "*Quand je veux savoir ce que pense la France, je m'interroge.*"[7] (When I want to know what France thinks, I ask myself.)

Leaders are apt to have other blind spots. They are often unable, as Cartwright has noted, to recognize that the very possession of power is enough to pose threats to those subject to that power.[8] But subordinates know that even the most benevolent of leaders can make things hard for them. As a result, they are more sensitive to the behavior of their superiors than superiors often are to the behavior of their subordinates. These differentials in sensitivity explain why leaders so often find even their best intentions being interpreted as malevolent. As possessors of power, leaders are perennially subject to being experienced as sources of danger.

Related to both the "law" of oligarchy and differentials in sensitivity to behavior between leaders and led is the observed tendency for communication within groups to become less open as the same leadership continues. Just as with biological systems, though for different reasons, long-lived social systems of leadership are subject to hardening of the arteries of communication. There is a fundamental reason for this. Experiments have found that people tend to see what is congenial to them and to insulate themselves from uncongenial opinions and ideas. Confronted with pleasant objects, the size of pupil dilates significantly: confronted with unpleasant objects, it contracts. All this suggests that long-enduring leaders who would also be effective ones will make a special effort to keep lines of communication open and particularly with those who do not see things as they themselves do.

Another pathology of leadership is found in the excess multiplication of rules in social systems. Rules can accumulate to the point of paralyzing needed innovation. It has been found that the number and specificity of rules increase as an adaptation to conflict between leaders and rank and file. What is equally in point, the reverse process has also been observed: the rapid growth of regulations, which often work at cross-purposes, goes along with a greater potential for conflict. These observations provide a social diagnostic. If you find yourself in an organization that is multiplying rules at a rapid rate, you are being given a sociological warning signal. There is more conflict in that system than may at first meet the eye.

Another ailment of organizational leadership was long since diagnosed by Chester Barnard as "the dilemma of time-lag."[9] By this phrase, he referred to the problem of discrepancy between organizational requirements for immediate adaptive action and the slow process of obtaining democratic approval for it. This is an authentic dilemma. Democratically organized groups can cope with this dilemma only by having their members come to recognize in advance that, remote as they are from the firing line of daily decision, there will be occasions in which decisive action must be taken before it can be fully explored and validated by the membership. This comes hard for democratic organizations which often prefer to pay the price of maladaptation in order to avoid having their leadership converted into Caesarism or Bonapartism.

That leadership is of various kinds, that it works its ways variously under various conditions, that it has its distinctive requirements and its processes, that it has, too, its pathologies—all this means that leadership is not simply a mystique. Slowly our understanding of leadership grows and sometime, perhaps, it will emerge from the sociological twilight into the full light of day.

References

1. Aristotle. *Politics* Book I, Chap. 5.
2. Mann, R. D. A review of the relationships between personality and performance in small groups. *Psychol. Bull.* 56:241-270. July, 1959.
3. Stogdill, R. M. Leadership, membership and organization, *Psychol. Bull.* 47:1-14. Jan., 1950.
4. Boulding, Kenneth. *Conflict and Defense.* New York, Harper and Row, 1961, p. 192.
5. Fiedler, F. E. A contingency model of leadership effectiveness. In *Advances in Experimental Social Psychology,* ed. by Leonard Berkowitz. New York, Academic Press, 1964, pp. 149-190.
6. Michels, Robert. *Political Parties; a Sociological Study of the Oligarchical Tendencies of Modern Democracy,* translated by Eden Paul and Cedar Paul. New York, Dover Publications, 1959.
7. Monane, J. H. *Sociology of Human Systems.* New York, Appleton-Century-Crofts, 1967, p. 55.
8. Cartwright, Dorwin. Influence, leadership, control. In *Handbook of Organizations,* ed. by James G. March. Chicago, Ill., Rand McNally and Co., 1965, p. 36.
9. Barnard, Chester. *The Functions of the Executive.* Cambridge, Mass., Harvard University Press, 1938, p. 8.

Managers and leaders: are they different?

ABRAHAM ZALEZNIK

What is the ideal way to develop leadership? Every society provides its own answer to this question, and each, in groping for answers, defines its deepest concerns about the purposes, distributions, and uses of power. Business has contributed its answer to the leadership question by evolving a new breed called the manager. Simultaneously, business has established a new power ethic that favors collective over individual leadership, the cult of the group over that of personality. While ensuring the competence, control, and the balance of power relations among groups with the potential for rivalry, managerial leadership unfortunately does not necessarily ensure imagination, creativity, or ethical behavior in guiding the destinies of corporate enterprises.

Leadership inevitably requires using power to influence the thoughts and actions of other people. Power in the hands of an individual entails human risks: first, the risk of equating power with the ability to get immediate results; second, the risk of ignoring the many different ways people can legitimately accumulate power; and third, the risk of losing self-control in the desire for power. The need to hedge these risks accounts in part for the development of collective leadership and the managerial ethic. Consequently, an inherent conservatism dominates the culture of large organizations. In *The Second American Revolution,* John D. Rockefeller, 3rd, describes the conservatism of organizations:

"An organization is a system, with a logic of its own, and all the weight of tradition and inertia. The deck is stacked in favor of the tried and proven way of doing things and against the taking of risks and striking out in new directions."[1]

Out of this conservatism and inertia organizations provide succession to power through the development of managers rather than individual leaders. And the irony of the managerial ethic is that is fosters a bureaucratic culture in business, supposedly the last bastion protecting us from the encroachments and controls of bureaucracy in government and education. Perhaps the risks associated with power in the hands of an individual may be necessary ones for business to take if organizations are to break free of their inertia and bureaucratic conservatism.

MANAGER VS. LEADER PERSONALITY

Theodore Levitt has described the essential features of a managerial culture with its emphasis on rationality and control:

"Management consists of the rational assessment of a situation and the systematic selection of goals and purposes (what is to be done?); the systematic development of strategies to achieve these goals; the marshalling of the required resources; the rational design, organization, direction, and control of the activities required to attain the selected purposes; and, finally, the motivating and rewarding of people to do the work."[2]

In other words, whether his or her energies are directed toward goals, resources, organization structures, or people, a manager is a problem solver. The manager asks himself, "What problems have to be solved, and what are the best ways to achieve results so that people will

1. John D. Rockefeller, 3rd., *The Second American Revolution* (New York, Harper-Row, 1973), p. 72.
2. Theodore Levitt, "Management and the Post Industrial Society," *The Public Interest,* Summer, 1976, p. 73.

continue to contribute to this organization?'' In this conception, leadership is a practical effort to direct affairs; and to fulfill his task, a manager requires that many people operate at different levels of status and responsibility. Our democratic society is, in fact, unique in having solved the problem of providing well-trained managers for business. The same solution stands ready to be applied to government, education, health care, and other institutions. It takes neither genius nor heroism to be a manager, but rather persistence, tough-mindedness, hard work, intelligence, analytical ability and, perhaps most important, tolerance and good will.

Another conception, however, attaches almost mystical beliefs to what leadership is and assumes that only great people are worthy of the drama of power and politics. Here, leadership is a psychodrama in which, as a precondition for control of a political structure, a lonely person must gain control of him or herself. Such an expectation of leadership contrasts sharply with the mundane, practical, and yet important conception that leadership is really managing work that other people do.

Two questions come to mind. Is this mystique of leadership merely a holdover from our collective childhood of dependency and our longing for good and heroic parents? Or, is there a basic truth lurking behind the need for leaders that no matter how competent managers are, their leadership stagnates because of their limitations in visualizing purposes and generating value in work? Without this imaginative capacity and the ability to communicate, managers, driven by their narrow purposes, perpetuate group conflicts instead of reforming them into broader desires and goals.

If indeed problems demand greatness, then, judging by past performance, the selection and development of leaders leave a great deal to chance. There are no known ways to train ''great'' leaders. Furthermore, beyond what we leave to chance, there is a deeper issue in the relationship between the need for competent managers and the longing for great leaders.

What it takes to ensure the supply of people who will assume practical responsibility may inhibit the development of great leaders. Conversely, the presence of great leaders may undermine the development of managers who become very anxious in the relative disorder that leaders seem to generate. The antagonism in aim (to have many competent managers as well as great leaders) often remains obscure in stable and well-developed societies. But the antagonism surfaces during periods of stress and change, as it did in the Western countries during both the Great Depression and World War II. The tension also appears in the struggle for power between theorists and professional managers in revolutionary societies.

It is easy enough to dismiss the dilemma I pose (of training managers while we may need new leaders, or leaders at the expense of managers) by saying that the need is for people who can be *both* managers and leaders. The truth of the matter as I see it, however, is that just as a managerial culture is different from the entrepreneurial culture that develops when leaders appear in organizations, managers and leaders are very different kinds of people. They differ in motivation, personal history, and in how they think and act.

A technologically oriented and economically successful society tends to depreciate the need for great leaders. Such societies hold a deep and abiding faith in rational methods of solving problems, including problems of value, economics, and justice. Once rational methods of solving problems are broken down into elements, organized, and taught as skills, then society's faith in technique over personal qualities in leadership remains the guiding conception for a democratic society contemplating its leadership requirements. But there are times when tinkering and trial and error prove inadequate to the emerging problems of selecting goals, allocating resources, and distributing wealth and opportunity. During such times, the democratic society needs to find leaders who use themselves as the instruments of learning and acting, instead of managers who use their accumulation of collective experience to get where they are going.

The most impressive spokesman, as well as exemplar of the managerial viewpoint, was Alfred P. Sloan, Jr. who, along with Pierre du Pont, designed the modern corporate structure. Reflecting on what makes one management successful while another fails, Sloan suggested that "good management rests on a reconciliation of centralization and decentralization, or 'decentralization with coordinated control' ".[3]

Sloan's conception of management, as well as his practice, developed by trial and error, and by the accumulation of experience. Sloan wrote:

"There is no hard and fast rule for sorting out the various responsibilities and the best way to assign them. The balance which is struck . . . varies according to what is being decided, the circumstances of the time, past experience, and the temperaments and skills of the executive involved."[4]

In other words, in much the same way that the inventors of the late nineteenth century tried, failed, and fitted until they hit on a product or method, managers who innovate in developing organizations are "tinkerers." They do not have a grand design or experience the intuitive flash of insight that, borrowing from modern science, we have come to call the "breakthrough."

Managers and leaders differ fundamentally in their world views. The dimensions for assessing these differences include managers' and leaders' orientations toward their goals, their work, their human relations, and their selves.

3. Alfred P. Sloan, Jr., *My Years with General Motors* (New York: Doubleday & Co. 1964), p. 429.
4. Ibid., p. 429.

ATTITUDES TOWARD GOALS

Managers tend to adopt impersonal, if not passive, attitudes toward goals. Managerial goals arise out of necessities rather than desires, and, therefore, are deeply embedded in the history and culture of the organization.

Frederic G. Donner, chairman and chief executive officer of General Motors from 1958 to 1967, expressed this impersonal and passive attitude toward goals in defining GM's position on product development:

". . . To meet the challenge of the marketplace, we must recognize changes in customer needs and desires far enough ahead to have the right products in the right places at the right time and in the right quantity.

"We must balance trends in preference against the many compromises that are necessary to make a final product that is both reliable and good looking, that performs well and that sells at a competitive price in the necessary volume. We must design, not just the cars we would like to build, but more importantly, the cars that our customers want to buy."[5]

Nowhere in this formulation of how a product comes into being is there a notion that consumer tastes and preferences arise in part as a result of what manufacturers do. In reality, through product design, advertising, and promotion, consumers learn to like what they then say they need. Few would argue that people who enjoy taking snapshots *need* a camera that also develops pictures. But in response to novelty, convenience, a shorter interval between acting (taking the snap) and gaining pleasure (seeing the shot), the Polaroid camera succeeded in the marketplace. But it is inconceivable that Edwin Land responded to impressions of consumer need. Instead, he translated a technology (polarization of light) into a product, which proliferated and stimulated consumers' desires.

The example of Polaroid and Land suggests how leaders think about goals. They are active

5. Ibid. p. 440.

instead of reactive, shaping ideas instead of responding to them. Leaders adopt a personal and active attitude toward goals. The influence a leader exerts in altering moods, evoking images and expectations, and in establishing specific desires and objectives determines the direction a business takes. The net result of this influence is to change the way people think about what is desirable, possible, and necessary.

CONCEPTIONS OF WORK

What do managers and leaders do? What is the nature of their respective work?

Leaders and managers differ in their conceptions. Managers tend to view work as an enabling process involving some combination of people and ideas interacting to establish strategies and make decisions. Managers help the process along by a range of skills, including calculating the interests in opposition, staging and timing the surfacing of controversial issues, and reducing tensions. In this enabling process, managers appear flexible in the use of tactics: they negotiate and bargain, on the one hand, and use rewards and punishments, and other forms of coercion, on the other. Machiavelli wrote for managers and not necessarily for leaders.

Alfred Sloan illustrated how this enabling process works in situations of conflict. The time was the early 1920s when the Ford Motor Co. still dominated the automobile industry using, as did General Motors, the conventional water-cooled engine. With the full backing of Pierre du Pont, Charles Kettering dedicated himself to the design of an air-cooled engine, which, if successful, would have been a great technical and market coup for GM. Kettering believed in his product, but the manufacturing division heads at GM remained skeptical and later opposed the new design on two grounds: first, that it was technically unreliable, and second, that the corporation was putting all its eggs in one basket by investing in a new product in-

stead of attending to the current marketing situation.

In the summer of 1923 after a series of false starts and after its decision to recall the copper-cooled Chevrolets from dealers and customers, GM management reorganized and finally scrapped the project. When it dawned on Kettering that the company had rejected the engine, he was deeply discouraged and wrote to Sloan that without the "organized resistance" against the project it would succeed and that unless the project were saved, he would leave the company.

Alfred Sloan was all too aware of the fact that Kettering was unhappy and indeed intended to leave General Motors. Sloan was also aware of the fact that, while the manufacturing divisions strongly opposed the new engine, Pierre du Pont supported Kettering. Furthermore, Sloan had himself gone on record in a letter to Kettering less than two years earlier expressing full confidence in him. The problem Sloan now had was to make his decision stick, keep Kettering in the organization (he was much too valuable to lose), avoid alienating du Pont, and encourage the division heads to move speedily in developing product lines using conventional water-cooled engines.

The actions that Sloan took in the face of this conflict reveal much about how managers work. First, he tried to reassure Kettering by presenting the problem in a very ambiguous fashion, suggesting that he and the Executive Committee sided with Kettering, but that it would not be practical to force the divisions to do what they were opposed to. He presented the problem as being a question of the people, not the product. Second, he proposed to reorganize around the problem by consolidating all functions in a new division that would be responsible for the design, production, and marketing of the new car. This solution, however, appeared as ambiguous as his efforts to placate and keep Kettering in General Motors. Sloan wrote: "My plan was to create an independent pilot operation under the sole jurisdiction of Mr. Kettering, a kind of copper-cooled-car division. Mr. Kettering would designate his own chief engineer and his production staff to solve the technical problems of manufacture."[6]

While Sloan did not discuss the practical value of this solution, which included saddling an inventor with management responsibility, he in effect used this plan to limit his conflict with Pierre du Pont.

In effect, the managerial solution that Sloan arranged and pressed for adoption limited the options available to others. The structural solution narrowed choices, even limiting emotional reactions to the point where the key people could do nothing but go along, and even allowed Sloan to say in his memorandum to du Pont, "We have discussed the matter with Mr. Kettering at some length this morning and he agrees with us absolutely on every point we made. He appears to receive the suggestion enthusiastically and has every confidence that it can be put across along these lines."[7]

Having placated people who opposed his views by developing a structural solution that appeared to give something but in reality only limited options, Sloan could then authorize the car division's general manager, with whom he basically agreed, to move quickly in designing water-cooled cars for the immediate market demand.

Years later Sloan wrote, evidently with tongue in cheek, "The copper-cooled car never came up again in a big way. It just died out, I don't know why."[8]

In order to get people to accept solutions to problems, managers need to coordinate and balance continually. Interestingly enough, this managerial work has much in common with what diplomats and mediators do, with Henry Kissinger apparently an outstanding practitioner. The manager aims at shifting balances of power toward solutions acceptable as a compromise among conflicting values.

What about leaders, what do they do? Where managers act to limit choices, leaders work in the opposite direction, to develop fresh approaches to long-standing problems and to open issues for new options. Stanley and Inge Hoffmann, the political scientists, liken the leader's work to that of the artist. But unlike most artists, the leader himself is an integral part of the aesthetic product. One cannot look at a leader's art without looking at the artist. On Charles de Gaulle as a political artist, they wrote: "And each of his major political acts, however tortuous the means or the details, has been whole, indivisible and unmistakably his own, like an artistic act."[9]

The closest one can get to a product apart from the artist is the ideas that occupy, indeed at times obsess, the leader's mental life. To be effective, however, the leader needs to project his ideas into images that excite people, and only then develop choices that give the projected images substance. Consequently, leaders create excitement in work.

John F. Kennedy's brief presidency shows both the strengths and weaknesses connected with the excitement leaders generate in their work. In his inaugural address he said, "Let every nation know, whether it wishes us well or ill, that we shall pay any price, bear any burden, meet any hardship, support any friend, oppose any foe, in order to assure the survival and the success of liberty."

This much-quoted statement forced people to react beyond immediate concerns and to identify with Kennedy and with important shared ideals. But upon closer scrutiny the statement must be seen as absurd because it promises a position which if in fact adopted, as in the

6. Ibid. p. 91.
7. Ibid. p. 91.
8. Ibid. p. 93.

9. Stanley and Inge Hoffman, "The Will for Grandeur: de Gaulle as Political Artist," *Daedalus*, Summer 1968, p. 849.

Viet Nam War, could produce disastrous results. Yet unless expectations are aroused and mobilized, with all the dangers of frustration inherent in heightened desire, new thinking and new choice can never come to light.

Leaders work from high-risk positions, indeed often are temperamentally disposed to seek out risk and danger, especially when opportunity and reward appear high. From my observations, why one individual seeks risks while another approaches problems conservatively depends more on his or her personality and less on conscious choice. For some, especially those who become managers, the instinct for survival dominates their need for risk, and their ability to tolerate mundane, practical work assists their survival. The same cannot be said for leaders who sometimes react to mundane work as to an affliction.

RELATIONS WITH OTHERS

Managers prefer to work with people; they avoid solitary activity because it makes them anxious. Several years ago, I directed studies on the psychological aspects of career. The need to seek out others with whom to work and collaborate seemed to stand out as important characteristics of managers. When asked, for example, to write imaginative stories in response to a picture showing a single figure (a boy contemplating a violin, or a man silhouetted in a state of reflection), managers populated their stories with people. The following is an example of a manager's imaginative story about the young boy contemplating a violin:

Mom and Dad insisted that junior take music lessons so that someday he can become a concert musician. His instrument was ordered and had just arrived. Junior is weighing the alternatives of playing football with the other kids or playing with the squeak box. He can't understand how his parents could think a violin is better than a touchdown.

After four months of practicing the violin, junior has had more than enough, Daddy is going out of his mind, and Mommy is willing to give in reluc-

tantly to the men's wishes. Football season is now over, but a good third baseman will take the field next spring.[10]

This story illustrates two themes that clarify managerial attitudes toward human relations. The first, as I have suggested, is to seek out activity with other people (i.e. the football team), and the second is to maintain a low level of emotional involvement in these relationships. The low emotional involvement appears in the writer's use of conventional metaphors, even clichés, and in the depiction of the ready transformation of potential conflict into harmonious decisions. In this case, Junior, Mommy, and Daddy agree to give up the violin for manly sports.

These two themes may seem paradoxical, but their coexistence supports what a manager does, including reconciling differences, seeking compromises, and establishing a balance of power. A further idea demonstrated by how the manager wrote the story is that managers may lack empathy, or the capacity to sense intuitively the thoughts and feelings of others. To illustrate attempts to be emphatic, here is another story written to the same stimulus picture by someone considered by his peers to be a leader:

This little boy has the appearance of being a sincere artist, one who is deeply affected by the violin, and has an intense desire to master the instrument.

He seems to have just completed his normal practice session and appears to be somewhat crestfallen at his inability to produce the sounds which he is sure lie within the violin.

He appears to be in the process of making a vow to himself to expend the necessary time and effort to play this instrument until he satisfies himself that he is able to bring forth the qualities of music which he feels within himself.

With this type of determination and carry through,

---

10. Abraham Zaleznik, Gene W. Dalton, and Louis B. Barnes, *Orientation and Conflict in Career*, (Boston: Division of Research, Harvard Business School, 1970), p. 316.

this boy became one of the great violinists of his day.[11]

Empathy is not simply a matter of paying attention to other people. It is also the capacity to take in emotional signals and to make them mean something in a relationship with an individual. People who describe another person as ''deeply affected'' with ''intense desire,'' as capable of feeling ''crestfallen'' and as one who can ''vow to himself,'' would seem to have an inner perceptiveness that they can use in their relationships with others.

Managers relate to people according to the role they play in a sequence of events or in a decision-making *process,* while leaders, who are concerned with ideas, relate in more intuitive and empathetic ways. The manager's orientation to people, as actors in a sequence of events, deflects his or her attention away from the substance of people's concerns and toward their roles in a process. The distinction is simply between a manager's attention to *how* things get done and a leader's to *what* the events and decisions mean to participants.

In recent years, managers have taken over from game theory the notion that decision-making events can be one of two types: the win-lose situation (or zero-sum game) or the win-win situation in which everybody in the action comes out ahead. As part of the process of reconciling differences among people and maintaining balances of power, managers strive to convert win-lose into win-win situations.

As an illustration, take the decision of how to allocate capital resources among operating divisions in a large, decentralized organization. On the face of it, the dollars available for distribution are limited at any given time. Presumably, therefore, the more one division gets, the less is available for other divisions.

Managers tend to view this situation (as it affects human relations) as a conversion issue:

11. Ibid. p. 294

how to make what seems like a win-lose problem into a win-win problem. Several solutions to this situation come to mind. First, the manager focuses others' attention on procedure and not on substance. Here the actors become engrossed in the bigger problem of *how* to make decisions, not *what* decisions to make. Once committed to the bigger problem, the actors have to support the outcome since they were involved in formulating decision rules. Because the actors believe in the rules they formulated, they will accept present losses in the expectation that next time they will win.

Second, the manager communicates to his subordinates indirectly, using ''signals'' instead of ''messages.'' A signal has a number of possible implicit positions in it while a message clearly states a position. Signals are inconclusive and subject to reinterpretation should people become upset and angry, while messages involve the direct consequence that some people will indeed not like what they hear. The nature of messages heightens emotional response, and, as I have indicated, emotionally makes managers anxious. With signals, the question of who wins and who loses often becomes obscured.

Third, the manager plays for time. Managers seem to recognize that with the passage of time and the delay of major decisions, compromises emerge that take the sting out of win-lose situations; and the original ''game'' will be superseded by additional ones. Therefore, compromises may mean that one wins and loses simultaneously, depending on which of the games one evaluates.

There are undoubtedly many other tactical moves managers use to change human situations from win-lose to win-win. But the point to be made is that such tactics focus on the decision-making process itself and interest managers rather than leaders. The interest in tactics involves costs as well as benefits, including making organizations fatter in bureaucratic and political intrigue and leaner in direct, hard activity and warm human relationships. Consequently, one often hears subordinates characterize managers as inscrutable, detached, and manipulative. These adjectives arise from the subordinates' perception that they are linked together in a process whose purpose, beyond simply making decisions, is to maintain a controlled as well as rational and equitable structure. These adjectives suggest that managers need order in the face of the potential chaos that many fear in human relationships.

In contrast, one often hears leaders referred to in adjectives rich in emotional content. Leaders attract strong feelings of identity and difference, or of love and hate. Human relations in leader-dominated structures often appear turbulent, intense, and at times even disorganized. Such an atmosphere intensifies individual motivation and often produces unanticipated outcomes. Does this intense motivation lead to innovation and high performance, or does it represent wasted energy?

SENSES OF SELF

In *The Varieties of Religious Experience,* William James describes two basic personality types, "once-born" and "twice-born."[12] People of the former personality type are those for whom adjustments to life have been straightforward and whose lives have been more or less a peaceful flow from the moment of their births. The twice-borns, on the other hand, have not had an easy time of it. Their lives are marked by a continual struggle to attain some sense of order. Unlike the once-borns, they cannot take things for granted. According to James, these personalities have equally different world views. For a once-born personality, the sense of self, as a guide to conduct and attitude, derives from a feeling of being at home and in harmony with one's environment. For a twice-born, the sense of self derives from a feeling of profound separateness.

12. William James, *Varieties of Religious Experience* (New York: Mentor Books, 1958).

A sense of belonging or of being separate has a practical significance for the kinds of investments managers and leaders make in their careers. Managers see themselves as conservators and regulators of an existing order of affairs with which they personally identify and from which they gain rewards. Perpetuating and strengthening existing institutions enhances a manager's sense of self-worth: he or she is performing in a role that harmonizes with the ideals of duty and responsibility. William James had this harmony in mind—this sense of self as flowing easily to and from the outer world—in defining a once-born personality. If one feels oneself as a member of institutions, contributing to their well-being, then one fulfills a mission in life and feels rewarded for having measured up to ideals. This reward transcends material gains and answers the more fundamental desire for personal integrity which is achieved by identifying with existing institutions.

Leaders tend to be twice-born personalities, people who feel separate from their environment, including other people. They may work in organizations, but they never belong to them. Their sense of who they are does not depend upon memberships, work roles, or other social indicators of identity. What seems to follow from this idea about separateness is some theoretical basis for explaining why certain individuals search out opportunities for change. The methods to bring about change may be technological, political, or ideological, but the object is the same: to profoundly alter human, economic, and political relationships.

Sociologists refer to the preparation individuals undergo to perform in roles as the socialization process. Where individuals experience themselves as an integral part of the social structure (their self-esteem gains strength through participation and conformity), social standards exert powerful effects in maintaining the individual's personal sense of continuity, even beyond the early years in the family. The line of development from the family to schools, then to career is cumulative and reinforcing. When the line of development is not reinforcing because of significant disruptions in relationships or other problems experienced in the family or other social institutions, the individual turns inward and struggles to establish self-esteem, identity, and order. Here the psychological dynamics center on the experience with loss and the efforts at recovery.

In considering the development of leadership, we have to examine two different courses of life history: (1) development through socialization, which prepares the individual to guide institutions and to maintain the existing balance of social relations; and (2) development through personal mastery, which impels an individual to struggle for psychological and social change. Society produces its managerial talent through the first line of development, while through the second leaders emerge.

DEVELOPMENT OF LEADERSHIP

The development of every person begins in the family. Each person experiences the traumas associated with separating from his or her parents, as well as the pain that follows such frustration. In the same vein, all individuals face the difficulties of achieving self-regulation and self-control. But for some, perhaps a majority, the fortunes of childhood provide adequate gratifications and sufficient opportunities tofind substitutes for rewards no longer available. Such individuals, the ''once-borns,'' make moderate identifications with parents and find a harmony between what they expect and what they are able to realize from life.

But suppose the pains of separation are amplified by a combination of parental demands and the individual's needs to the degree that a sense of isolation, of being special, and of wariness disrupts the bonds that attach children to parents and other authority figures? Under such conditions, and given a special aptitude, the origins of which remain mysterious, the person becomes deeply involved in his or her inner world at the expense of interest in the outer

world. For such a person, self-esteem no longer depends solely upon positive attachments and real rewards. A form of self-reliance takes hold along with expectations of performance and achievement, and perhaps even the desire to do great works.

Such self-perceptions can come to nothing if the individual's talents are negligible. Even with strong talents, there are no guarantees that achievement will follow, let alone that the end result will be for good rather than evil. Other factors enter into development. For one thing, leaders are like artists and other gifted people who often struggle with neuroses; their ability to function varies considerably even over the short run, and some potential leaders may lose the struggle altogether. Also, beyond early childhood, the patterns of development that affect managers and leaders involve the selective influence of particular people. Just as they appear flexible and evenly distributed in the types of talents available for development, managers form moderate and widely distributed attachments. Leaders, on the other hand, establish, and also break off, intensive one-to-one relationships.

It is a common observation that people with great talents are often only indifferent students. No one, for example, could have predicted Einstein's great achievements on the basis of his mediocre record in school. The reason for mediocrity is obviously not the absence of ability. It may result, instead, from self-absorption and the inability to pay attention to the ordinary tasks at hand. The only sure way an individual can interrupt reverie-like preoccupation and self-absorption is to form a deep attachment to a great teacher or other benevolent person who understands and has the ability to communicate with the gifted individual.

Whether gifted individuals find what they need in one-to-one relationships depends on the availability of sensitive and intuitive mentors who have a vocation in cultivating talent. Fortunately, when the generations do meet and the self-selections occur, we learn more about how to develop leaders and how talented people of different generations influence each other.

While apparently destined for a mediocre career, people who form important one-to-one relationships are able to accelerate and intensify their development through an apprenticeship. The background for such apprenticeships, or the psychological readiness of an individual to benefit from an intensive relationship, depends upon some experience in life that forces the individual to turn inward. A case example will make this point clearer. This example comes from the life of Dwight David Eisenhower, and illustrates the transformation of a career from competent to outstanding.[13]

Dwight Eisenhower's early career in the Army foreshadowed very little about his future development. During World War I, while some of his West Point classmates were already experiencing the war first-hand in France, Eisenhower felt "embedded in the monotony and unsought safety of the Zone of the Interior . . . that was intolerable punishment."[14]

Shortly after World War I, Eisenhower, then a young officer somewhat pessimistic about his career chances, asked for a transfer to Panama to work under General Fox Connor, a senior officer whom Eisenhower admired. The army turned down Eisenhower's request. This setback was very much on Eisenhower's mind when Ikey, his first-born son, succumbed to influenza. By some sense of responsibility for its own, the Army transferred Eisenhower to Panama, where he took up his duties under General Connor with the shadow of his lost son very much upon him.

In a relationship with the kind of father he would have wanted to be, Eisenhower reverted to being the son he lost. In this highly charged situation, Eisenhower began to learn from his mentor. General Connor offered, and Eisenhower gladly took, a magnificent tutorial on the military. The effects of this relationship on Eisenhower cannot be measured quantitatively, but, in Eisenhower's own reflections and the unfolding of his career, one cannot overestimate its significance in the reintegration of a person shattered by grief.

As Eisenhower wrote later about Connor, "Life with General Connor was a sort of graduate school in military affairs and the humanities, leavened by a man who was experienced in his knowledge of men and their conduct. I can never adequately express my gratitude to this one gentleman. . . . In a lifetime of association with great and good men, he is the one more or less invisible figure to whom I owe a incalculable debt.[15]

Some time after his tour of duty with General Connor, Eisenhower's breakthrough occurred. He received orders to attend the Command and General Staff School at Fort Leavenworth, one of the most competitive schools in the army. It was a coveted appointment, and Eisenhower took advantage of the opportunity. Unlike his performance in high school and West Point, his work at the Command School was excellent; he was graduated first in his class.

Psychological biographies of gifted people repeatedly demonstrate the important part a mentor plays in developing an individual. Andrew Carnegie owed much to his senior, Thomas A. Scott. As head of the Western Division of the Pennsylvania Railroad. Scott recognized talent and the desire to learn in the young telegrapher assigned to him. By giving Carnegie increasing responsibility and by providing him with the opportunity to learn through close personal observation, Scott added to Carnegie's self-confidence and sense of achievement. Because of his own personal strength and achievement, Scott did not fear Carnegie's aggressiveness. Rather, he gave it

13. This example is included in Abraham Zaleznik and Manfred F. R. Kets de Vries, *Power and the Corporate Mind* (Boston: Houghton Mifflin, 1975).

14. Dwight D. Eisenhower, *At Ease: Stories I Tell to Friends* (New York: Doubleday, 1967), p. 136.

15. Ibid. p. 187.

full play in encouraging Carnegie's initiative.

Mentors take risks with people. They bet initially on talent they preceive in younger people. Mentors also risk emotional involvement in working closely with their juniors. The risks do not always pay off, but the willingness to take them appears crucial in developing leaders.

CAN ORGANIZATIONS DEVELOP LEADERS?

The examples I have given of how leaders develop suggest the importance of personal influence and the one-to-one relationship. For organizations to encourage consciously the development of leaders as compared with managers would mean developing one-to-one relationships between junior and senior executives and, more important, fostering a culture of individualism and possibly elitism. The elitism arises out of the desire to identify talent and other qualities suggestive of the ability to lead and not simply manage.

The Jewel Companies Inc. enjoy a reputation for developing talented people. The chairman and chief executive officer, Donald S. Perkins, is perhaps a good example of a person brought along through the mentor approach. Franklin J. Lunding, who was Perkins's mentor, expressed the philosophy of taking risks with young people this way: "Young people today want in on the action. They don't want to sit around for six months trimming lettuce."[16]

This statement runs counter to the culture that attaches primary importance to slow progression based on experience and proved competence. It is a high-risk philosophy, one that requires time for the attachment between senior and junior people to grow and be meaningful, and one that is bound to produce more failures than successes.

The elitism is an especially sensitive issue. At Jewel the MBA degree symbolized the elite. Lunding attracted Perkins to Jewel at a time when business school graduates had little interest in retailing in general, and food distribution in particular. Yet the elitism seemed to pay off: not only did Perkins become the president at age 37, but also under the leadership of young executives recruited into Jewel with the promise of opportunity for growth and advancement, Jewel managed to diversify into discount and drug chains and still remain strong in food retailing. By assigning each recruit to a vice president who acted as sponsor, Jewel evidently tried to build a structure around the mentor approach to developing leaders. To counteract the elitism implied in such an approach, the company also introduced an "equalizer" in what Perkins described as "the first assistant philosophy." Perkins stated:

Being a good first assistant means that each management person thinks of himself not as the order-giving, domineering boss, but as the first assistant to those who 'report' to him in a more typical organizational sense. Thus we mentally turn our organizational charts upside-down and challenge ourselves to seek ways in which we can lead . . . by helping . . . by teaching . . . by listening . . . and by managing in the true democratic sense . . . that is, with the consent of the managed. Thus the satisfactions of leadership come from helping others to get things done and changed — and not from getting credit for doing and changing things ourselves.[17]

While this statement would seem to be more egalitarian than elitist, it does reinforce a youth-oriented culture since it defines the senior officer's job as primarily helping the junior person.

A myth about how people learn and develop that seems to have taken hold in the American culture also dominates thinking in business. The myth is that people learn best from their peers. Supposedly, the threat of evaluation and even humiliation recedes in peer relations because of the tendency for mutual identification

---

16. "Jewel Lets Young Men Make Mistakes," *Business Week,* January 17, 1970, p. 90.

17. "What Makes Jewel Shine so Bright," *Progressive Grocer,* September, 1973, p. 76.

and the social restraints on authoritarian behavior among equals. Peer training in organizations occurs in various forms. The use, for example, of task forces made up of peers from several interested occupational groups (sales, production, research, and finance) supposedly removes the restraints of authority on the individual's willingness to assert and exchange ideas. As a result, so the theory goes, people interact more freely, listen more objectively to criticism and other points of view and, finally, learn from this healthy interchange.

Another application of peer training exists in some large corporations, such as Philips, N.V. in Holland, were organizational structure is built on the principle of joint responsibility of two peers, one representing the commercial end of the business and the other the technical. Formally, both hold equal responsibility for geographic operations or product groups, as the case may be. As a practical matter, it may turn out that one or the other of the peers dominates the management. Nevertheless, the main interaction is between two or more equals.

The principal question I would raise about such arrangements is whether they perpetuate the managerial orientation, and preclude the formation of one-to-one relationships between senior people and potential leaders.

Aware of the possible stifling effects of peer relationships on aggressiveness and individual initiative, another company, much smaller than Philips, utilizes joint responsibility of peers for operating units, with one important difference. The chief executive of this company encourages competition and rivalry among peers, ultimately appointing the one who comes out on top for increased responsibility. These hybrid arrangements produce some unintended consequences that can be disastrous. There is no easy way to limit rivalry. Instead, it permeates all levels of the operation and opens the way for the formation of cliques in an atmosphere of intrigue.

A large, integrated oil company has accepted the importance of developing leaders through the direct influence of senior on junior executives. One chairman and chief executive officer regularly selected one talented university graduate whom he appointed his special assistant, and with whom he would work closely for a year. At the end of the year, the junior executive would become available for assignment to one of the operating divisions, where he would be assigned to a responsible post rather than a training position. The mentor relationship had acquainted the junior executive firsthand with the use of power, and with the important antidotes to the power disease called *hubris* —performance and integrity.

Working in one-to-one relationships, where there is a formal and recognized difference in the power of the actors, takes a great deal of tolerance for emotional interchange. This interchange, inevitable in close working arrangements, probably accounts for the reluctance of many executives to become involved in such relationships. *Fortune* carried an interesting story on the departure of a key executive, John W. Hanley, from the top management of Proctor & Gamble, for the chief executive officer position at Monsanto.[18] According to this account, the chief executive and chairman of P&G passed over Hanley for appointment to the presidency and named another executive vice president to this post instead.

The chairman evidently felt he could not work well with Hanley who, by his own acknowledgement, was aggressive, eager to experiment and change practices, and constantly challenged his superior. A chief executive officer naturally has the right to select people with whom he feels congenial. But I wonder whether a greater capacity on the part of senior officers to tolerate the competitive impulses and behavior of their subordinates might not be healthy for corporations. At least a greater tol-

---

18. "Jack Hanley Got There by Selling Harder," *Fortune*, November, 1976.

erance for interchange would not favor the managerial team player at the expense of the individual who might become a leader.

I am constantly surprised at the frequency with which chief executives feel threatened by open challenges to their ideas, as though the source of their authority, rather than their specific ideas, were at issue. In one case a chief executive officer, who was troubled by the aggressiveness and sometimes outright rudeness of one of his talented vice presidents, used various indirect methods such as group meetings and hints from outside directors to avoid dealing with his subordinate. I advised the executive to deal head-on with what irritated him. I suggested that by direct, face-to-face confrontation, both he and his subordinate would learn to validate the distinction between the authority to be preserved and the issues to be debated.

To confront is also to tolerate aggressive interchange, and has the net effect of stripping away the veils of ambiguity and signaling so characteristic of managerial cultures, as well as encouraging the emotional relationship leaders need if they are to survive.

Chapter 7

COMMUNICATION AND GROUP PROCESS

Straight from the shoulder: leveling with others on the job

ROBERT B. MORTON, Ph.D.

Straight from the shoulder . . .

Like many other words in the English language, the verb *level* has a variety of meanings. One of them is "to deal frankly and without artifice; to speak candidly and openly," and this comes closest to the definition of *leveling* when it refers to the technique used in training laboratories—a technique that has also proved effective in actual work situations.

The principles that are operative in communicating simple, concrete information are not always adequate when we are faced with the problem of communicating information that affects the feelings and personal values of subordinates and co-workers. It is in this area that leveling can be of great value. We must realize, however, that this kind of leveling is more complex than the kind of leveling implied in the colloquial phrase "to level with someone." It does not mean, for example, to say just anything we feel like to a man—to let him have it with both barrels. This approach obviously breeds resentment and hostility. On the other hand, it doesn't mean confining remarks to polite and "safe" topics, either, for this leaves the important and pertinent things unsaid. The kind of leveling we are talking about involves

Reprinted by permission of the publisher from *Personnel*, November-December, 1966. Copyright 1966 by American Management Association, Inc., New York, N.Y.

saying the things we feel are most significant about current problems in the work or in personal relationships, with the intention of helping a colleague to learn.

Four factors determine the effectiveness of leveling: the conditions under which leveling occurs, the speaker's behavior, the listener's behavior, and the expectations of the listener.

EXTERNAL CONDITIONS

The conditions that influence the effectiveness of leveling are content, timing, and climate. Content, of course, is the subject under discussion and what is being said about it. The use of vague or abstract terms—such as "You have an inferiority complex" or "You are authoritarian"—makes it hard for the other man to understand what he has done to give such an impression, and leaves wide latitude for misinterpretation of what the speaker is trying to convey. This misinterpretation, in turn, is likely to produce a defensive reaction.

The speaker should not talk in terms of what he thinks the motivations of the other might be; rather, he should speak about the other man's behavior, and how he sees the consequences of this behavior. If he does want to interpret what's behind the behavior, the interpretation should be in terms of what it indicates to the speaker, not in judgments about the other's motivation.

When the man on the receiving end is told about specific behavior, as well as how the other is affected, he can understand what he has done and how it affects another person who is significant to him. If he wishes, he can check the validity of the conclusions he draws with others in his work group, and validate or invalidate openly and objectively the information he has received. Until what he has done and how others are affected are clear to him, however, he cannot make any worthwhile decisions about a change in his behavior.

As for timing, the information should be current. We often hear that in any emotional situation people should postpone the discussion of problems until after a cooling-off period. But this forbearance often becomes procrastination, and to the degree that there is a delay in the communication of pertinent information, there is forgetting—often the forgetting of significant factors that would facilitate the desired change in behavior.

The climate in which leveling occurs is very important, but frequently overlooked. When there is a great deal of distrust, so that the need for politeness is felt strongly, it is extremely difficult for the speaker to get his point across, and for the other man to respond affirmatively. Ironically, it is in this very kind of situation that leveling is most urgently needed. One begins to break down distrust by selecting areas in which the facts are objective and definable and the intentions of the leveler are clear and open. Once leveling has begun to develop, even with relatively insignificant kinds of information, trust begins to be enhanced, and as trust develops, leveling becomes more significant and effective.

THE SPEAKER'S BEHAVIOR

The behavior of the man who is giving information is of prime importance in leveling. It is extremely important that the giver understand his own intentions. No learning, or at least not the intended learning, is likely to come about if the speaker is bent on laying out the other fellow, cutting him down to size, humiliating him, or in any other way depreciating him. In this case, the only result will be greater defensiveness, increased hostility, and a rejection of the information that has been passed on. Conversely, a greater probability for learning occurs if it is clear that the only goal of the speaker is to help the other learn from his own experience and the consequences of what he has done. It is the responsibility of the speaker to help the other man understand what he is telling him; he has implicitly joined in a contract to help the man in an exercise of change through learning, often in areas of considerable importance to the man's career.

Giving advice is a pitfall to be avoided. There are times when a little advice can be helpful, but a little can go a long way. Usually, when one gives advice he is saying what he would do if he were in the other person's shoes. The familiar "if I were you" is really meaningless, because the "I" and "you" are unique personalities. Most people don't know enough about the other person's situation to give sound advice. They have different skills, different backgrounds, different goals, and their reactions and methods of operating may be entirely different. The best advice about giving advice is: Keep it to yourself.

A much more valuable service is performed by helping the man to look at alternatives and seek his own solutions, thereby gaining a better understanding of the conditions that contribute to the problems. Admittedly, the problem-solving approach requires skill, but it can be acquired by practice. The person who learns to ask questions that stimulate a search for alternatives may at the same time clarify his own assumptions and learn something himself.

THE LISTENER'S BEHAVIOR

The way a man being given this kind of information reacts can have a great influence on the leveling process. The significance of the information given often increases as he shows his willingness to accept the information and facilitates the process by being a good listener. It is difficult, of course, to be a good listener when what we are hearing threatens our own conception of ourselves. But this is the very kind of information that has the greatest potential for learning, because it concerns the effects of behavior in which we have a heavy investment.

The more support a person can offer to someone who is trying to explain the effects of his behavior, the more clearly the other will be able to communicate his thoughts. One way the listener can help is by asking questions. The most useful questions are those that bring out examples of behavior supporting the information being transmitted. They should be questions that clarify, not questions that belittle, discredit, or punish the person who is giving the information. Once the speaker begins to see a smoke screen, a distorting perceptual filter, he will tend to avoid explicit information and to generalize, to get himself out of the uncomfortable situation.

EXPECTATIONS

The amount of change in a person is very definitely related to his opinion about the degree of impact his behavior has on events. Some people are inclined to feel that what happens to them depends not so much on their own actions as on luck, chance, or the control of others who are more powerful. Or they see events as unpredictable because of the great complexity of the surroundings. In any case, they think there is small probability that what they do makes much difference. On the other hand, some feel strongly that what happens is contingent on what they do—that they contribute significantly or do nothing, the consequences will be modified considerably.

It has been found that inefficient behavior persists much longer when people believe that the consequences of their efforts are related to others more powerful or to chance occur-

rences, instead of being subject to their own control. When a man is convinced that what happens afterward will be determined by his own actions, leveling will be more successful and greater learning will take place.

GUIDES FOR LEVELING

The following ten suggestions will help the manager develop and use the techniques of leveling:

1. Focus on behavior rather than the person. It is important to refer to what a person does, rather than to comment on what you imagine he *is*. Use adverbs (which relate to actions) rather than adjectives (which relate to qualities) when referring to a person. Thus, it is better to say that a person "talked a good deal in the meeting" than to call him a "loud-mouthed person."

2. Focus on observations rather than inferences. Observations refer to what you can see or hear of the behavior of another person, or its effect on you. Inferences are interpretations of the behavior ("You were defensive" or "You are a driver"). The sharing of inferences may be valuable, but it is important that they be so identified.

3. Focus on description rather than judgment. Describing is reporting what has occurred. Judging is evaluating in terms of good or bad, right or wrong, pleasant or unpleasant. Judgments come out of a personal frame of reference or values, whereas description is more neutral.

4. Focus on descriptions of behavior in terms of "more" or "less," rather than either-or. The more-or-less terminology stresses quantity, which is objective and measurable, rather than quality, which is subjective and judgmental. Thus, a person's participation may be anywhere from low to high, rather than good or bad. To think in terms of categories—for instance, authoritarian or permis-

sive—rather than in terms of more or less easily leads to the conversion of a description into a casual interpretation: "He behaves this way because he is authoritarian."

5. Focus on behavior related to a specific situation—preferably to the here and now—rather than on behavior in the abstract. What people do is always tied in some way to time and place, and understanding of behavior is sharpened by keeping it tied to time and place. Information is most meaningful when given as soon as appropriate after the observation or reactions occur.

6. Focus on the sharing of ideas and information rather than on giving advice. When ideas and information are shared, the receiver is freer to decide for himself, in the light of his own goals, in a particular situation and at a particular time, how to use the ideas and information. When you give advice you tell him what to do with the information, and thus restrict his freedom to determine for himself the most appropriate course of action. You also reduce his personal responsibility for his own behavior, since he is doing what someone else told him to do.

7. Focus on exploration of alternatives. The more attention given to the possible alternatives for the attainment of a par-

ticular goal, the greater the probability that the best solution to any problem will be found. It is all too easy to carry around a collection of set answers and courses of action, which we automatically apply to every problem that arises.

8. Focus on the "contract" that exists between persons in any significant relationship. The information provided should serve the needs of the recipient rather than the needs of the giver. Help and feedback should be given and perceived as an offer, not an imposition.

9. Focus on the amount of information that the person receiving it can use, rather than on the amount that you have and might like to give. To overload a person with information is to reduce the possibility that he may use what he receives effectively. When we give more than can be profitably used, we are actually satisfying some need of our own, instead of helping the other person.

10. Focus on what is said rather than why it is said. The aspects of information that relate to the *what, how, when,* and *where* are observable characteristics. The *why* of what is said, however, goes from the observable to the inferred, and brings up questions of motive. To make assumptions about the motives of the person may prevent him from hearing or lead him to distort what you are saying.

How to diagnose group problems
LELAND P. BRADFORD, Ph.D., DOROTHY STOCK, Ph.D., and MURRAY HORWITZ, Ph.D.

A group has two things in common with a machine or with any organism anywhere.
  1. It has something to do.
  2. It must be kept in running order to do it.

Reprinted with permission from *Adult Leadership*.

These twin functions require continual attention. Groups show their concern for the first—their specific jobs, goals, activities—by establishing procedures, rules of order, expected leadership responsibilities. But sometimes the rules a group sets up for itself fail to take into account its maintenance needs. When this happens the group finds itself bogging down.

The importance of the maintenance function is immediately recognized in other situations. Airlines require the services of maintenance crews as well as navigators. An automobile, a sewing machine, a typewriter, or a whistling peanut wagon that has no care paid to its upkeep soon begins to break down.

We can't, of course, carry the analogy too far. Among the important ways in which groups differ from machines, consider this: A new machine has its peak of efficiency at the beginning of its life. A new group, on the other hand, is likely to be more inept and less efficient at the beginning than it is later. If it is healthy, a group grows and changes, becoming more cohesive, more productive, more capable of helping its individual members in specific ways. The problem of maintenance, therefore, is inseparable from the process of growth.

This article will analyze the causes and symptoms of some common problems that interfere with group growth and productivity, and describe some methods of diagnosis.

GROUP PROBLEMS

Three of the most common group problems are:

1. Conflict or fight
2. Apathy and nonparticipation
3. Inadequate decision-making.

Fight. We don't necessarily mean a heavyweight bout. Fight here means disagreement, argumentation, the nasty crack, the tense atmosphere, conflict.

Some ways in which fight can be expressed are:

a) members are impatient with one another
b) ideas are attacked before they are completely expressed
c) members take sides and refuse to compromise
d) members disagree on plans or suggestions
e) comments and suggestions are made with a great deal of vehemence

f) members attack one another on a personal level in subtle ways
g) members insist that the group doesn't have the know-how or experience to get anywhere
h) members feel the group can't get ahead because it is too large or too small
i) members disagree with the leader's suggestions
j) members accuse one another of not understanding the real point
k) members hear distorted fragments of other members' contributions

The following are several possible reasons for such fight behavior:

1. *The group has been given an impossible job and members are frustrated because they feel unable to meet the demands made of them.* This frequently happens when the group is a committee of a larger organization. Perhaps the committee has a job which is impossible because it doesn't have enough members. Or perhaps the job is impossible because it is ambiguous—the task for the committee has not been clearly defined by the larger group. (Under these circumstances the committee has no way of knowing to what extent alternative plans are appropriate or will be acceptable to the larger group.) For whatever reason, an impossible task can easily produce frustration and tension among the members of a group, and this may be expressed in bickering and attack.

2. *The main concern of members is to find status in the group.* Although the group is ostensibly working on some task, the task is being used by the members as a means of jockeying for power, establishing alignments and cliques, or trying to suppress certain individuals or cliques. Under such circumstances certain members may oppose one another stubbornly on some issue for reasons which have nothing to do with the issue. Or there may be a lot of attack on a personal level which is intended to deflate and reduce the prestige of another member. This kind of power struggle may involve

the leader. If it does, the attack will include him, perhaps in the form of refusing to understand or to follow his suggestions (if members can show that the leader is not a good leader, then he should be deposed).

3. *Members are loyal to outside groups of conflicting interests.* This can happen when the members of a committee are each representing some outside organization. They have an interest in getting a job done within the committee but they also have a loyalty to their own organization. This situation creates conflicts within each individual so that he doesn't know whether he should behave as a member of this committee or as a member of another group. His behavior may be inconsistent and rigid and his inner confusion may burst out as irritation or stubbornness. His loyalty to his own organization may make him feel that he has to protect its interests carefully, keep the others from putting something over on him, be careful not to give more than he gets. This may lead to a refusal to cooperate, expressions of passive resistance, etc.

4. *Members feel involved and are working hard on a problem.* Members may frequently express impatience, irritation, or disagreement because they have a real stake in the issue being discussed. They fight for a certain plan because it is important to them—and this fight may take the form of real irritation with others because they can't "see" or won't go along with a suggestion which—to the member—is obviously the best one. As long as there is a clearly-understood goal and continuing movement on a problem, this kind of fight contributes to good problem-solving.

These are not intended to be *all* the possible reasons for fight behavior, but they are some, and they are quite different from one another. The obvious question arises: How can a member or leader tell which diagnosis is appropriate to a specific situation? If the fourth situation obtains, then fight is operating in the service of work and should not worry a group. If fight is interfering with getting things done on the work

task, as it is in the other three situations, then it is important to know which description fits the group so that the underlying causes can be attacked.

The solution to this diagnostic problem lies in the need to understand the context in which the symptom has occurred. That is, one cannot understand fight, or any other symptom, by looking at the symptom only. It is necessary to broaden one's view and look at the syndrome—all the other things which are going on in the group at the same time.

Let's re-examine our four descriptions of symptoms, this time in terms of possible diagnoses:

If
—every suggestion made seems impossible for practical reasons,
—some members feel the committee is too small,
—everyone seems to feel pushed for time,
—members are impatient with one another,
—members insist the group doesn't have the know-how or experience to get anywhere,
—each member has a different idea of what the committee is supposed to do,
—whenever a suggestion is made, at least one member feels it won't satisfy the larger organization,

Then
—the group may have been given an impossible job and members are frustrated because they feel unable to meet the demands made of them, or the task is not clear or is disturbing.

If
—ideas are attacked before they are completely expressed,
—members take sides and refuse to compromise,
—there is no movement toward a solution of the problem,
—the group keeps getting stuck on inconsequential points,
—members attack one another on a personal level in subtle ways,
—there are subtle attacks on the leadership,
—there is no concern with finding a goal or sticking to the point,
—there is much clique formation,

Then

—the main concern of members may be in finding status in the group. The main interest is not in the problem. The problem is merely being used as a vehicle for expressing interpersonal concerns.

If

—the goal is stated in very general, non-operational terms,
—members take sides and refuse to compromise,
—each member is pushing his own plan,
—suggestions don't build on previous suggestions, each member seeming to start again from the beginning,
—members disagree on plans or suggestions,
—members don't listen to one another, each waiting for a chance to say something,

Then

—each member is probably operating from a unique, unshared point of view, perhaps because the members are loyal to different outside groups with conflicting interests.

If

—there is a goal which members understand and agree on,
—most comments are relevant to the problem,
—members frequently disagree with one another over suggestions,
—comments and suggestions are made with a great deal of vehemence,
—there are occasional expressions of warmth,
—members are frequently impatient with one another,
—there is general movement toward some solution of the problem,

Then

—probably, members feel involved and are working hard on a problem. The fight being expressed is constructive rather than destructive in character and reflects real interest on the part of members.

Apathy. An apathetic membership is a frequent ailment of groups. Groups may suffer in different degrees from this disease. In some cases members may show complete indifference to the group task, and give evidences of marked boredom. In others, apathy may take the form of a lack of genuine enthusiasm for

the job, a failure to mobilize much energy, lack of persistence, satisfaction with poor work.

Some ways in which apathy may be expressed:

a) frequent yawns, people dozing off
b) members lose the point of the discussion
c) low level of participation
d) conversation drags
e) members come late; are frequently absent
f) slouching and restlessness
g) overquick decisions
h) failure to follow through on decisions
i) ready suggestions for adjournment
j) failure to consider necessary arrangements for the next meeting
k) reluctance to assume any further responsibility

A commonly held idea is that people require inspirational leadership in order to maintain a high level of interest and morale and to overcome apathy. An outgrowth of this belief is the prescription of pep talks which, unfortunately, have only momentary effects, if any, and become less and less effective the more often they are used. To overcome or prevent apathy, we must treat the causes rather than the symptoms.

Here are some of the common reasons for apathy:

1. *The problem upon which the group is working does not seem important to the members, or it may seem less important than some other problem on which they would prefer to be working.* The problem may be important to someone. Perhaps to some outside part, perhaps to the total organization of which the group is a part, perhaps to the group leader, or even to a minority of the members. But it fails to arouse positive feelings or "involvement" on the part of the apathetic members.

Sometimes problems will be considered because of tradition. Again, members may find it difficult to express themselves freely enough to call for reconsideration of an unsatisfactory group goal. Sometimes, in organizational settings, problems are assigned, and the members haven't enough information to judge why the problem is important, except that "somebody upstairs" thinks it is. Again, the problem may be important to the leader or to some dominant member, and the group is coerced by these individuals into working on the problem as if it were really its own. In all of these cases the members will feel that they have had no part in initiating the problem, but that it has been imposed upon them. The basic feature of such imposed, "meaningless" tasks is that they are not related to the present needs of the members.

2. *The problem may seem important to members, but there are reasons which lead them to avoid attempting to solve the problem.* If members both desire to achieve the goal and fear attempting to achieve it, they are placed in a situation of conflict which may lead to tension, fatigue, apathy. Where subordinates feel they will be punished for mistakes, they will avoid taking action, hoping to shift responsibility to someone higher up the line of organizational authority. Similar fears, and similar desires to avoid working on particular problems, may stem from hostile feelings to other individuals, or to subgroups within the group. Sometimes the group atmosphere is such that members avoid exposing themselves to attack or ridicule, and feel insecure, self-conscious or embarrassed about presenting their ideas.

3. *The group may have inadequate procedures for solving the problem.* Inadequacies in procedure arise from a variety of sources. There may be lack of knowledge about the steps which are necessary to reach the goal. There may be poor communication among members within the group based on a failure to develop mutual understanding. There may be a poor coordination of effort so that contributions to the discussion are made in a disorganized, haphazard way, with a failure of one contribution to build upon previous ones. Members may not have the habit of collecting facts against which to test decisions, so that decisions turn out to be unrealistic and unrealizable.

4. *Members may feel powerless about influencing final decisions.* Although none of the

apathy-producing conditions described above exists, it is possible that any decisions they arrive at are "meaningless." If the decisions will have no practical effects, the activity of problem-solving becomes only an academic exercise. Examples of this may be found in committees within an organization which are assigned some job, where members feel that their recommendations will get lost somewhere up the line. Or, perhaps they may feel that the top personnel in the organization are pretending to be "democratic," and are only making a show of getting participation, but will in all likelihood ignore their suggestions. In such cases groups tend to operate ritualistically, going through the required motions, without involvement.

The same effect may occur if within the group there is a domineering leader, who is recognized by other members as making all the decisions. Again it is pointless for the members to invest their emotional energy in attempting to create solutions to their problem. Apathy may also arise because individual members are passed by while a smoothly functioning subgroup forces quick decisions, not giving the slower members opportunity to make decisions. Status differences within the group will frequently have the same effect. People with lower status may find it difficult to get an opportunity to be heard by other members, with the result that they come to feel that their contributions will have little effect upon the outcome.

5. *A prolonged and deep fight among a few members has dominated the group.* Frequently two or three dominant and talkative members of a group will compete with one another or with the leader so much that every activity in the group is overshadowed by the conflict. Less dominant members who feel inadequate to help solve the conflict become apathetic and withdraw from participation.

In considering these five types of causes for apathy, it seems clear we have to direct our attention to underlying conditions, rather than symptoms. Measures which are taken directed at the symptom itself—pep-talks, for example, may be completely off the mark. It should also be borne in mind that while a single explanation may largely account for the apathetic behavior, this is not necessarily the case. Any of the suggested reasons may apply, in any combination, and in varying degrees. To determine whether a given reason applies to a particular group situation, it is sometimes helpful to look for the set of symptoms, the syndrome—which may be associated with each cause. Not all the symptoms under each set need be present to indicate that the disease is of a given type, but if several can be observed, it is probably a good bet that the particular diagnosis applies.

If

- questions may be raised about what's really our job, what do *they* want us to do,
- members fail to follow through on decisions,
- there is no expectation that members will contribute responsibly, and confused, irrelevant statements are allowed to go by without question,
- members wonder about the reason for working on this problem,
- suggestions are made that we work on something else,
- the attitude is expressed that we should just decide on anything, the decision doesn't really matter,
- members seem to be waiting for a respectable amount of time to pass before referring the decision to the leader, or to a committee,
- members are inattentive, seem to get lost and not to have heard parts of the preceding discussion,
- suggestions frequently "flop," are not taken up and built on by others,
- no one will volunteer for additional work,

Then

- the group goal may seem unimportant to the members.

If

- there are long delays in getting started, much irrelevant preliminary conversation,

- the group shows embarrassment or reluctance in discussing the problem at hand,
- members emphasize the consequences of making wrong decisions, imagine dire consequences which have little reference to ascertainable facts,
- members make suggestions apologetically, are over-tentative, and hedge their contributions with many *if's* and *but's,*
- solutions proposed are frequently attacked as unrealistic,
- suggestions are made that someone else ought to make the decision—the leader, an outside expert, or some qualified person outside the group,
- members insist that we haven't enough information or ability to make a decision, and appear to demand an unrealistically high level of competence,
- the group has a standard of cautiousness in action,
- numerous alternative proposals are suggested, with the group apparently unable to select among them,

Then

- members probably fear working toward the group goal.

If

- no one is able to suggest the first step in getting started toward the goal,
- members seem to be unable to stay on a given point, and each person seems to start on a new tack,
- members appear to talk past, to misunderstand one another, and the same points are made over and over,
- the group appears to be unable to develop adequate summaries, or restatements of points of agreement,
- there is little evaluation of the possible consequences of decisions reached, and little attention is given to fact-finding or use of special resources,
- members continually shift into related, but off-target, tasks,
- complaints are made that the group's job is an impossible one,
- subgroups continually form around the table, with private discussions held off to the side,

—there is no follow-through on decisions or disagreement in the group about what the decisions really were,

—complaints are made that you can't decide things in a group anyway, and the leader or somebody else should do the job,

Then

—the group may have inadequate problem-solving procedures.

If

—the view is expressed that someone else with more power in the organization should be present in the meeting, that it is difficult to communicate with him at a distance,

—unrealistic decisions are made, and there is an absence of sense of responsibility for evaluating consequences of decisions,

—the position is taken that the decision doesn't really matter because the leader or someone outside the group isn't really going to listen to what we say,

—there is a tendency to ignore reaching consensus among members, the important thing being to get the leader to understand and listen,

—the discussion is oriented toward power relations, either within the group, jockeying to win over the leader, or outside the group, with interest directed toward questions about who really counts in the organization,

—doubts are voiced about whether we're just wasting our efforts in working on this program,

—members leave the meeting feeling they had good ideas which they didn't seem to be able to get across,

Then

—members feel powerless about influencing final decisions.

If

—two or three members dominate all discussion, but never agree,

—conflict between strong members comes out no matter what is discussed,

—dominant members occasionally appeal to others for support, but otherwise control conversation,

—decisions are made by only two or three members,

Then

—a conflict among a few members is creating apathy in the others.

Inadequate decision-making. Getting satisfactory decisions made is often a major struggle in the group. . . . Here is a list of common symptoms of inefficient decision-making.

If

—the group swings between making too rapid decisions and having difficulty in deciding anything,

—the group almost makes the decision but at the last minute retreats,

—group members call for definition and redefinition of minute points,

—the discussion wanders into abstraction,

Then

—there has been premature calling for a decision, or the decision is too difficult, or the group is low in cohesiveness and lacks faith in itself.

If

—the group has lack of clarity as to what the decision is,

—there is disagreement as to where consensus is,

—a decision is apparently made but challenged at the end,

—group members refuse responsibility,

—there is continued effort to leave decision-making to leader, subgroup or outside source,

Then

—the decision area may be threatening to the group, either because of unclear consequences, fear of reaction of other groups, or fear of failure for the individuals.

IMPROVING GROUP EFFICIENCY

Today guided missiles have a feedback mechanism built into them that continuously collects information about the position of the target in relation to the flight of the missile. When the collected information indicates a shift of the target or a discrepancy in the arc of flight of the missile the feedback mechanism corrects the flight of the missile.

Most houses with central heating today have a small feedback mechanism, called a thermostat. When the information collected by it indicates the temperature is below a certain point, the mechanism signals the furnace to turn itself on. When information collected by the thermostat indicates that the temperature is too high, it signals the furnace to stop.

Groups need to build in feedback mechanisms to help in their own steering. Such a process of feedback calls for collecting information on the discrepancy between what the group wants to do (its target) and what it is doing (reaching its target) so that it can make corrections in its direction.

DIAGNOSIS AND FEEDBACK

Human beings, and therefore groups, not only need continuous self-correction in direction but also (and here they differ from machines) need to learn or grow or improve. Collecting adequate data and using this information to make decisions about doing things differently is one of the major ways of learning.

There are three basic parts to the process of changing group behavior:

1. Collecting information
2. Reporting the information to the group
3. Making diagnosis and decisions for change.

WHO SHOULD DIAGNOSE?

If a member of a group strives to improve his own behavior in the group so that he can make more useful contributions, he will need to make his own personal observations and diagnoses about the group and about his behavior in it. Each member has this individual responsibility.

If the group as a whole is to make decisions about changing its procedures or processes, then the entire group must assume responsibility for collaborative diagnoses of its difficulties and its effectiveness. If the leader takes over this function, he continues to direct and dominate the group—leading them like sheep. If only the leader analyzes group difficulties and acts upon them, only he learns. Similar problems arise if diagnosis is left to any group member; he may too readily use this job to steer the group in the direction he desires.

Each member and the leader may guide and encourage the group toward diagnosis, but the responsibility for self-steering and the opportunities to learn and to grow must remain with the group if it is to improve its operational effectiveness.

COLLECTING INFORMATION

While analysis and evaluation of information and decision about what to do should be carried out by the total group, the collecting of information may be delegated. A number of patterns of delegation are possible.

1. The leader, serving also as observer, can report to the group certain pertinent observations he has made about problems and difficulties of group operation. However, although the leader may have more experience with groups, to add the function of observer to his leadership responsibilities complicates his job and also tends to create greater dependency upon him.

   But when the group is unfamiliar with the process of observation, the leader may play an informal observer role for a few meetings, gradually getting other group members to assume this function.

2. The group may appoint one of its members, perhaps on a rotating basis, to serve as group observer, with the task of noting the manner in which the group works. While a group loses a member as far as work on its task is concerned, it can gain in the growth and improvement of the group.

   Frequently there is a leader-team made up of a discussion leader and observer. The leader and observer work together in behalf of the group, one helping to guide the group and making procedural suggestions, the other watching how it works.

   When a leader-team is formed, it makes possible team planning for each meeting. Between meetings the leader-observer team can look back at the past meeting from two vantage points, and look forward to the next meeting.

3. A third method calls for all group members to be as sensitive as they can, while participating actively, to the particular problems the group faces. Although in mature groups members may raise a question about group procedures or maintenance at any time as a normal contribution to the discussion, in new groups the leader may start a discussion looking at how the group has worked and what its problems are. This may occur at some time during the discussion, when the group has bogged down, or during the last fifteen minutes to half an hour as an evaluation of the entire meeting.

WHAT INFORMATION TO COLLECT?

Because of the many group problems and the many causes of these problems there is a wide range of information that a group may need at different points in time. General questions such as these may help get started:

1. What is our goal? Are we "on" or "off the beam"?
2. Where are we in our discussion? At the point of analyzing the problem? Suggesting solutions? Testing ideas?
3. How fast are we moving? Are we bogged down?
4. Are we using the best methods of work?
5. Are all of us working or just a few?

6. Are we making any improvement in our ability to work together?

In any observation of a group more can be seen than can possibly be used for steering, corrective or growth purposes. The following questions may help guide an observer in collecting data about a group.

1. What basic problems does the group seem to have for which information is needed?
2. What is the most important or pertinent information? What information will lead the group into stray paths?
3. What is the essential minimum of material the group needs?

METHODS OF OBSERVATION

Just as there are many areas of information about group behavior, so there are many possible guides and scales for observation. Frequently groups develop such scales to fit their particular needs. Three techniques of observation are given, each useful for collecting a different kind of information.

1. Who talks to whom

The number of lines made by the observer on this form indicates the number of statements made in a fifteen-minute period—20. Four of these were made to the group as a whole, and so the arrows go only to the middle of the circle. Those with arrows at each end of a line show that the statement made by one person to another was responded to by the recipient.

We see that one person, Harold, had more statements directed toward him than did any-

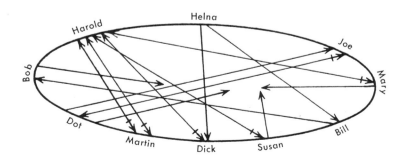

one else and that he responded or participated more than anyone else. The short lines drawn at the head of one of the pair of arrows indicates who initiated the remark. Harold, the leader, in other words had remarks directed at him calling for response from four other people.

This record makes possible the quick rating not only of who talked, but the type of contribution. Individuals in the group are given numbers which are listed at the top of columns. At the end of a time period it is possible to note the frequency and type of participation by each member.

2. Who makes what kinds of contributions*

Member No.	1	2	3	4	5	6	7	8	9	10
1. Encourages										
2. Agrees, accepts										
3. Arbitrates										
4. Proposes action										
5. Asks suggestion										
6. Gives opinion										
7. Asks opinion										
8. Gives information										
9. Seeks information										
10. Poses problem										
11. Defines position										
12. Asks position										
13. Routine direction										
14. Depreciates self										
15. Autocratic manner										
16. Disagrees										
17. Self-assertion										
18. Active aggression										
19. Passive aggression										
20. Out-of-field										

*Based upon observation categories discussed in *Interaction Process Analysis,* by Robert F. Bales. Cambridge, Mass.: Addison-Wesley Press, 1950.

3. What happened in the group?

1. What was the general atmosphere in the group?

Formal	_____	Informal	_____
Competitive	_____	Cooperative	_____
Hostile	_____	Supportive	_____
Inhibited	_____	Permissive	_____

Comments: _____

2. Quantity and quality of work accomplished

Accomplish-ment:	High	_____	Low	_____
Quality of production:	High	_____	Low	_____
Goals:	Clear	_____	Vague	_____
Methods:	Clear	_____	Vague	_____
	Flexible	_____	Inflexible	_____

Comments: _____

3. Leader behavior

Attentive to group needs	_____		
Supported others			
Concerned only with topic	_____	Took sides	_____
Dominated group		Helped group	_____

Comments: _____

4. Participation

Most people talked	_____	Only few talked	_____
Members involved	_____	Members apathetic	_____
Group united	_____	Group divided	_____

Comments: _____

This form can be used as a checklist by an observer to sum up his observations, or it can be filled out by all group members to start an evaluation discussion. Forms 1 and 2 can be used only by a full-time observer.

REPORTING INFORMATION TO THE GROUP

The second step is feeding back pertinent information to the entire group. Whether the information is collected and reported by the leader or by the observer, it is very easy to hurt the group rather than help it. The following cau-

tions are particularly pertinent in reporting to the group.

1. Be sensitive to what information the group is ready to use—what will be most helpful to the group now, rather than what was the most interesting point observed.
2. Don't "avalanche" the group with information. If too much information is given it can't be used. Select only two or three observations which will stimulate thinking and discussion. Let the group ask for more information as it needs it.
3. Don't praise the group too much. Learning doesn't take place by being told only when we are "on the beam." Mentioning accomplishments is desirable as it helps difficulties get honestly faced.
4. Don't punish or preach or judge. The observer can't play the role of God. He says, "It was interesting that participation was less widespread today than yesterday." He doesn't say, "Some of you dominated the discussion today."
5. It is easier to discuss role behavior than people's behavior. "What role did the group need filled at that time," rather than, "That behavior is bad."
6. Go lightly on personality clashes. It is usually better to discuss what helped and what hindered the whole group.

EVALUATING INFORMATION AND DECIDING ABOUT CHANGE

The third stage is diagnosis from the information reported and the consideration of what the group and its members will do differently in the future. Usually this has a number of steps.

1. The members assess the observations, relate them to their experiences, test to see whether they agree with the report.
2. The group examines the reasons. What caused a thing to happen? Could we have recognized it earlier?
3. The group moves to a decision of what to do. What can be done in future similar

circumstances? What can individual members do earlier to help? What methods or procedures should be changed? What new directions sought?

This stage is the crucial one if the group is to benefit from its feedback activities. Unless the members are able to gain new insights into the functioning of the group, and are able to find new ways of behaving, the group will not improve its processes and continue in its growth and development.

It is very easy for the time of the discussion to be consumed by the first two steps in this procedure. The leader, as well as the members, needs to be sensitive to this danger and encourage the group to move into the third step of decision. Although the decisions which are made may be quite simple, agreement on future action sets up common expectations for the next meeting and gives a point to the evaluation.

Cog's Ladder: a model of group growth

GEORGE O. CHARRIER

Models of human behavior are criticized as being too simplistic. However, models help conceptualize abstract relationships, provide a point of departure from which to draw similarities and differences, and help the serious researcher to formulate meaningful experiments. Models, such as Johari's Window, are especially useful in teaching basic courses in applied behavioral science.

The original Cog's Ladder model as discussed in this article was developed in 1965. It has been tested in T-Groups, Grid groups, intercultural workshops, and weekend seminars. Men and women have participated equally. Students from over 30 foreign cultures were included to determine whether the model is limited or modified by culture. Over 1,000 people have contributed to the data including businessmen, students, engineers, secretaries, nurses, lawyers, priests, teachers, contemplative religious, teenagers, and others. Mem-

bers of different professions placed emphasis on different parts of the model, but the model generally reflected the growth of all groups. Training sessions which were designed on the model were notably more successful than training sessions which violated the model.

THE MODEL

Franklyn S. Haiman (1951) suggested that a group goes through a process of growth similar to the maturation process of individuals. Zenger (1970) developed the analogy of group and individual maturation. During the past eight years, I have been researching this single question. In 1965, I developed an hypothesis which has been only slightly modified over the years to a coherent, concise model. This model of group growth consists of five steps.

The first step is called the "polite stage." In this phase, group members are getting acquainted, sharing values and establishing the basis for a group structure. The group members need to be liked.

The second step is "why are we here?" During this phase the group members define the objectives and goals of the group.

Reprinted, by permission of the publisher, from *S.A.M. Advanced Management Journal* January, 1972, © 1972 by Society for Advancement of Management a division of American Management Associations. All rights reserved.

The third step consists of a "bid for power." On this step of the ladder to maturity, the group is composed of individuals attempting to influence other group members by changing each other's ideas, values, or opinions. This stage is characterized by competition for attention, recognition, and influence.

The fourth step is cooperative. It is the "constructive" stage. In this phase, group members are open minded, listen actively and accept the fact that others have a right to different value systems. This stage might be referred to as the "team action" stage.

The fifth and final step is one of unity, high spirits, mutual acceptance and high cohesiveness. It is the *esprit* stage.

This model is referred to as a ladder and is called "Cog's Ladder."

Polite phase

The first step of Cog's Ladder is the "Polite" step. The initial item on every group's agenda is to get acquainted, whether or not the leader of the group allows time for it. Generally, a T-Group will begin with members introducing themselves. Name tags are provided to other groups to aid in the process of "getting to know you." Polite conversation includes information-sharing which helps group members anticipate each other's future responses to group activities.

During this phase, some group members rely on stereotyping to help categorize other group members. A group establishes an emotional basis for future group structure. Cliques are formed which will become important in later phases. The items on the hidden agenda of group members stay hidden and do not usually affect behavior at this time. The need for group approval is strong. The need for group identity is low or completely absent. Group members participate actively, though unevenly, and usually agree that getting acquainted is important to the group. Conflict is usually absent in this phase. The rules of behavior seem to be: keep ideas simple; say things that will be acceptable to all group members; avoid controversy; avoid serious topics; if you share feeling, keep feedback to a minimum; avoid disclosure.

The best exercises to accelerate the polite stage are non-verbal. By eliminating words, group members respond only to non-verbal behavior. When conversation and bodily gestures transmit conflicting signals, the polite stage slows down and group members must spend time to sort out the signals from the noise.

There is a cultural emphasis which is important. Asian and Latin cultures seem to want to prolong the Polite phase of group growth. Edward T. Hall (1959) outlined the cultural patterns of getting acquainted in Latin America. He described days or even weeks during which groups of businessmen relate to each other over dinner, soccer games or polite conversation before getting down to serious business. During this interpersonal by-play, the American businessman in a Latin milieu often becomes impatient to "get on" with the job at hand. It has been observed that an American relating with his fellow Americans will greatly shorten the Polite phase and sometimes eliminate it entirely.

All groups participating in the study of Cog's Ladder displayed an expectation for getting acquainted, and group members took an active part in this initial phase of group maturity. In groups where the Polite phase was omitted, this study found that the group members were uncomfortable and had difficulty relating. In groups which broke up and reconvened, this Polite phase invariably re-occurred. Even when a fully mature group reconvened, the group members started the group process with a few minutes of polite interaction.

Groups I have studied usually allotted 1-5% of their expected life to the Polite phase. T-Groups scheduled for 2 weeks usually spend 1-5 hours sharing names, backgrounds, interests, hobbies, professions, etc. In a 2 week advanced human relations laboratory the trainers decided to extend the usual non-verbal exercise from several hours to several days. Although the group showed dramatic progress through the Polite stage, strong reactions from group members occurred when the exercise was prolonged to 3½ days, significantly in excess of the 1-5% expectation of the group for step one of Cog's Ladder.

Why we're here

When a group is ready to grow beyond the Polite stage, it usually enters the "why we're here" stage. Group members want to know the group's goals and objectives.

Some members demand a written agenda. A branch of managerial science (Management by Objectives) focuses on this step of group maturity. A task-oriented group needs to spend more time in this phase than a personal growth group. For example, while T-groups will usually discuss establishing a purpose but will not agree on one, a Blake Grid group[1]* finds that agreement on goals is essential to group success.

In the second phase cliques start to wield influence. Cliques grow and merge as clique members find common purpose. Hidden agenda items begin to be sensed as group members try to verbalize group objectives most satisfying to themselves.

Identity as a group is still low. The need for group approval declines from what it was in the Polite step as group members begin taking risks and displaying commitment. There is usually active participation from all members.

Many groups will look to another group for a purpose during this phase. In a T-Group, it is not uncommon for trainees to look to the trainer to supply a group goal or objective. Structure appears to evolve in this phase.

The time spent in this phase varies widely. Some groups omit this phase completely while a few groups will spend most of the allotted time in this phase. Much seems to depend on

---

*All footnote references appear at the end of this article.

the task to be done. The easier it is to define objectives, the faster a group appears to agree on them. When purpose comes from outside the group, the members will still discuss it in order to gain understanding and to build commitment. The group also needs to know that the purpose agreed on is important.

Some groups can function for years without advancing to the second stage, e.g. some neighborhood discussion groups or neighborhood bridge clubs. In such groups, it appears that group members have agreed not to grow or that they are simply content to relate in the Polite phase.

Bid for power

The third stage of the model is characterized by competition. I call it the "Bid for Power" stage.

In this phase a group member tries to rationalize his own position, and to convince the group to take the action he feels is appropriate. Members are closed-minded and are accused of not listening. Conflict in the group rises to a higher level than in any other stage of group growth. A struggle for leadership occurs which involves active participation by all subgroups. Typical attempts to resolve this struggle involve voting, compromise, or seeking arbitration from an outside group.

The group does not feel a strong team spirit during this phase. Rather, some members may feel very uncomfortable as latent hostility is expressed. I have noticed some group members, who contribute willingly in phase I and II, remain completely silent in this phase. Other members relish the opportunity to compete and will attempt to dominate the group. In T-Groups these members may be accused of "bulldozing."

Cliques, or subgroups, take on greatest importance in this phase. Through cliques, the group members find they can wield more power.

Hidden agenda items cause a behavior change in this phase. Members who easily concealed their hidden agenda in earlier stages now find that other group members are becoming aware of it.

Feedback from T-Groups in this phase can have a sting to it. Disclosure is cautiously attempted. The need for group approval declines below the level it had in step two. Group members are willing to go out on a limb and risk the censure of the group. In all groups, creative suggestions fall flat[2] because the group projects the feeling that the author wants credit (Power) for the suggestion.

The group still does not build an identity in this phase. The range of participation by group members is the highest of any phase. That is, the difference between the air time of the least and most talkative will be numerically higher in this phase than in any other phase.

The need for structure will be strong. In T-Groups the content during this phase may well be whether to elect a rotating chairman, recording secretary, or a group leader. The process is, in reality, a bid for power and is the third step of a group's ascent to maturity.

Roles are important in third phase activity. The group building and maintenance roles are most important. The harmonizer, the compromiser, the gate-keeper and the follower try to maintain an acceptable balance between the needs of individual group members and the needs of the group. The level of conflict is reduced by the harmonizer to offset the tendency for conflict levels to rise due to the aggressor.

Some groups never mature past this stage. Nevertheless, these groups can fulfill their task. My data indicate, however, that solutions arising out of third phase activity are not optimum solutions. Also, the solutions never satisfy all group members and, at best, are products of compromise. Dr. Blake's 9-1 managerial[1] style typifies the active group member who enjoys relating in third phase activity.

Constructive phase

The transition from third stage (Power) to fourth stage (Constructive) is characterized by an attitude change. Group members give up their attempts to control and substitute an attitude of active listening.

In the constructive stage, group members are willing to change preconceived ideas or opinions based on facts presented by other group members. You hear group members actively asking questions of each other. A team spirit starts to build. Cliques begin to dissolve. Real progress toward the group's goals becomes evident. Leadership becomes a "shared leadership." Group identity starts becoming important to the group members. The range of participation by members narrows. When conflict arises it is dealt with as a mutual problem rather than as a win-lose battle. At this point in a group's growth, it may be increasingly difficult to bring in a new member.

Depending on the talents of the group members and the problem to be solved, an optimum solution can result from fourth phase interaction. This optimum solution can be better than any solution offered by single group members. For this reason some businesses are attempting to organize for fourth phase "team" group activity.

McGregor's theory X (1960) would seem to apply to a group positioned at step three on Cog's Ladder while his theory Y would seem to apply more to a group in phase four.

The important difference between phase four (Constructive) and phase three (Power) is the willingness of group members to listen and to change based on what they hear. Because of this willingness, a group in phase four will often use the talents of any individual who can contribute effectively. In phase four practical creativity can be high because the group is willing to accept creative suggestions from group members. Furthermore, creative suggestions are solicited by the group, listened to, questioned, responded to and, if appropriate, acted on. For this reason, group decisions arising out of phase four activity are almost always better than decisions proposed by a single group member[3].

Any group exercises which enhance the basic values of group cooperativeness are proper for groups in this phase. Exercises based on sharing, helping, listening, anticipating group needs, questioning, and building are all appropriate. Competitive exercises here will tend to be disruptive of group growth as they will apply gentle pressure to regress back to phase three (Power).

Group leaders can be most effective in phase four by asking constructive questions, summarizing and clarifying the group's thinking, trusting the group to achieve its maximum potential, trying to blend in with the group as much as possible, and refraining from making any comments tending to reward or punish other group members. An effective group leader will also recognize that group members will vary widely in their abilities to contribute to the group's goals. The effective group leader will be tolerant of this variety.

Esprit phase

The fifth and final phase of group growth is the *esprit* phase. Here the group feels a high group morale. Relationships between individuals are empathetic. The group feels an intense group loyalty. The need for group approval is absent because each group member approves of all others and accepts them as individuals. Both individuality and creativity are high. The overall feeling is "we don't always agree on everything but we do respect each other's views and agree to disagree." From this flows a non-possessive warmth and freedom of the group member to express his individuality. Cliques are absent.

The group may demand an identity symbol. The members participate as evenly as they ever will. The need for structure depends on whether the group is an action group or a learning group. Learning groups have no need for structure if they have evolved to phase five.

In phase five, there is a strong closedness of the group. It is impossible to bring a new member into a phase five group without destroying the feeling of camaraderie and grou esprit. A period of group regression sets in while the group must grow from an earlier stage back up to the *esprit* stage, carrying the new member with it.

A group in phase five continues to be constructive and productive. In fact, such a group usually achieves more than is expected or than can be explained by the apparent talents of the group members. Examples of unusually high performance coupled with high *esprit* are legion in the world of team sports such as football, baseball, hockey, etc. It has been suggested that the difference between an average professional football coach and the coach of the national champion is his ability to encourage the group to grow "beyond" stage four (play football) and to grow into stage five (identify as an intensely loyal team).

Although hidden agenda items are present in phase five, they do not seem to detract from the *esprit* and group loyalty. One reason which has been suggested to explain this is that group members have granted to each other, including to themselves, the *right* to have hidden agenda provided it is productive. Group members then work to make their hidden agenda items productive not only for themselves but for the group. Another reason may be that the trust level has risen so high by phase five that the group trusts each member not to misuse the group loyalty. Still another reason may be that, by this time, the group is well aware of each member's hidden agenda and the group matured to phase five because it saw no threat from anyone's personal hidden agenda.

INTER-RELATIONSHIPS

The step from the Polite phase to the Why We're Here phase seems to occur when any single group member desires it. Simply by saying "Well, what's on the agenda today?" the group will usually move to phase two.

The transition from phase four (Constructive)

to phase five *(Esprit),* however, seems to require unanimous agreement among group members. This study has not observed any group in phase five which had not included *all* group members.

The transition from phase three (Power) to phase four (Constructive) can be permanently blocked by a strong competitive group member or by his clique. Conversely, the bridge between these two phases is the ability to listen. This ability to listen has been found to be the most important human trait in helping groups move from phase three to phase four. There have been cases where the group as a whole desired to relate in fourth phase while several members stayed rooted in third phase. Some groups have been observed to reject members for this behavior.[4]

Every group studied moved from one phase to another in an uneven, sometimes fitful flow. Many task-oriented groups regressed from a later stage to phase two for a better definition of the problem. In one 20 minute exercise, 8 regressions from phase three to phase two occurred.

In most groups studied there appeared to be a dominant group phase with other members relating in adjacent phases. Many observations made were of groups where most members would be relating in phase three (Power) while two group members would form a small clique and be discussing purpose (phase two-Why We're Here) or even engaging in polite conversation such as weather or vacations (phase one-Polite). Group cohesiveness seems to depend on how well the group members are in the same phase at the same time.

A group will grow through these five stages only to the extent that its members are willing to grow. Therefore, it seems appropriate to discuss the interrelationships between group growth and individual willingness to allow the group to grow based on what each member has to give up at each stage. To grow from stage one (Polite) to stage two (Why We're Here),

each member must give up the comfort of discussing non-threatening topics. He must now risk the possibility of conflict. To grow from stage two (Why We're Here) to stage three (Power) he gives up continued discussion of the purpose and he risks commitment to a purpose with which he may not be in complete agreement. He must now further risk personal attacks which he knows occur in phase three.

To grow from phase three (Power) to phase four (Constructive) requires individuals to give up the comfort of defending one's own views and risking the possibility of being wrong. Phase four demands some humility. To grow from phase four (Constructive) to phase five *(Esprit)* demands trusting oneself and trusting other group members. To trust is to risk a breach of trust. It has been noted in this study that groups find it difficult to grow much beyond phase three (Power).

The emphasis by profession on different steps of the Ladder is interesting. Scientific professions were notably in the fourth phase (Constructive) except for groups who felt incompetent, out of their field or unchallenged. They typically became third phase (Power). Members of religious groups, priests and nuns, etc., were almost universally interested in phase five *(Esprit)* and how to achieve it. Teenagers and some non-professionals were most interested in phase one (Polite). College students seemed to place most emphasis on phase two (Why We're Here).[5]

Members of the teaching profession and politicians related well in phase three (Power), while businessmen varied widely from phase one (Polite) to phase five *(Esprit).* Salesmen seemed to be comfortable in phase one, while outstanding managers understood the Cog process intuitively and, by example, led their group through the necessary steps to achieve phase five.

This study could find no correlation between educational level and need to relate in any given phase. In other words, each of over 1,000 people involved in this study naturally gravitated to a phase most comfortable for that person but there appeared to be no connection between phase number and educational level of the participants.

CONCLUSIONS

In designing a group session, the model of Cog's Ladder is helpful. During this study when certain phases were deliberately skipped or suppressed, the groups invariably became disoriented. Skipping phase one (Polite) can be especially harmful to a group.

The design of group sessions should be flexible, but should chart a course up Cog's Ladder with each group exercise proper for the phase the group is in at the time. For example, introducing a structured listening exercise[6] early in phase one might not be as effective as waiting until the group is ready to mature to phase four (Constructive).

The degree or intensity of the feeling in phase five *(Esprit)* is directly proportional to the group's accomplishments in phase four (Constructive). The more a group feels it has accomplished in phase four, the greater the *esprit*. Managers who gauge the productivity of their businesses by "morale" are, therefore, using an apparently valid correlation.

Conversely, some groups have as their main purpose to develop *esprit* in the group. Without another purpose, such as personal growth, this is not possible. In other words, it is not possible to skip phase four (Constructive) and still grow in phase five *(Esprit)*.

Cog's Ladder may seem intuitive to a good leader; however, by developing cognitive awareness of the Ladder, group leaders can do a better job of planning group exercises. Cog's Ladder has been extremely valuable when used within volunteer groups. In any business, meetings can be planned which lead to more productive results when the leader is consciously aware of the steps in Cog's Ladder.

Organizational development in business concentrates on improving group effectiveness. A knowledge of the Cog Model can be especially useful in firms considering "Team Organization."

References

1. The Managerial Grid is a concept published by Doctors Blake and Mouton in 1964, which includes styles of management.
2. Typically, met with total silence.
3. The committee which is accused of designing the camel probably is a group which has matured only to phase three (power) and has stopped short of maturing to phase four (Constructive).
4. Del Vecchio (1970) demonstrates this dramatically in Lesson 5 of INTERACT.
5. During a two day weekend seminar, students from over 30 cultures expressed a strong need to stay in phase two (Why We're Here) for almost 1½ days.
6. The best listening exercises include both content and feelings and are designed to improve empathy.

Bibliography

1. Blake, Robert R. and Mouton, Jane S.; *The Managerial Grid;* Gulf Publishing Company; 1964.
2. Cartwright, Dorwin and Zander, Alvin; *Group Dynamics;* Harper & Row; 1953.
3. Culbert, Samuel A.; *The Interpersonal Process of Self-Disclosure: It Takes Two to See One;* NTL Institute of Applied Behavioral Science; 1968.
4. Del Vecchio, Dr. Anthony, and Maher, William; *Interact;* National Council of Catholic Men; 1970.
5. Haiman, Franklyn S.; *Group Leadership and Democratic Action;* Houghton Mifflin Company; 1950.
6. Hall, Edward T.; *The Silent Language in Overseas Business;* Harvard Business Review; May-June, 1960.
7. Luft, J.; *Group Processes: An Introduction to Group Dynamics;* National Press; 1963.
8. McGregor, Douglas; *The Human Side of Enterprise;* McGraw-Hill Book Company; 1960.
9. Pfeiffer, J. William, and Jones, John E.; *A Handbook of Structured Experiences for Human Relations Training,* Vol. I and II; University Associates Press; 1969.
10. Zenger, John H.; *A Comparison of Human Development with Psychological Development in T-Groups;* Development Journal; July, 1970.
11. Tuckman, Bruce W.; *Developmental Sequence in Small Groups,* Psychological Bulletin; Vol. 63, No. 6, 384-399; 1965.

Identifying blocks to communication in health care settings and a workshop plan

CECILIA M. SMITH, R.N., M.S.

Several months ago I was approached by a director of staff development working in a health care center for the aged. She identified the main problem as one of difficulties with interpersonal communication among staff members. Certainly her problem is not unique to that setting. A growing body of theory in the area of communication attests to the fact that there is a major concern in this area and an increasing interest in discerning ways to deal with problems being encountered. The following discussion will focus upon three aspects for consideration: (1) an approach to the identification of stumbling blocks to communication; (2) a view of how more effective means of communication might be facilitated; and (3) an outline of a workshop that was conducted to promote more effective communication among staff members.

What are some of the stumbling blocks to the communication process? Barna,[1] in his discussion of intercultural communication, listed five which he felt caused communication breakdown: lack of common understanding of the language, differences in relating to the sensory world, high levels of anxiety, the presence of preconceptions and stereotypes, and the tendency to evaluate the actions of others. He further indicated that the solution to the problem lies in sensitizing people to the kinds of things that need to be taken into account. Margaret Mead and Edward Stewart[2,3] supported this view. These authors were concerned with the communication process as it occurs between

Reprinted with permission from the *Journal of Continuing Education in Nursing*, vol. 8, November, 1977.

individuals of different ethnic and cultural backgrounds. Here an interesting parallel might be drawn. These factors may also play a large part in the difficulties encountered in interpersonal relationships in health care settings. Let us examine each of the factors and their applicability.

LANGUAGE

All disciplines have specialized words which have been vested with meanings that are shared by the members of those disciplines. Thus, for example, all nurses know what STAT means. PRN, qid, and intake and output are no mysteries. For a new aide on the floor, however, they may indeed be "foreign" until that aide has had the chance to validate her perceptions with others. Some words which may have been understood by all may have changed in their intent. Thus, "good nursing care" to a nurse of 25 years ago may be interpreted quite differently today, and may encompass quite different skills. "See if you can do anything to make the patient comfortable" might have involved straightening the bed clothes and giving a backrub. Today, that might include sitting beside the patient and listening to what is bothering him.

Not only may there be problems affecting communication within one group with specialized training, there may also be difficulties encountered in working with other members of the health care team. At a recent dinner attended by physicians and nurse educators, one physician was overheard asking a nurse to tell him exactly what was meant by "nurse-patient relationship." A lack of familiarity with the jargon can block communication, cause misunderstandings, and lead to misconceptions regarding roles.

THE SENSORY WORLD

Anthropological studies have shown that individuals with different cultural backgrounds tend to stress the use of a variety of perceptual skills. Thus, for people whose survival is dependent upon visual acuity, this skill will be highly developed. Within our own culture there are individual differences. Hill[4] and his colleagues have found that there are a variety of ways by which individuals prefer to search for meaning. They may be strongly oriented qualitatively to any of the sensory modes. Thus, a nurse might be very conscious of a variety of odors and be able to identify aspects of a patient's condition not obvious to another member of the health team. We have all been aware of the individual who just "doesn't hear a thing I've said." Not only may this cause difficulties in working with others on the team, it may also prevent effective communication between the patient and the nurse. Perhaps it is the individual who is oriented to many qualitative modes who would be judged to be proficient in communicative skills. This could prove to be an interesting and fruitful area for research.

HIGH ANXIETY

It is a recognized fact that a high level of anxiety reduces productivity. Individuals operating in situations in which they are extremely anxious tend not to hear or see as much as when their tension is reduced. Although one would hope that the hospital setting would not be conducive to such anxiety, it is conceivable that certain sections, such as the operating room or the intensive care unit, could be potentially tension producing. This might be particularly true for the individual who is new to that area or has had limited practice using the necessary skills. Here the process may be circular in that the anxiety may block communication, which

in turn will increase rather than decrease the level of anxiety.

PRECONCEPTIONS AND STEREOTYPES

All of us operate with certain preconceptions. In order for people to make sense out of his world, they categorize perceptions and experiences. Repeated experiences lead individuals to certain expectations of behavior. It is when we operate on the assumption that our preconceptions and stereotypes are invariable that we can adversely affect the communication process. A nurse might, for example, believe that all hospital administrators know little about nursing care and are mainly concerned about maintaining a cost effective operation, and therefore, hesitate to approach an administrator with an innovative proposal to which the administrator might well be amenable.

As Signell[5] has indicated, individuals may stereotype on the basis of one of any number of characteristics. These may include sex, age, ethnic origin, and position. It is not uncommon to perceive individuals stereotyping patients by diagnosis — "old crocks" with low back pain or "drunken bums" with alcoholic problems, for example. Preconceptions and stereotypes predispose individuals to communicate in limited ways based upon their expectations. They limit the possibilities of actualizing the potentialities of individual differences.

TENDENCY TO EVALUATE

A tendency to evaluate the actions of others is probably the most common block to the communication process. Involved in this is the use of the expression, "but I told her." Here the assumption is made that the message as communicated by the sender was received and perceived as identically the same. Without feedback to the sender, this assumption cannot be made.

Mention has been made of some of the factors, such as lack of familiarity with the jargon, that can cause a breakdown in communication. By indicating that the message has been sent and that the receiver has failed to act in an expected manner, the sender, who in this instance might be the supervisor, places a value judgment on a resultant action with insufficient information. The following account presents an example of this problem.

A head nurse was assigning a patient who was scheduled for surgery to a new aide. She instructed her to go down to his room and to see if the patient was ready for surgery. The aide looked in at the patient. He had been medicated and was sleeping. The side rails were up. His water had been removed. He "looked" ready for surgery. When the patient arrived in the operating room it was discovered that his dentures had not been removed. Following the surgery the physician communicated his displeasure to the head nurse who replied, "But I *told* Miss Jones to see if he was ready for surgery." The aide had interpreted her orders to mean that she should look in on the patient and *see* if he was ready to go. Since she couldn't see his dentures, she did not include removing them among her repertoire of necessary activities. Rather than checking with the aide to determine her perceptions of what was involved, the head nurse evaluated the actions of the aide and placed blame, thereby discouraging communication.

FACILITATING COMMUNICATIONS

Once some of the stumbling blocks to communication have been identified such as: (1) lack of common understanding of the language; (2) differences in relating to the sensory world; (3) high anxiety; (4) the preconceptions and stereotypes; and (5) the tendency to evaluate others, how can one go about the process of sensitizing individuals in the health care setting, if indeed this is the basic principle involved in facilitating communication?

First, one must recognize that the range of personality characteristics differs greatly from institution to institution. Individuals responsible for facilitating communication, as well as those who hopefully will benefit from some intervention, are unique individuals with their own values, beliefs, and habit patterns. In addition, the health care settings themselves constitute a variety of social systems. They may differ in size, location, amount of interdependence upon other institutions, and in structure within the particular setting itself. Not only are there differences in organizational structures, *i.e.,* lines of responsibility, but there may also be a wide variety of "social climates" operating therein. In institutions where an "authoritarian" climate prevails, there may be too little flexibility for the expression of new ideas or attempts to facilitate change. On the other end of the continuum, in a "laissez faire" situation there may be a complacency with the status quo and little interest in a follow-through to assess results of the intervention, should one be instituted.

In the process of sensitizing individuals, one concept, that of participation, seems to assume major importance. It is a well-known fact that people learn and retain knowledge or acquire skills better if they are actively involved in the learning process.[6] Sensitization is a learning process in every sense of the word. The methods used in the process of sensitizing individuals to communication blocks and suggesting new ways to facilitate communication may be varied. That which may be effective in one setting, with one group of individuals, may be less effective in another. The following is an example of a workshop which was conducted.

COMMUNICATION WORKSHOP

As indicated earlier, the main problem in a health care center for the aged, related to staff communication problems. As a means of solving the problem, it was decided that two nurse educators would be responsible for conducting a workshop to be held in that institution. From the beginning, in the initial phase of identifying the problems and planning a course of action, the director of staff development for the health care center was involved. It was felt that this would provide some continuity after the workshop, in that she would be knowledgeable in the rationale for the section of certain experiences. In addition, her sharing in some of the leadership functions might enable staff personnel to perceive her as an individual to whom they could relate in the future should further communication difficulties arise.

Keeping in mind some on the potential areas blocking effective communication, a variety of experiences were discussed. It was decided that the workshop would be held for four hours a day, with two sessions one week apart. This would provide an opportunity for a one-week "practice session" for participants. The workshop would be repeated one month later for staff unable to attend the first series. Objectives were outlined, and plans were made for a variety of activities, involving the total group as well as small groups.

Activities of the first session

In light of difficulties in the area of language, preconceptions, and stereotypes, a list of words was given to the participants to define. These words included some terms with emotional overtones such as "good," "adequate," and "normal," and other terms such as "communicate" and "nursing." In this way, it was hoped that commonalities as well as differences in individual interpretations could be illustrated. The plan called for a sharing in small groups, followed by an analysis of the words as barriers to communication, in the total group.

To facilitate effective communication during the workshop, it was next felt appropriate to share definitions of the words to be used during the workshop. Terms such as "communication," "perception," "listening," "role playing," and "perceptual validation" were discussed in order to provide workshop leaders and participants with a common frame of reference.

The next planned activity, relating to both common understanding of language as well as differences in relating to the sensory world, involved a set of three drawings. These drawings consisted of simple sets of geometric designs, *i.e.,* rectangles, triangles, and circles, placed in different configurations for each of the three pictures. Participants were divided into three groups and directed to separate parts of the room. One individual in each group was selected to describe the drawings to three persons, who were unable to view the pictures. They were then given descriptions of the first drawing by the "narrator" and asked to reproduce it. They were not allowed to obtain any feedback by asking questions. The second drawing was then described. Questions which could be answered either "yes" or "no" were allowed. Any question could be asked about the third drawing. Following this exercise, participants were allowed to compare and contrast the results and discuss the implications in terms of communication in their respective positions.

The final exercise for the first session related to perceptual validation. This concept was described as a process of confirmation of what was perceived — in this instance verbally. The demonstration illustrated the process by which one could validate what was heard by such expressions as: "As I understand it you mean . . . ," "Are you saying that . . .?" or "Do you mean . . .?" until both the sender of a message as well as the receiver arrived at a commonality of meanings. Participants were then presented with printed statements and divided into groups of three for a practice session. It was interesting to note that although they began with the prepared sentences, they soon devised their own and continued to practice the exercise. In sharing the experience with the total group, some individuals expressed discomfort and stated that they felt that it was "unnatural." This was not an unusual or unexpected response. Exaggerated practice in which the participants were engaged leads to greater facility with a technique which can then be utilized by individuals with their own unique styles.

An assignment was then presented. Participants were asked to practice perceptual validation during the following week. This was not restricted only to the hours in which they were on duty but elsewhere as well, if they so desired. They were asked to bring back three examples of these interactions for the next week's session. A short question and answer period concluded the first session.

Activities of the second session

The first activity of the second session involved a follow-up on the perceptual validation exercise practiced by the participants during the preceding week. Examples of interactions were reproduced on transparencies and a lively discussion of the relative effectiveness of the technique followed.

The next exercise for this session was termed a "listening workshop." It involved the introduction of a topic for discussion, *e.g.,* the gasoline shortage and how it should be handled, which was of great concern at that time. This related again mainly to the area of perceptual validation. Individuals were encouraged to express their views; however, other participants were not allowed to state their opinions until they had confirmed that they had correctly interpreted what had been stated by the speaker. Although the groups had once again been divided, a total group discussion followed.

Three additional major activities were planned for the second session. These were: the viewing of a film, a role playing session, and individual delineation of personal goals by participants. The film, "Confronting Conflict," demonstrated a situation in which members of an organization discussed their evaluations of the actions of each individual as he performed the duties of his respective position. An additional dimension, which was identified by the group in the discussion that followed, was a percep-

tion of role stereotyping, which workshop participants felt was well illustrated.

Although Barna does not allude specifically to proxemics of man's spatial relations, this aspect, as has been documented by such authors as Hall[7] and Watson,[8] can effect interpersonal communications. For this reason, the next workshop exercise consisted of a series of three role playing situations. In one example, participants were instructed to simulate an office confrontation between a supervisor and staff member with the supervisor assuming a variety of poses at varying distances from the staff member. Given the opportunity to practice the situations, participants identified district differences in their emotional reactions.

For the final exercise, participants were provided with a list of guidelines for improving skills in face-to-face communication. They then identified those specific areas which they felt they would like to concentrate on for the purpose of improving their communication skills.

EVALUATION

As with any workshop, the process of evaluation is of vital importance. Not only must an assessment be made of how well the objectives have been met, but also there are decisions to be made about whether or not there might be merit in repeating various aspects, with or without modifications.

In the workshop that has been described, participants were asked for their reactions at the conclusion of the final session.

Responses indicated a high degree of satisfaction with the activities in which the participants engaged, and an expressed commitment to practice the techniques proposed for facilitating communication. Although circumstances did not permit the program planners to return to the health care facility to personally engage in the follow-up evaluation, the director of staff development arranged for this activity. It was felt that this function could well be assumed by her since she had been involved throughout all stages of the planning and implementation. A meeting of participants was scheduled six weeks following the conclusion of the workshop. A number of interesting observations were identified during the interim period, as well as at the six weeks follow-up session.

The director of staff development perceived that initially the staff utilized the suggested techniques for facilitating communication to a significant degree. There was also an increase in the amount of interdepartmental communication.When interacting with staff personnel, the director of staff development perceived the communication as being one in which messages were transmitted more clearly and effectively.

Approximately one-fourth of the participants attended the follow-up session. At that time some of the participants indicated that they did not recall the areas identified as problems on which they wished to focus. Some stated that they had experienced definite benefits in improving their abilities to communicate.

Perhaps one of the most significant observations of the director of staff development was that of the degree to which she perceived the effects of the workshop to be sustained. Admittedly, this observation was subjective judgment on her part. She reported that the first group to experience the workshop appeared to demonstrate a higher degree of interest and application of learned skills over a longer period of time than the second group. There are a number of variables which may be hypothesized to affect this phenomenon. Assuming that both workshops were similar in content and presentation, the individuals attending each were different. Specific differences were noted in represented roles, *e.g.,* the assistant administrator attended the second session. The fact that some staff interacted with a number of individuals participating in the activity prior to their own involvement may have influenced their expectations and perceptions of the experience. The extent to which external conditions

and events affected the participants is also an unknown factor which may have influenced the degree to which the effects of the workshop appeared to be sustained. Although an overall decrease in the utilization of specific mechanisms to facilitate communication was noted, it was felt that the demonstrated increase in communication skills persisted at a more proficient level than was experienced prior to the workshop.

Based upon the entire experience, including the evaluation, a number of recommendations can be delineated. It should be recognized that if a workshop is repeated, perceived interest in and commitment to the practice of communication skills may differ for each participant group. This may be the only way to schedule the experience in order to provide maximum participation given staffing patterns. Opportunity should be provided for participants to share their expectations and preconceived ideas about the objectives and anticipated outcomes. It may be necessary to modify the scheduled activities on the basis of identified differences in the participants' perceptions.

It appears that it would also be beneficial to have a number of scheduled periodic follow-up sessions to provide feed-back for reinforcement to participants. Research has shown that feedback is a positive factor influencing learning.

Finally, instructors involved in presenting workshops should be directly involved in the evaluation process. This would enable them to individualize the follow-up sessions based upon the perceived needs and provide support to the facility personnel responsible for assisting staff in their efforts to improve interpersonal relationships through effective communication.

CONCLUSION

Although all blocks to communication were not addressed at the workshop, *e.g.,* high levels of anxiety, the content of the exercises planned for the participants was tailored to meet the needs identified by the director of staff development and appropriate objectives which were subsequently developed. Individuals attending this particular workshop presented a variety of levels of staff personnel, including the assistant administrator, supervisors, nursing personnel, and members of housekeeping and maintenance departments. Since individual characteristics, roles, and institutions and their goals differ, certain aspects of any planned workshop must also differ.

This paper has presented one conceptualization of how blocks to communication may be viewed. Differences among individuals and within institutions as social systems were discussed. The workshop is an example of one method of dealing with some of the factors which may hinder effective interpersonal communication and encourage creative efforts to improve skillful communication.

References

1. Barna LM: Stumbling blocks in interpersonal intercultural communications. *In* Samovar LA, Porter RE (eds): Intercultural Communication: A Reader. Belmont, Wadsworth Publishing Co, Inc, 1972, pp 242-244.
2. Mead M: The cultural perspective. *In* Capes M (ed): Communication or Conflict. Association Press, 1960.
3. Stewart EC: American Culture Patterns: A Cross-cultural Perspective. Pittsburg, Regional Council for International Education, University of Pittsburg, April 1971, p 14.
4. Hill JE: The educational sciences. Unpublished manuscript, Oakland Community College, 1968.
5. Signell KA: The development of cognitive structure in inference about other persons and nations. Unpublished doctoral dissertation, University of Colorado, 1964.
6. Chickering AW: Education and Identity. San Francisco, Jossey-Bass, Inc, 1972, p 325.
7. Hall ET: Proxemics: Man's Spatial Relations. *In* Samovar LA, Porter RE (eds): Intercultural Communication: A Reader. Belmont, Wadsworth Publishing Company, Inc, 1972, pp 203-220.
8. Watson, OM: Symbolic and expressive uses of space: an introduction to proxemic behavior. Addison-Wesley Modular Publications, Module 20, 1972, pp 1-18.

A cognitive transactional approach to communication

JAMES S. DeLO, Ph.D., and WILLIAM A. GREEN

The present situation of the appearance of black and white people together in new work and social settings suggests that there is a real need for the development of an approach to black-white relations which could help improve communication. To date, major interventional approaches brought to bear on the problem have not dealt directly with the need to increase the effectiveness of face-to-face black-white communication, which is referred to in this article as "transracial communication." The major interventional approaches that have had his-

Reprinted with permission from *Social Casework,* May, 1977.

torical significance may be identified as: (1) the sociolegal approach, (2) the socioeconomic approach, and (3) the educative-emotive approach.

The sociolegal approach depends on economic and social pressure to bring about equality through change in the judicial structure. The socioeconomic approach insists that differences between blacks and whites are economic, and that blacks, if they have the means, would model after white middle-class America and resolve their differences. The educative-emotive approach underlines the irrationality of prejudice and attempts to persuade white America to give up the emotionality connected with their beliefs and to accept reason. All of these approaches have been effective and have resulted in some positive changes in the institutional structure, thereby expediting equitable distribution of goods, services, and opportunities.

Despite the progress made by these approaches, however, they have significant limitations. First, they have a negative side effect in that they have the inherent message that black people must depend upon white people to relinquish power before progress can be made. This message has a demeaning effect, in that blacks must entreat rather than act in their own behalf. Second, these three existing approaches are further limited in that equal opportunity before the law does not equalize employment if black individuals are deprived of the opportunity to acquire the skills to compete; equal distribution of economic resources does not compensate for cultural differences; and traditional educational techniques do not necessarily convince people to give up biased emotional beliefs, especially if there are social and economic rewards associated with their maintenance.

The purpose of this article is to introduce a new approach which focuses on the problem of black-white communication, but at the same time circumvents many of the problems inherent in the three traditional approaches. This approach is designed to provide a workable interventional system that can help ameliorate many of the problems generated when blacks and whites meet each other in work and social situations. Although frequently some kind of equilibrium is established in these situations, there is evidence to suggest that it is superficial. This phenomenon was observed in a study done by William Green[1] with a number of professional white interviewers. It was found that although the whites felt they had done a creditable job with black applicants, the blacks felt there had been scarcely any communication at all. When confronted with this disparity, neither group could accurately assess what had gone wrong. This study underlines the crucial need to improve the quality of communication between blacks and whites. Because both blacks and whites are responsible for interactional effects in their communication, a focus on transracial communication demands that each group accept responsibility for its actions. In contrast to the traditional approaches described, the cognitive transactional approach to transracial communication described in this article insists that blacks, as well as whites, are equal partners in the task of improving relations between them.

A COGNITIVE TRANSACTIONAL APPROACH TO HUMAN LEARNING

Most, if not all, psychological activity is essentially transactional in nature. It is well established that the human organism from earliest infancy is actively engaged in the complex task of transacting with and mastering his environment. Much of this learning involves interpersonal relationships with others. In this process the infant develops a repertoire of perceptual responses. This process eventuates certain behavioral modes or adaptive responses to the environment in terms of needs or wants. These needs or wants are not biological and therefore are not essential to survival, but they may be psychologically necessary for the reduction of conflict. Such felt needs include approval and acceptance. From this standpoint, most adult responses are taken from the ''cues'' which have been learned over a long period of time and have been cyrstallized into habitual styles of perceiving and adapting to and transacting with the social environment. The same is often true of ethnic or racial

---

[1] William Green, Some Effects of Racism in Job Interviews (Paper presented at the American Personnel and Guidance Association Convention, Chicago, Illinois, April 1974).

stances and is reflected in habitual ways of transacting. In this sense, a positive or negative racial stance is primarily a product which has been acquired through interaction with significant others. This kind of learning can occur so early in life that it antedates any real capacity for judgment and is therefore accepted without question. This early learning may be maintained through a social system that supports such a stance through informal interactions with others and formal interactions with institutional structures.

George A. Kelly[2] points out that the individual uses a cognitive process to develop personal constructs that account for the organization and direction of behavior. The end product —his behavior—is dependent upon the manner in which the individual conceptualizes his experiences. According to this interpretation, the individual seeks information which will help support his personal construct system. This action leads to behavioral choices which further support his personal constructs, and leads him to anticipate events. This cycle of events usually has an intense overlay due to a strong vested interest in maintaining personal constructs. It leads to a lack of awareness appearing as social constrictiveness which can lead to deficient or dishonest transaction.

Assuming that individuals act in such a manner as to validate personal constructs, it must be expected that transactions are influenced by the cognitive set of the participants. Due to cultural separation experienced historically by blacks and whites in this society, it may be assumed that blacks and whites approach each other with totally different sets of constructs which they wish to validate. This difference sets up a situation for deficient transactions in which both actors, "black and white," seek to validate their own constructs at the expense

of the other. Therefore, black-white transactions can take on a kind of "games" quality which frequently results in one or both individuals being put down.

The technique of intervention in black-white communication described in this article is called a cognitive transactional approach. The term cognitive is included because the authors have concerned themselves not only with the dishonest games that blacks and whites play with each other, but also with the kinds of constructs and stereotypes that both blacks and whites bring with them and that inevitably influence the nature of black-white transactions.

A TRANSACTIONAL PARADIGM
Honest transactions versus dishonest games

A transaction is defined as that which takes place between two or more actors, either verbally or nonverbally, that concludes in a given effect, which is generally satisfying to one or all the actors. Honest transactions are characterized by open and genuine communication. Dishonest transactions, however, are characterized by a "game" quality in which ultimately one or both individuals is "put down." In order to clarify the number of possible interactional effects of transactions between members of majority and minority groups, the following paradigm has been constructed. The cells in the paradigm represent transactions between two or more actors. The capital letters "B" and "W" are used to represent black or white individuals who experience satisfaction as a result of a transaction without loss of self-esteem. The small letters "b" and "w" represent black or white individuals respectively who do not experience satisfaction and lose self-esteem as a result of the transaction. In interpreting the transactions identified in the cells of the paradigm, the first letter in the pair is designated as the individual who initiates the transaction. As shown in the figure on p. 136, there are sixteen possible interactions

[2]George A. Kelly, *The Psychology of Personal Constructs,* Vol. 2 (New York: W. W. Norton, 1955), pp. 560-65.

	W	w	B	b
W	W W	W w	W B*	W b*
w	w W	w w	w B*	w b*
B	B W*	B w*	B B	B b
b	b W*	b w*	b B	b b

Cells with an * indicate a transracial interaction..

Fig. I. Transactional paradigm.

that can occur between pairs of black and white individuals. Eight of these interactions involve transactions between whites and blacks without involving "transracial" communication. Eight of these transactions, however, may be called transracial interactions because they actually involve communication between blacks and whites. Attention was not focused on transactions between members of the same racial group. Intraracial transactions have significant influence in the development of attitudinal sets, and are worthy of investigation. Because they are not transracial units that occur between blacks and whites, however, they are not dealt with in this article.

The actual units of transactions between whites and blacks as identified by the paradigm are as follows:

1. W-B. A white individual initiates the transaction. Neither individual in the transaction is put down. Both individuals communicate with each other in an honest and direct fashion.
2. W-b. A white individual initiates the transaction which ends with the black individual being put down.
3. b-W. A black individual begins a transaction and is put down by a white.

4. w-B. A white individual initiates the transaction which ends with him being put down by a black individual.
5. B-W. Similar to a W-B transaction with the exception that a black individual initiates the transaction.
6. B-w. A black individual initiates a transaction which ends with a white person being put down.
7. b-w. A black initiates a transaction in the context of which they put each other down, take loser positions, and are stalemated.
8. w-b. A white initiates a transaction in the context of which both individuals are put down and stalemated.

Blacks and whites enter into transaction with constructs (reflecting cognitive sets and stereotypes) that influence the manner in which they transact with each other. It is not necessary for individuals to be aware of the operation of these cognitive sets in order for them to influence transactions. In fact, to the contrary, many individuals report that they are totally lacking in prejudice, but at the same time they may be observed to act out of cognitive sets that unconsciously support racism and preclude honest communication. In order to illustrate the difference between honest transactions and dishonest games, a number of critical incidences was compiled. Some of these critical incidences have been included for purposes of illustration in the following section.

B-W and W-B transactions

The following is an example of an effective transaction in which both individuals communicate honestly with each other.

Mr. Black plans to open a service station in partnership with Mr. White. Both men agree to share the responsibility for the business. Because the business is to be located in a racially troubled area of town they discuss the possibility of damage to their new station and decide to delay the opening for several weeks.

This transaction is considered to be B-W honest communication. Although racially oriented material is discussed, both men approach the problem with what they believe to be a realistic view of the situation. Although it is possible that some may disagree with their conclusion, the salient quality of respect for each other in approaching a common goal makes this an effective transaction. Although there is no assurance that each individual will act upon the conclusions reached in honest transactions, the stage is set for behavorial action. These subsequent actions are really the "acid test" of honest transactions.

A W-B transaction is similar except that a white individual initiates the transaction. For example:

Mr. White and Mr. Black are discussing problems in their church congregations. Mr. White complains that his congregation will not allow any blacks to join the church. Mr. Black replies that perhaps Mr. White should drop his membership as a protest. Mr. White replies that he thought of this action but decided it would be more helpful if he stayed and worked with his church congregation, hoping eventually to change the congregation's attitude.

Again, as in the previous transaction, both individuals interact honestly and treat each other with respect. Again, some may not like the conclusion that the men reached, but the quality of directness and honesty is present in the transaction.

W-b and B-w games

In W-b and B-w games the initiator may begin the game with a conscious intent to put the other person down. In most cases, however, the initiator will not be aware of the cognitive construct that is the impetus for moving the transaction to a negative conclusion. The following examples are illustrative of W-b and B-w transactional games that conclude with the initiator putting down the recipient. The following

game, "Token," is illustrative of a W-b transaction.

Mr. Black, an unmarried man, has been the only black teacher in the high school for several years. The school principal, in order to improve racial balance, hired Miss Black, also unmarried. Mrs. White, who is handling the arrangements for the faculty Christmas party makes it a point to place Mr. and Miss Black place cards together so they can get better acquainted. Mr. and Miss Black acquiesce to the situation.

It is clear to most blacks that the white woman in question is reacting to the token quality of the presence of both black teachers rather than to an awareness of them as separate people. It may be assumed that Mrs. White does not wish to convey hostility, but is acting on a cognitive set that people of the same color should be classified together rather than be accepted as separate persons. In most cases, a transaction such as this one is concluded with the white actor being unaware or vaguely aware that the transaction has ended with the black individuals being in a put-down state.

Other games are played in which a black individual begins the transaction and ends it by closing off communication and putting down the white participant. The following is an example of a B-w transaction which ends in the white individual being put down. This game is called, "You are not like me."

A group of whites and blacks are talking about problems with their teen-age daughters. Mrs. Black takes the opportunity to tell them of the problems that her own daughter is having in dating situations. The whites in the group are dismayed and ask her for clarification because they do not quite understand what she is talking about.

In this transaction the assumptive construct is that people who appear to be different cannot have similar life concerns. This construct negates the fact that black children and black parents experience similar kinds of problems in growth and development. A construct that implies qualitative differences in human emotion and concerns is easily converted into meaning "less than me." This tendency of whites to inferiorize blacks has been reported on by William H. Grier and Price M. Cobbs.[3] In a setting such as the one described, whites may not be aware of the impact of this transaction on a black person and may even rationalize that their questions are purely intellectual.

Conversely, an example of a w-B transaction is reflected in the following transaction. This game is called, 'You can't get to me.''

Mr. White is giving a talk to a mixed group of whites and blacks concerning quality public education. During the question-and-answer period at the end of the talk one of the blacks interjects, "I'm from the Ghetto! You'll have to break it down for me!''

As indicated in the preceding transaction, it is assumed that the white individual is attempting to deal with the problem of quality education in an honest manner. It is conceivable that some of his comments may be inappropriate or even identified as racist by black participants. The put down from the black participant, however, restricts further communication and does not deal directly and honestly with either the problem of education for blacks or problems in communication between the speaker and the participants. The put down may be interpreted as an extension of a cognitive set that presupposes that white intellectuals are not really knowledgeable about black problems. An effective transaction should, in contrast, require that the black individuals deal honestly and directly with the white individual and the material he is presenting.

Stalemated transactions

Some transactions end in a negative stalemate where each participant ends the transac-

---

[3]William H. Grier and Price M. Cobbs, *Black Rage* (New York: Basic Books, 1968). pp. 12-31, 152-67.

tion in a diminished position. These transactions are designated as w-b, b-w games. Some w-b, b-w games are played in such a way that the participants are not aware that their counterpart has initiated a put down. If each participant falsely believes that he is one up, these games will tend to be repeated because of their pay-off to the participants. An example of a b-w transaction that would tend to be repeated is the following game, "Ya-Suh, Mr. Charlie.''

Mr. Black goes through a red light in a small town. He is stopped by Mr. White, a policeman. Mr. Black gets out of his car and goes back to Mr. White's car. Mr. Black expresses astonishment and bewilderment. When Mr. White reprimands him, he says over and over, 'Ya-Suh, Ya-Suh, I'll never do that again.'' Mr. White finally finds the situation humorous and decides to let Mr. Black go without a citation.

Both individuals enter this transaction with cognitive sets which reflect stereotypes toward individuals of different racial groups. The white policeman validates his cognitive construct that blacks are amusing and dumb and should be treated like children. The black individual in question believes that white policemen as a group have this construct, act accordingly and use it to avoid receiving a citation. This action in turn validates his own construct that white authority figures are rigid, opinionated, and easily fooled.

Other examples of b-w, w-b games occur in settings where both individuals know they have been put down. These situations are painful to participants and tend not to be repeated. They are characterized by anger and frustration in the context of which neither party participates in a playful or challenging game, but each sets out to transact in such a manner to hurt the other individual. These w-b, b-w transactions are particularly stressful to participants because anger generated in one transaction may increase in intensity in the next and can escalate to the point of actual physical or verbal assault. This situation is likely to prohibit productive communication in the immediate future. An example of a b-w transaction where each individual ends up short is the following game, "I want the last word."

A white meter maid is in the process of writing a parking citation for a black driver when he arrives. He confronts her by saying that she would not have given him the citation if he were white. She responds angrily by saying, "White people pay taxes," and proceeds to write the ticket.

Both individuals approach each other with cognitive sets that produce an ineffectual transaction which is mutually harmful. The black man assumes that white meter maids are prejudiced toward blacks. The white woman in question operates out of a set which holds that blacks tend to be dishonest and avoid responsibility. Each individual, if he takes the other seriously, is diminished as a result of the transaction.

A COGNITIVE TRANSACTIONAL MODEL

The task has been to provide a situation in which both blacks and whites can deal with the personal constructs that underpin their belief systems. As Kelly indicates,[4] an image is changed or can be changed through the provision of experiences that are both *new and assimilable* (authors' italics) in terms of existing, accessible cognitive categories. Similar to organ rejection in medical organ transplants, cognitive categories provide a hostile environment for new belief systems. A vested personal belief system cannot be bullied or forced into change; it tends to reject or resist experiences that do not seem to have a "natural fit." In order to deal with this phenomenon, an interventional model was devised that permitted an expansion of boundary categories through recognition of deficient transactions and the

constructs that support them. These new experiences can then be used to alter categorical constructs without undue threat. In contrast to the three approaches outlined in the beginning of this article, there is no attempt to modify behavior by empathizing the culpability of whites. Neither are blacks encouraged to "blow their cover" and express pent-up anger they may be experiencing. Although these approaches may be helpful in some situations, it is not felt that they bring about long-term behavioral change. The assumption is made that whites and blacks both contribute in playing dishonest games with each other. It is stressed that all human beings have something to say to each other that frequently, for a variety of reasons, does not get said.

The model described involves the presentation of a series of critical incidences that are representative of transactions between blacks and whites. These presentations have the effect of stimulating cognition and lead workshop participants to generalize to other transactional experiences in their lives. In the process, there is exploration of the cognitive personal constructs that determine the nature of transactions. Interventional strategies which rely solely on guilt and, or, anger inadvertently get bogged down when it becomes necessary to translate insights into action for social change. The complexity and pervasiveness of institutional racism is overwhelming to many individuals. Although feeble promises may be made for future action, individuals are easily disillusioned. In contrast, a cognitive transactional model focuses on realistic changes that are within the individual's capacity to produce with some sense of immediacy. A participant's first trial runs at honest communication can be made within the context of a workshop with little personal threat to himself or to others.

The utilization of this model has been highly effective in stimulating cognitive change which influences the individual's capacity to recognize transactional games and the cognitive

---

[4]Kelly, *The Psychology of Personal Constructs*, p. 562.

sets that set them in motion. This recognition has the effect of enabling both black and white participants to be aware of the existence of transactional games. This recognition can lead to actual behavioral change, which is in effect the "acid test" of the validity of the approach. It has been learned through experience that this model is sufficiently flexible to be utilized in a variety of settings. Examples of critical transactional incidents have been expanded to include business and employment, social settings, educative institutional settings, and therapeutic interactions between therapists and clients. This approach has been utilized in presentations and in extended workshop for public and private educational settings, and in social work staffs and groups formed to promote black progress. In each of these settings almost all participants reported a positive change in their ability to recognize and alter defective transactions.

Although the authors' activities have been confined to black-white transactions, the cognitive transactional approach and the corresponding paradigm presented in this article should also hold for understanding other majority-minority group interactions. A similar transactional paradigm could be constructed to help explain deficient transactions between men and women, disabled and non-disabled, ethnic groups and "wasps," and so forth.

CONCLUSION

This article has underlined the fact that there are subtleties in transracial transethnic communication that are manifested in game playing and the resultant maintenance of social distance. The model described in this article has identified interactional effects in communication between whites and blacks. This article has also explored the part that cognition plays in the development of personal constructs which determine the quality of transactions. Experience applying this model indicates that personal constructs can be modified and resultant transracial communication improved if individuals are made aware of deficient transactions and the constructs that support them. This indication leads to the conclusion that it is possible for whites and blacks to learn to communicate honestly and effectively with each other and begin to bridge gaps that have been created by numerous years of cultural separation.

Chapter 8

CONFLICT, MOTIVATION, AND JOB SATISFACTION

Management by objectives and its subsystems

LEO B. OSTERHAUS, Ph.D.

Management by objectives is sometimes interpreted as a simple approach to conducting annual performance rating and review. This article presents the system of management by objectives in a larger context than that of a mere appraisal procedure. It regards appraisal as only one of several sub-systems operating within the larger system. The larger system of management embraces the major principles of management, with better appraisal of performance being a tangible result.

The major principles of management by objectives can be stated as follows:

1. Hospital management takes place within an economic and social system that provides an environmental situation for the individuals and groups within the hospital. This environment is continually changing and, consequently, goals must be updated.

2. Management objectives are aimed at meeting the new requirements of the changing environment. Learning the operations of the various subsystems of management by objectives is a preliminary step to increasing productivity and achieving successful management.

3. Management by objectives assumes that

managerial behavior is more important than managerial personality. This behavior should be defined in terms of specific results measured against specific goals established for an individual.

4. This type of management identifies participation as highly desirable in goal-setting and decision-making but recognizes that such participation may subordinate production to social and political values.

5. Once organizational goals are identified, orderly procedures are established to distribute responsibilities to individual managers at various levels.

6. By giving managers the right to delegate performance evaluation standards, management by objectives regards them as managers of the situation. Performance standards are determined by the purpose of the organization and the managerial behavior best calculated to achieve that purpose.

Hospital administrators are under three pressures today: To lower costs, to provide better patient care, and to achieve greater efficiency. Although these three pressures are seldom wholly compatible, they appear to be parts of a total system having overlapping subsystems. If hospitals can increase efficiency and productivity, they can reduce costs and in turn provide

Reprinted with permission from *Hospital Progress*, December, 1970, and the author.

better patient care. To understand this interrelation, it is helpful to look more closely at some of the underlying factors.

PRODUCTIVITY

Increased productivity is assumed to be a primary goal of the hospital. Galbraith[1] decries the further accumulation of gadgets, and argues, instead, for social balance. He feels that more of the national income should be allocated to hospitals, parks, and education; to things which emphasize human dignity, individuality, and worth which make life more pleasant and satisfying.

The efficiency of the hospital must be judged in terms of human happiness and health. Likert[2] emphasizes the importance of this factor in measuring organizational performance and human assets:

Decentralization and delegation are powerful concepts based on sound theory. But there is evidence that, as now utilized, they have a serious vulnerability which can be costly. This vulnerability arises from the measurements being used to evaluate and reward the performance of those given authority over decentralized operations.

This situation is becoming worse. While companies have during the past decade made greater use of work measurements and measurements of end results in evaluating managers, and also greater use of incentive pay in rewarding them, only a few managements have regularly used measurements that deal directly with the human assets of the organization—for example, measurements of loyalty, motivation, confidence, and trust. As a consequence, many companies today are encouraging managers of departments and divisions to dissipate valuable human assets of the organization. In fact, they are rewarding these managers well for doing so!

Productivity is defined for our purpose as output per man per hour, quality considered. It is necessary to realize that output per man hour results not from man's efforts alone but from all the factors of production: Labor, management, money, machines, raw materials, etc. Increased productivity depends upon or is determined by technical factors (technology, raw materials, job layout, and methods) and human factors (job performance, needs, desires).

Hospital productivity is not determined solely by how hard and how well people work. The technical factors play a role, sometimes an overwhelmingly important one, sometimes only a minor one. Making available the best designed machines and equipment, hospital and job layouts, and standard methods reduces time, waste, and spoilage and often encourages employes to work harder.

Since the hospital is an organization with many employes and little automation, productivity is likely to be determined largely by what employes do. The human contribution is determined by employes' job performance, which is a result of ability and motivation or, more accurately, ability times motivation. Ability results from knowledge and skill. Knowledge is achieved through education, experience, training, and interest. Skill is affected by aptitude and personality, as well as by education, training, experience, and interest.

MOTIVATION

Motivation is determined by an individual's needs and desires, the physical conditions of the job, and the social conditions of the job. Satisfying an individual's needs does not necessarily motivate him to improve his performance and contribute to greater productivity. Several case studies found that when an employe's needs were met his productivity increased, but other cases found that, even when morale was high because of individual need satisfaction, output was limited. The relationship between need satisfaction, morale, job performance, and productivity is very complex.

First, it might be assumed that employes are not aware of different kinds and levels of needs. Maslow[3] identifies five categories of needs: Physiological, safety, love, esteem, and self-actualization. Physiological needs include such essentials as food, water, housing, and clothing. In this society, these needs are likely to be well satisfied, and therefore are not normally motivators of behavior.

Social needs can be satisfied by contact with others, such as fellow employes, the supervisor, or friends off the job. Social needs provide for friendship, identification with the group, and teamwork, but often do not motivate the individual to greater productivity.

Egoistic needs are the needs an individual has for a high evaluation of himself. They include such things as knowledge, achievement, competence, independence, self-respect, status, and recognition.[4] When satisfied, these needs cease to motivate. However, research by Argyris,[5] McClelland,[6] Likert,[7] and Herzberg[8] seems to indicate that ego needs are never completely satisfied and continue to motivate. Likert's principle of supportive relationships is as follows: "The leadership and other processes of the organization must be such as to ensure a maximum probability that in all interactions and all relationships with the organization each member will, in the light of his background, values, and expectations, view the experience as supportive and one which builds and maintains his sense of personal worth and importance."

The highest level of needs are those of self-actualization or self-fulfillment. These needs are felt less by nonprofessional employes than they are by professional employes. They are considered the highest motivators, and the opportunity to fulfill them should be provided for any employe who desires it.

Need, satisfaction, motivation, employe performance, and productivity are interrelated. Hospital productivity will depend upon both employe performance and on technology. Employe performance will depend upon both the employe's motivation and ability. High motivation alone cannot increase employe performance or productivity; it must be combined with ability and the required technology.

The relationship between need satisfaction and motivation is not as clear. Although it

might seem as if high level need satisfaction would invariably produce a high level of motivation and low level of need satisfaction would invariably produce a low level of motivation, this is not necessarily true. Research studies indicate that the patterns may crisscross: High need satisfaction may be accompanied by low motivation, low need satisfaction by low motivation, or low need satisfaction by high motivation.

High need satisfaction is usually accompanied by high motivation when the employe's physiological and social needs have been satisfied, his egoistic needs have been activated but not satisfied, and his need for self-fulfillment on the job motivates him to perform well.

Low need satisfaction is usually accompanied by low motivation when physiological and social needs have been activated but not satisfied, and when the employe's egoistic needs have been activated but he feels his efforts are neither recognized nor appreciated. In such cases, the employe is usually discouraged from giving his best effort and only does enough to get by, yet keep his job.

High need satisfaction with low motivation occurs when the individual satisfies his needs off the job. There may be no motivation for him to perform on the job. The employe may also achieve need satisfaction by being a member of an informal cohesive group. The existence of this group might hamper the hospital achieving its goal of increased productivity. The individual who works hard at first and makes a favorable impression on his boss but then coasts doing just enough to get by is another example of an employe with high need satisfaction but low motivation. Some research indicates that a state of stress and tension encourages greater achievement. On the other hand, total satisfaction of needs may lead to contentment without initiative.

HIGH MOTIVATION

Low need satisfaction with high motivation often occurs when a worker is beginning a career. He is usually guided by goals set by his superiors and hopes to get ahead even though his physiological and social needs are not met. In addition, motivation may be high, even though needs are not satisfied, when unemployment is high. If the employe does not know where he can get another job, he may work hard to keep from being laid off. If physiological needs are being met during widespread unemployment, social and egoistic needs do not seem too important. Another case of low need satisfaction with high motivation occurs when the individual's need is not satisfied but he belongs to a cohesive group whose production goals are high. As a result, he is under constant pressure to conform to the expectations of his peers.

Need satisfaction, employe performance, and higher productivity all seem to be related to and supportive of each other. Reward is a key factor in improved performance and increased productivity. If an employe's improved performance is not recognized or rewarded, either monetarily, or non-monetarily, his need satisfaction could diminish. March and Simon[9] emphasize that the expected value of rewards determines the individual's satisfaction. The expected reward may raise his aspiration, which in turn may make him less satisfied with results.

In summary, the chances of motivating an employe to perform well and, thus, of contributing to higher productivity over a period of time are greater if:

1. Employes' physiological and social needs are generally satisfied.

2. Employes' egoistic needs are activated and fairly well-satisfied on a continuing basis, or

3. Employes' egoistic and self-fulfillment needs are not being satisfied, but they feel that their present progress will lead to such need satisfaction in the future.

PARTICIPATION

Because participative management seems to be an essential step in training for management by objectives, it would be well to consider some of the results of the research that has been done in this area. Advocates of power equalization favor the system of management by objectives because of the possibilities it holds for the exercise of participative management.

Douglas McGregor[10] said: "Genuine commitment is seldom achieved when objectives are externally imposed. Passive acceptance is the most that can be expected, indifference or resistance is the most likely consequence."

Likert[11] reports: "Where men are free to set their own pace, their department is probably higher producing than when closer supervision exists."

Kahn,[12] in a study of clerical operation, found that high goals and an enthusiastic supervisor who shows a lot of interest in his people lead to high productivity.

In the railroad industry Katz, Macoby, Gurin, and Floor[13] reported that high-producing foremen tended to ignore the mistakes of their men, whereas low-producing foremen punished them.

Vroom[14] feels that the effects of participation in decision-making depend upon certain personality characteristics of the participants. For example, independent people perform better when they have high participation. Highly authoritarian personalities, on the other hand, perform better when they do not participate but are simply told what to do, when to do it, and how to do it.

A valid conclusion is that neither tight nor loose supervision is the sole controlling variable, and that, of itself, participation cannot guarantee high productivity. There is some evidence that a strong orientation toward shared goal determination, coupled with leader enthusiasm and ample rewards for achieving goals, will unite people in a move toward greater productivity.

Participative management seems to have several advantages. This kind of management should be considered in the following situations:

1. When subordinates (for example, profes-

sional and scientific personnel) expect to participate. In such cases, it would be unproductive to bar participation.

2. When one member of the group proves to be habitually inattentive to his work, careless in his relations, or productive with foolish suggestions. His peer group can bring to bear on him organizational or cultural values, and his performance will tend to improve to meet expectations of his peers.

3. When a wide scope of ideas, especially those having social implications, is needed in making decisions in areas such as race relations, government and civic affairs, hiring the handicapped, etc.

Social scientists argue for universal participation on the grounds that it leads to increased productivity. Although their research data indicates that participative management probably does no harm, it is, nevertheless, somewhat biased. For example:

1. It is heavily weighted with values, such as power equalization and democracy-at-work, that are ethical and normative but not scientific.

2. It is heavily weighted with abstract ideas, such as Theory X or Theory Y, dictatorial versus permissive, autocratic versus participative management.

3. It relies on the power of generalizations. Results of studies conducted in laboratories at universities, insurance companies, etc., have been extrapolated to businesses, shops, hospitals, and the military.

It seems that, in general, most individuals can respond to the work situation and do a job well whether they participate or not. The employe can be paid for the job he does, based on his behavior, and still retain his own personal privacy and satisfy his own basic needs.

PERFORMANCE EVALUATION

What values should be included in managerial performance standards? The problem inherent in this question is how to set fair and accurate standards that do not result in conformity. Today, most appraisal systems in hospitals are based on standards that make it easy for a supervisor to fill out a checklist and use the results to force subordinates to conform.

In the past, appraisal systems have relied upon the following techniques and standards for performance.

1. Measuring a man against a list of personality traits. Research in this area indicates a degree of uncertainty as to what traits are necessary in a manager. It seems nearly impossible for the layman to identify, let alone apply, relative values to the traits against which he is supposed to rate his subordinates. Moreover, such rating cannot be done much better in a group evaluation than individually.

2. Sorting out a group of people according to their worth and ability and ranking them from highest to lowest. Again the standards used in this system, called the man-to-man technique, are unclear. In a medium or larger size group of employes such a ranking system can distinguish between only the very good and the very poor. It is difficult to help an employe improve when all that can be said is that he is not quite as good as Mr. Jones, but better than Mr. Smith. However, such ranking does have value in merit-rating and salary administration.

3. Using a master scale of managerial performance to describe the general characteristics required on a job and checking the performance of employes against the qualities listed. This system is somewhat arbitrary because the standards fluctuate with raters, and the system assumes that managers know what good performance for a manager is. It also relies on people who are not necessarily good managers to rate the managerial competence of others who may have real ability.

POTENTIAL VS. PERFORMANCE

4. Combining performance appraisal with potential in order to rate employes. This system tends to combine the two objectives, making neither evaluation very accurate. An employee's past performance is only one factor to be considered in analyzing potential value. Native

intelligence, aptitudes, interest, desires, availability, supply of candidates, and over-all personal inventory should also be considered. The danger of discussing potential and performance in the same evaluation is that the evaluation of potential may overshadow the urgent matter of improving present performance.

It seems clear that the appraisal problem can be solved by devising better performance standards for each job. A supervisor must sit down with each of his subordinates and discuss with him the conditions that should exist if the subordinate's job is to be done well. Together, they can develop objective performance standards. At the end of six months or a year, the mutually agreed-upon objectives can be reviewed and the results of the employee's performance can then be measured against the standards.

This procedure eliminates the confusion inherent in attempting to measure traits. It obviates the need for man-to-man rating, because each employee's work results are measured against his agreed-upon objectives. It eliminates the need to define the limits of good managerial ability and the need to measure potential. In addition, it simplifies the problem of counseling, because it involves factual work results rather than abstract ideas on the shortcomings of a human being.

Despite the many advantages of management by objectives, there are some limitations: 1. It does not appraise or completely identify potential, but deals instead only with performance on the present job. 2. It presumes that supervisors and their employes will work together to establish suitable goals that will serve the hospital. 3. It assumes that supervisors will accept the limits of their authority and refrain from "playing God." 4. It stresses results alone and does not provide for methods of achieving them.

Management by objectives attempts to create a climate conducive to achievement motivation, to goal-mindedness. The organization that uses this managerial system must provide opportunities for responsible behavior, for positive rewards, and positive interpersonal relations without undue fear of punishment. This sort of climate and this kind of supervision requires the hospital and all its members to become self-aware, to know themselves as individuals, and to understand their role in furthering organizational objectives. The system presupposes an effective, understandable procedure for identifying hospital goals; a meaningful technique for establishing personal goals; and a system for achieving personal and hospital goal interaction.

References

1. John Galbraith, *The Affluent Society,* Houghton Mifflin Company, Boston, 1958, p. 280.
2. Rensis Likert, "Measuring Organizational Performance," *Harvard Business Review,* March-April, 1958, pp. 41-50.
3. A. H. Maslow, *Motivation and Personality,* Harper and Brothers, New York, 1954, pp. 80-106.
4. Douglas McGregor, *The Human Side of Enterprise,* McGraw-Hill Book Co., New York, 1960, p. 36.
5. Chris Argyris, *Personality and Organization,* Harper & Row, Publishers, Inc., New York, 1957, pp. 49-53.
6. David C. McClelland, *The Achievement Motive,* Appleton-Century-Crofts, Inc., New York, 1953.
7. Rensis Likert, *New Patterns of Management,* McGraw-Hill Book Co., New York, 1961, chapter 8, pp. 97-106.
8. Frederick Herzberg, *Work and the Nature of Man,* the World Publishing Company, Cleveland, 1966.
9. James G. March and Herbert A. Simon, *Organizations,* John Wiley and Sons, Inc., New York, 1958, p. 49.
10. Douglas McGregor, *op. cit.*
11. Rensis Likert, *New Patterns of Management,* McGraw-Hill Book Co., New York, 1961.
12. D. Katz and R. Kahn, "Leadership Practices in Relation to Productivity and Morale," in D. Cartwright and A. Zander (Eds.), *Group Dynamics Research Theory,* New York, Harper & Row, 1968, p. 301.
13. Daniel Katz, N. Macoby, G. Gurin, and L. Floor, *Productivity, Supervision, and Morale Among Railroad Workers,* The University of Michigan Press, 1951.
14. Victor Vroom, *Work and Motivation,* John Wiley and Sons, Inc., New York, 1964, pp. 181-185.

Motivation in task-oriented groups

AMARJIT CHOPRA, B.Sc., S.B.

Over the past eleven years we have studied several thousand managers, supervisors, and their subordinates. Our purpose in studying such groups was to learn about what makes some of them more successful than others in accomplishing what they set out to do.* Not surprisingly, a characteristic of the more successful groups was their high degree of motivation, which was evident in their enthusiasm and high level of interest and commitment. What was surprising was that the nature of the task did not seem to affect this motivation to any great extent. Rather, the members of such groups were motivated to *work with each other*. They seemed to find working with each other to be enough of a satisfying experience and they were willing and able to tackle almost any problem.

How well a group functions in a given setting is influenced by many things, including the hierarchial relationships that exist within it and the organizational climate in which they work. By themselves, however, these factors are not sufficient to explain what makes one group function more effectively than another. A team from an organization considered to have low morale and a poor working climate may work well together. A group from a company thought to have good working conditions and organizational climate may not be able to function together at all. Also, it does not seem to be necessary for a group to have worked with each other for any given length of time to perform successfully as a team. A group of persons who have

never worked with each other before can develop into an effective team at their very first meeting. And this is true of individuals from any organization, whether it be industrial, government, hospital, or educational.

Our observations lead us to believe that a factor which *is* critical to the success of any group is the way in which the members *interact* with each other. Especially important is the way the manager or other person with the most authority behaves toward the others in the group.

THE ANATOMY OF INTERACTIONS

Most persons are not fully aware, at a conscious level, of how they interact with others—why, for example, they respond as they do in a given instance or what effect their response might have on another person. This is understandable, since most of us tend to concentrate on the problem or task we happen to be working on and not on *how* we go about it. When asked, managers and supervisors of successful teams find it difficult to explain just what it is they do that seems to work; they just do it "naturally." Much of our work has been aimed at finding out which of the things the members do naturally help the group, as well as what they do that hinders the group.

One of the basic tools in this research has been the tape recorder; audiotape when we first started and, more recently, videotape. The tapes provide a complete and accurate record of what goes on; they make it possible to look closely at the various interactions between group members and to study the effects of these interactions on the group's motivation and ability to accomplish its task.

To study interactions in a controlled way, we devised an experiment in which the group is

---

Reprinted with permission from *The Journal of Nursing Administration,* January-February, 1973.

*We define a group simply as two or more persons; for example, a supervisor and one or more subordinates. Most of the groups we work with consist of four to ten individuals.

given a "standard" problem to work on and is asked to develop one or more workable solutions within a given time limit.[1] The group's discussion is taped, and the time limit is varied from fifteen minutes to several hours. We have also varied the make-up of the groups, from individuals who have worked together for years to individuals who have just met. The group's membership has included high school dropouts, corporation presidents, blue collar workers, doctors, nurses, and scientists. At times the groups have known that they were being taped while in other instances they have not known. Regardless of these variations, a number of observations were consistent.

Some basic observations

What the tapes reveal is interesting. There are about seven basic ideas for solving the standard problem, and most groups will bring up two or more of these ideas during their discussion. Roughly one in ten groups will take these ideas and develop them into workable solutions. These are the successful and motivated groups. The other nine, starting with the same ideas, will somehow "lose them in the shuffle." The difference thus does not lie in a lack of ideas in some groups as compared to others. It lies in how the individuals treat each other's ideas.

For example, one person will bring up an idea. Most ideas are not born fully developed, however. They need considerable attention and work before they can be considered even partially feasible as solutions. In a motivated group the idea will get this attention and work. Other group members will spend a lot of time and energy trying to fully understand the idea, exploring its implications and suggesting ways to overcome its limitations. In other words, members of the group work *with* the person who offered the idea and try to help him or her strengthen it. This kind of behavior, reasonable as it may sound, is not common. More typically, as soon as the idea is brought up, other

group members will begin to devote their talents to finding reasons why it will not work. This is justified later by the group members as realism. After all, ideas need to be evaluated; what better way to do this than to point out the flaws in it so that the group can go on to something else? At first glance, this seems to be a reasonable approach to take, one that would help the group to accomplish its task. It was only by contrast to the behavior observed in the successful groups that we began to question this assumption. And, we asked ourselves, if looking for and pointing out flaws in each other's ideas *does not* serve the group's task objective but is still a widely observed behavior, what other purpose might it serve? We began to take a closer look at the tapes.

More than one objective

Before they have looked at their own tapes, most individuals believe that they spend most if not all of their time and energy working on the stated purpose of the group—to solve a problem, for example, or to decide on a course of action. The tapes, however, show that this is true only for the roughly one in ten successful and motivated groups. The other nine groups spend much more time on something else.

Here is a sequence we have observed over and over. A offers an idea. Group member B points out why it won't work. A seems to accept this judgment, at least outwardly. A few minutes later B will make a suggestion. A will immediately start raising objections to it and will display considerable satisfaction if he manages to dispose of it.

There are many variations on this theme. A may bring up his idea several times before he is persuaded to drop it. And, if B happens to be the supervisor or boss, A will be much more careful in his attempts to dispose of B's ideas. Or, instead of retaliating, A may just drop out of the discussion. The remarkable thing is the degree of talent individuals can bring to this kind of interaction; they often display considerable ingenuity in inventing reasons why someone else's idea will not work. This suggests that it is not that the individuals in most groups are not motivated. Rather, it's a question of *what* they are motivated to work on—the group's common goal, or some other, personal objective.

One personal objective that can divert a great deal of a person's energy has to do with the strong emotional investment each of us has in his own work or ideas. Our ideas are an extension of ourselves, a reflection of our worth as individuals. To a considerable extent, we depend on the reactions of other persons to form a picture of who we are. These reactions form a kind of mirror—a changing, often distorted mirror—in which we view ourselves. A part of this image consists of reactions to our external selves, our physical appearance. To complete the picture, we also need feedback about the other things that make up our total worth, such as our minds and egos. And this comes from reactions to what we say or do.

The shift from one objective to the other

Because we see our work and ideas as extensions of ourselves, a response to what we have done or suggested carries a dual message. One message conveys information about the problem or decision we happen to be working on, the other message tells us something about ourselves. And if we perceive that our worth is being called into question, we will begin to devote our talents and energies to protecting and defending ourselves. Our motivation shifts allegiance, from the group's task objective to the personal objective. This shift can be triggered by relatively small stimuli—an interruption in the middle of explaining a point of view, or being told, for the third time, that an idea is "no good."

The ability to detect and react to such seemingly small stimuli is not limited to a few unduly sensitive individuals. Although the in-

tensity of the reaction may vary widely, from losing one's temper to raising an eyebrow, the ability to pick up the signal and respond to it seems to be universal. Most individuals, however, tend to deny that they own such sensitive antennae until they themselves see the evidence on the tapes. When asked, for example, whether having an idea shot down caused any reaction, an individual is likely to say, "Oh no, that didn't really bother me. It's just part of the normal give and take between people," or, "Well, we're all grownups here. Wouldn't last long if I let that kind of thing get to me." Somehow, letting "something like that" bother us is inconsistent with the image we like to have of ourselves as mature adults in full control of our actions. Indeed, to some extent, learning *not* to let too many things upset our equilibrium serves a useful purpose. It keeps us from being overwhelmed by the signals we are constantly bombarded with and it prevents us from reacting to the point of not being able to function in everyday situations. This is not all there is to it, however. We may learn to control our reactions to the point at which they are not obvious to others or even to ourselves. This does not mean that we have stopped detecting signals and reacting to them; the activity merely goes underground and continues to operate at a level below that of conscious awareness. Without being fully aware of it, we find sophisticated ways to make our reactions appear reasonable. In group after group, one can observe subtle and not so subtle forms of retaliation, withdrawal, and defensive behavior taking up the greater part of the available talent and energy.

Here is an example from one of our tapes: Two members of a group, Jim and Nancy, seem to have been engaged in a little contest of "who can shoot down the other's idea faster." Jim has been getting the better of it. He has managed to dispose of three of Nancy's ideas in quick succession, and Nancy has not taken part in the conversation for several minutes. At this point on the tape, Jim is proposing an idea and he appears to be winning the support of the group. Nancy chooses this moment to interrupt and point out to the group that they have not been following the procedure they had agreed on at the start of their meeting. They have not decided who should be taking notes and keeping track of time. This move diverts the group for the next five minutes or so, and by the time they decide that they don't really need a note taker, there no longer is much interest in Jim's idea.

In reviewing the tape, both Jim and Nancy were quick to see what had been going on, got a good chuckle out of it, and even complimented each other on the ingeniousness of their tactics. But both of them explained that during the meeting itself they had not been aware of their contest. Each of them felt, at the time, that they were genuinely trying to help the group accomplish this task. This is true in general. Except for rare instances, a person's conscious intent, when working with others, is to help get the job done. Group members do not actively set out to undermine each other's work and ideas, but because they are not aware of the great deal of investment they and others have in their ideas, they inadvertently send out messages that can trigger a reaction in others. When the other person reacts, again without being aware of having done so, it will most likely cause a counterreaction, and the game is on. The energy of the group members involved begins to be diverted away from their common task; their motivational allegiance shifts. This process, once started, is difficult to stop. It builds in a subtle chain reaction, and the usual result is a failure to accomplish the task as well as a feeling of frustration on the part of group members.

SOME ALTERNATIVES

Becoming aware of how individuals react does not, by itself, tell a supervisor what to do to motivate the persons he or she works with. The awareness is important, but only as a first step toward understanding behavior in every-day situations. What is also needed are alternative ways of interacting that can satisfy *both* the personal and the task objective. Without these alternatives, an awareness of what goes on can pose a problem for supervisors and managers. For example, a question that is often voiced is:

> But I have a job to get done. If someone is not doing proper work or makes an impractical suggestion, what am I supposed to do—worry about how the person might react or make sure the work gets done right?

This question reflects a real concern about the possible conflict between the two parts of a manager's responsibility, his people versus the job that has to be done. Fortunately this team versus task dilemma is more apparent than real, and this became clear as we studied the tapes of the more successful groups. We were able to identify the kinds of interactions that not only increased the group's probability of accomplishing the task, but also spoke to the investment the members had in their ideas and opinions.

Listening

One difference between successful and less successful groups has to do with the way group members listen to each other. In the more successful groups, there is a very high frequency of statements that indicate, first of all, a *willingness* to listen. We heard statements such as: "Jim, I think you were about to say something," or, "That sounds interesting, say some more about it."

The group members also spend a considerable amount of time trying to make certain that they understand each other. Fairly frequent are remarks such as: "I'm not sure I understand. Could you go over that again?" or, "If I hear you right, Claire, you mean that . . . ?" or, "What you're saying then is . . . is that right?"

Willingness to listen and understand increases the group's probability of success because it facilitates the flow of information among team members and it provides a check on the accuracy with which it has been received. It ensures that ideas and points of view have been understood *before* they are evaluated or otherwise acted upon. Further, it speaks to the personal investment aspect of ideas.When a person indicates a willingness to listen, he automatically sends out another message to the speaker. The message is "I wouldn't be interested in listening to you if I didn't think what you have to say is going to be of some value to me and the group." By its very nature, the act of listening reflects an image that values the other person.

Indicating a willingness to listen and checking one's understanding seems to be a simple matter, but it is something that can be extremely difficult to practice. Carl Rogers has described the many barriers that prevent us from listening with understanding.[2] A major barrier is our tendency to judge or evaluate what another person is saying *before* we fully understand him. This is especially true in situations in which our immediate impulse is to disagree with the other person. Often, a word or gesture can lead us to think that we know what the other person means, even before he or she has finished speaking. We read a meaning or intent behind a statement and react without checking it out with the speaker. It is surprising, when you do check, how often the other person really has something quite different in mind.

What seems to help members of successful groups to overcome these barriers is the basic assumption they are willing to make about each other. They are willing to assume that what the others have to say is somehow going to be useful, that they will get a fresh point of view or receive information that is going to help solve the problem at hand. Again, this is not an easy assumption to make. It seems that an individual needs to feel fairly secure about himself before he can assume value in others.

Evaluating work and ideas

Another noticeable difference between motivated and nonmotivated groups is the way in which the team members evaluate each other's work and ideas. In the more successful groups, both the advantages and the disadvantages of what someone has done or suggested are carefully examined. By recognizing and separating the useful elements in an idea from its potential drawbacks, for example, the team members are able to modify it so as to retain the advantages and eliminate the disadvantages. This is the process used by the successful groups in our experiment with a standard problem. As mentioned earlier, there are about seven basic ideas for solving the problem, and two or more of these ideas come up in almost every group's discussion. By carefully examining the advantages and disadvantages of these ideas, the successful groups are able to develop them into workable solutions. This is not, however, what happens in most groups. There is a much greater tendency to focus exclusively on the negative aspects of work and ideas. For many managers as well as their team members, evaluation or criticism seems to be synonymous with pointing out *only* what a person has done wrong or why his idea will not work. This may be because the negative elements are a source of anxiety; they seem to draw our attention and hold it so that we overlook or ignore the positive elements.

This kind of one-sided evaluation has consequences. First of all, the potentially useful parts of ideas get rejected along with the parts that might have caused problems. And, in criticizing someone's work, focussing exclusively on his mistakes does not provide the person with all of the information he needs to improve his performance. It tells him what he did wrong and therefore what to change, but it does not tell him what *not* to change—the portion of his work that he performed correctly or well. As a result, he may try to correct not only the mistake but also what he has been doing right.

Pointing out only the negative aspects of what a person has said or done also has motivational consequences. Not recognizing the useful aspects devalues the investment that he has in his work and ideas and is likely to trigger a defensive reaction on his part. He will be more concerned with protecting his investment than with learning from the evaluation.

An evaluation technique

The tendency to focus exclusively on the negative elements in our evaluation of a person's work or ideas appears to be a strong one in most of us. To counteract this tendency, we have formalized what successful groups do "naturally" into a technique that can be applied consciously. We call this technique the Itemized Response. It calls for the user to concentrate first on what might be *useful* in a person's work or idea, and to begin his evaluation by itemizing the merits he sees. Only after he has done this can he go on to list the negative elements. In addition, both the plus and the minus elements must be *specific*. Statements such as "yes, that's a good idea" or "no, that won't work" do not qualify. To qualify, the statement must explain clearly each advantage or disadvantage.

The Itemized Response is designed to provide complete information, to tell the complete truth about an idea or a piece of work. Because it specifies the useful elements along with the disadvantages, it is less likely to be perceived by the other person as a devaluation of his worth as an individual. If you are thorough in pointing out the merits in a person's idea, it becomes unnecessary for him to spend time and energy doing so. It is important to keep in mind that in order to get results from the Itemized Response, both from a task as well as a motivational point of view, the positive elements must consist of real task benefits. If the positive is merely "something nice to say before you let him have it," the technique will backfire, since most individuals are quite capable of picking up the real message ("I really don't think much of your idea"). More likely, the other person will perceive it as an attempt to manipulate him and will resent it. Also, an Itemized Response in which the positive or negative elements are not genuinely task related may provide confusing or conflicting information and reduce the probability of successful task completion.

In summary, the basic characteristics of the Itemized Response are as follows:

- it includes *both* positive and negative elements;
- the elements are *specific* rather than general;
- both positive and negative elements are *task related;*
- the positives *precedes* the negatives.

The characteristics listed above can be used as a mental checklist in responding to someone's work or idea. The Itemized Response, however, is more than just a verbal skill that requires the user to make his response fit a given pattern. It reflects a certain mental set on the part of the user; a mental set in which the user expects to find something of value in other people's work and ideas.

A question that is often asked about the use of the Itemized Response is: "But what if I can't find anything useful in what one of my people has done or proposed?" There are indeed times when it is very difficult to see any merit in someone's work or idea. In most cases, however, this is not because there actually is no merit, but because there is a negative that is causing so much concern that it is difficult to see beyond it. It is usually helpful in these cases to check your understanding, to make sure that you understand the other person's reasons for doing or suggesting what he did. It also helps to make a mental note of the negatives you are seeing and to reassure yourself that you are not going to forget to itemize them. This makes it easier, for the time being, to concentrate on the search for the useful elements. There will still be times when you either cannot find something useful or do not want to take the time and effort to do so. No one such instance, by itself, will greatly affect the task or someone's motivation. The overall effect depends on the relative frequency with which this occurs; for example, the relative frequency with which a supervisor either does or does not itemize his response to the work and ideas of the members of his work team. This does not mean that the supervisor should not make a conscious effort in each case, especially when he or she first begins to practice the technique. The tendency to focus on the negative is not easy to overcome. It constitutes a mental set or thinking habit, and like most habits it requires work to change it. Because it does require work, it is often tempting to think of exceptional situations in which this work may not be necessary. One such situation is when one is dealing with persons one knows well. The thought here is ''But I've worked with Jane for a long time. We understand and respect each other; surely I don't need to be formal with her.'' In this kind of situation, we recommend the following: The next time Jane makes a suggestion, go through a private Itemized Response in your own head to make sure that *you* don't overlook any useful elements. Then make a conscious decision, if you want, to *not* tell her about the plusses you see and itemize only the negatives, being fully aware of the effect this might have on Jane's investment in her idea.

CONCLUSION

Listening with understanding and using the Itemized Response are perhaps the two most important of the many factors that contribute to the degree of motivation and success of a group. In the groups we have observed, the most successful ones invariably exhibit a high proportion of interactions that involve listening and careful evaluation. At the same time, fewer symptoms are observed that would indicate that group members have shifted away from their task objective. If a group member does begin to be defensive about his or her idea, an Itemized Response from another team member appears to shift the person's energy back to the task. Few ideas are lost. Instead of being prematurely rejected, ideas tend to become developed into workable alternatives. In addition to being motivated to work on the group's task during the discussion, the members of successful groups also seem to be more committed to implementing the solutions or decisions that were the outcome of their discussion. We believe this happens as follows: When members of the group do not have to spend time defending their ideas or trying to be heard, they tend to use this energy more constructively. They begin to build on the useful components of the thoughts and suggestions of other members. As a result, each team member is likely to feel that a portion of his or her idea is a part of the outcome, that his or her ideas are *included* in any course of action that might have been arrived at as a result of the discussion. This is the case even though in most instances the final decision as to what is acceptable is not made by the group, but by one person, usually the manager or other person with the most authority in the group.

Whether in a formal group setting or in an informal discussion between a supervisor and one or more subordinates, the outcome of the discussion is influenced to a considerable extent by the supervisor's behavior. The supervisor, because of the power that goes with his or her position, has a greater influence on the team than any other member. Other members tend to model their behavior after that of the supervisor. And, the supervisor's feedback has a greater impact on a person's perception of his self-worth and therefore on whether or not that person will shift his motivational allegiance from the group's task to some other, personal objective.

References

1. Prince, G. M. *The Practice of Creativity*. New York: Harper and Row, 1970, pp. 12-27.
2. Rogers, C. *On Becoming a Person*. Boston: Houghton Mifflin, 1970, pp. 329-337.

Types and sources of conflict

ALAN C. FILLEY, Ph.D.

As humans we live our lives within a web of social relationships, most of which seem almost mechanical in their predictability and smoothness of function. We seek, establish, and maintain predictable patterns in our lives to avoid the anxiety of the unpredictable; such patterns, once established, require little conscious choice as they operate. We have predictable patterns for interacting with our family, for going to work in the morning, for performing in a job, for shopping at the market, and for socializing with others. Yet, because we are not solely mechanical, because we are social creatures in a social system, these patterns are not absolutely predictable.

We must also reckon with the elements of chance. While we can predict the movement of the solar system with relative certainty, we can only speak of the likelihood or probability of driving to work or of greeting the guard at the entrance. An accident or illness may have occurred to alter our usual routines. Finally, as human animals, we introduce a third element into our social systems, that of freedom (Boulding, 1964). We are capable of planning, of holding in our minds some picture of the future, and of altering our usual patterns of behavior.

Within our various social relationships are some which involve real or perceived differences between two or more parties. Where the interests of the parties are mutually exclusive — that is, where the gain of one party's goal is at the cost of the other's, or where the parties have different values — then the resulting social interaction between the parties contains fertile ground for conflict.

It is our freedom which allows us to learn

about our own social systems. We are able (1) to discover those elements of our systems which increase the likelihood of conflict, (2) to develop contingency plans when chance occurrences create disruptions, and (3) to produce and to improve systems for resolving conflict which maximize the benefits and minimize the costs to the parties involved. In this first chapter we shall be concerned with those characteristics of a system which increase the likelihood of conflict and with the system of conflict production. Such discussion permits us to organize in ways which minimize conflict, if that is the desired goal. Furthermore, by knowing the natural system of conflict production, we may adjust actions or conditions before conflicts take place, rather than wait for conflicts to develop before taking action.

In later chapters we shall focus on the conflict resolution process. Either because it may not be useful to avoid conflicts or because conflict develops as an unanticipated outcome, the resolution of conflict becomes necessary. We shall examine the various systems of resolution and suggest how they may be applied.

KINDS OF CONFLICT

Not all conflicts are of the same kind. Some, for example, follow definite rules and are not typically associated with angry feelings on the part of the parties, while others involve irrational behavior and the use of violent or disruptive acts by the parties. As a first step, therefore, we shall distinguish between conflicts which are *competitive* and those which are *disruptive*. In competitive situations there can be a victory for one party only at the cost of the opponent's total loss and the way in which the parties relate to each other is governed by a set of rules. The parties strive for goals which are mutually incompatible. The emphasis of each party is upon the event of winning, rather than upon the defeat or reduction of the opponent. The actions of each party are selected using criteria based on the probability of leading to successful outcomes, and the competition terminates when the result is obvious to both sides (Rapoport, 1960).

In the disruptive conflict, on the other hand, the parties do not follow a mutually acceptable set of rules and are not primarily concerned with winning. Instead, they are intent upon reducing, defeating, harming, or driving away the opponent. The means used are expedient, and the atmosphere is one of stress, anger or fear. In extreme cases, the parties in disruptive conflict will abandon rational behavior and behave in any manner necessary to bring about the desired outcome, the goal of defeat.

Experience tells us that conflicts are usually distributed along a continuum between those that are competitive and those that are disruptive. Anger arises in a game and causes disruption. A competitor changes his behavior from a rational pursuit of a stragety of winning to an irrational act of aggression. Thus, the motives of the parties and the degree of strategic control which each exhibits are important factors in determining the degree to which a conflict is competitive or disruptive.

For a further elaboration of the kinds of conflict, we may describe the interaction between the parties according to (1) their mutuality of interests and (2) their perception of resource availability. As seen in Table 1-1, when parties seek real or perceived scarce resources (for example, victory or a share of a fixed sum) and when they have a mutuality of interests, the relationship is one of competition. When they seek real or perceived scarce resources and have unlike interests, their relationship is likely to be characterized by fighting and disruption. When the parties seek abundant resources but have dissimilar interests, their interaction will contain disagreement. Finally, when the parties seek abundant resources and have similar interests, they will most probably resort to problem solving.

Competition, disruption, and disagreement all imply a win-lose outcome (or at least some degree of winning or losing by each of the parties). Problem solving, on the other hand, implies the development of an outcome which provides acceptable gain to both parties. Thus, if the focus of competition changes from a win-lose game to a situation involving enhancement of skill or knowledge by the parties, it becomes problem solving since the parties are now, in effect, asking each other, "How can we interact in a manner which increases the benefit to both of us?" Likewise, if opposing parties in a fight realize the mutuality of their interests and the existence of abundant resources or if debaters change their emphasis from argument to the achievement of a correct solution, then their interactions will also shift to a problem-solving mode.

The point in this classification scheme is that conflict has been defined in terms of incompatible goals and different values, but that such differences are frequently *perceived rather than real*. If opposing parties can change their perceptions of resources from scarce to abundant and can recognize the mutuality of their interests, it is often possible to change from a form of conflict to a form of problem solving.

We may summarize the characteristics of a conflict situation as follows:

1) At least two parties (individuals or groups) are involved in some kind of interaction.

Table 1-1. Elements of conflict

	Like interests	Unlike interests
Seek scarce resources	Competition/ games	Fights/disruption
Seek abundant resources	Problem solving	Disagreement/debate

2) Mutually exclusive goals and/or mutually exclusive values exist, in fact or as perceived by the parties involved.

3) Interaction is characterized by behavior designed to defeat, reduce, or suppress the opponent or to gain a mutually designated victory.

4) The parties face each other with mutually opposing actions and counteractions.

5) Each party attempts to create an imbalance or relatively favored position of power vis-à-vis the other.

THE VALUES OF CONFLICT

Conflict, a social process which takes various forms and which has certain outcomes, itself is neither good nor bad. The conflict process merely leads to certain results, and the value of those results as favorable or unfavorable depends upon the measures used, the party making the judgment, and other subjective criteria. Let us consider some of the possible positive values of conflict:

The diffusion of more serious conflict

Competitive situations such as games provide conflict processes and outcomes which are governed by rules. These types of conflict seem to provide entertainment value and tension release to the parties. Winning and losing are identified as events and may have little effect on the self-perception of any player. That is, to lose in a competitive event does not suggest that an individual is less important, has less status, or is less valued as a person. In addition, in competitive situations aggressive behavior can be channeled along socially acceptable lines.

Viewed another way, conflict processes which are institutionalized (that is, for which acceptable resolution procedures have been established) function as preventive measures against more destructive outcomes. Grievance systems, for example, permit the step-by-step adjudication of differences to avoid major clashes between parties such as labor and management. Similarly, systems which provide for participation by the members of an organization in decision making, while they are positively associated with the number of disuutes between parties, are negatively associated with the number of major incidents between them (Corwin, 1969). Thus, it might be accurate to say that intimacy between parties tends to result in disagreements which, in turn, reduce the likelihood of major fights and disruption.

The stimulation of a search for new facts or solutions

As pointed out earlier, at least some aspects of our social systems are automatic and predictable. Where social systems are functioning mechanically, however, there is little likelihood of creativity or change. On the other hand, when parties are involved in a disagreement the process may lead to a clarification of facts, thus facilitating the resolution of conflict. For example, if a wife tells her husband, "You are not doing your share of the housework," and the husband replies, "Yes, I am," then little may be resolved. However, if the husband replies, "What statements or behavior of mine have led to your conclusion that I am not assuming enough responsibility at home?" then the interaction is changed from a conflict to a problem-solving situation based on clarification of facts.

In another way, conflict can stimulate the search for new methods or solutions. When parties are in conflict about which of two alternatives to accept, their disagreement may stimulate a search for another solution mutually acceptable to both. In like manner, when both parties view themselves as seeking to gain an adequate share of scarce resources, they may actually find that their needs or goals can be met simultaneously with the development of creative solutions which neither had previously considered.

As these situations suggest, conflict can create tension which is reduced through problem solving. The tension acts as a stimulus to find new methods for its own reduction. This is the difference between *confrontation* and the way in which confrontation is resolved. The confrontations between labor and management, between students and college administrators, or between blacks and whites act as stimuli for change, stimuli which may lead to disruption or overt hostility or which may lead to new relationships between the parties and creative solutions to problems.

An increase in group cohesion and performance

Conflictive situations between two or more groups are likely to increase both the cohesiveness and the performance of the groups, although we must be careful to distinguish between effects during the conflict and those after the winner and loser have been identified. During the conflict members of each group close ranks and are united in their efforts. Members' evaluations of their own group improve (Blake and Mouton, 1961c); and each group judges its own solution as best. The positions of opponents are evaluated negatively, and there is little effort to understand them. Questions asked opponents are designed to embarrass or to weaken them rather than to generate facts and understanding. Perceptions of the group's own position are distorted, as is recognition of areas of common agreement with the opposing group. Even when the adversary's position is thought to be well understood by members of one group, research has shown that a real understanding is blocked by identification with the position of one's own group. In these circumstances intergroup resolution of conflict increases in difficulty since groups are most likely unaware of the distortions in factual knowledge that exist between them (Blake and Mouton, 1961a).

During the competitive period, levels of work and cooperation within each group are high. When competing groups select representatives to deal with other groups, they choose task leaders (hard-driving individuals who keep their own group on course) rather than individuals skilled in social facilitation. During conflict such leaders exhibit high loyalty to their group and tend to conform to group expectations rather than to focus upon the assigned problem (Blake and Mouton, 1961b).

Such conditions appear to be desirable, for the most part, and probably account for the popular belief that competition is valuable as a stimulus to work groups. But what actually happens when one group is declared the victor and the other the vanquished? For one thing, the leader of the winning group increases in status, while the leader of the losing group decreases in status. The leader in the losing group is blamed for the loss. The atmosphere in the groups also changes. The rate of tension, problem avoidance, fighting, and competitive feelings will increase in the losing group and decrease in the winning group. If the loss can be blamed on conditions beyond the control of the group, the result may be increased cohesion in the losing group (Lott and Lott, 1965). If the group does assume responsibility for the loss, it often analyzes the situation and prepares itself to fight better the next time. In contrast, the winning group merely says, "We did a good job. Let's knock off" (Blake and Mouton, 1961c, p. 432). Thus, heightened cooperation and effort by group members during the conflict may actually decrease once the conflict is resolved.

The measure of power or ability

Conflict provides a readily available method of measurement. If the ground rules for victory or defeat are identifiable to both parties, then the winner of a game or sports event can be easily determined. Such literal interpretation has cognitive value. In addition, while not precisely measurable, the relative power between parties may be identified through conflictive situations. Coercion, control, and suppression require clear superiority of power of one party over another, whereas problem solving requires an equalization of power among the parties. Thus, a party wishing to avoid overt suppression of the opponent must take action to provide a favorable power balance; suppression of the opponent can be avoided by employing problem-solving methods which insure a balance of power.

From the preceding discussion it should be clear that conflict is a process which itself is neither good nor bad, but which has elements and outcomes which may be judged favorably or unfavorably by those participating in or evaluating it. We shall now turn to the conflict process itself.

THE CONFLICT PROCESS

Conflict is defined in this book as a process which takes place between two or more parties.[1] By *parties* we may be referring to individuals, groups, or organizations. The six steps in the process are depicted in Figure 1-1.

1) Antecedent conditions are the characteristics of a situation which generally lead to conflict, although they may be present in the absence of conflict as well.
2) Perceived conflict is a logically and impersonally recognized set of conditions which are conflictive to the parties.
3) Felt conflict is a personalized conflict relationship, expressed in feelings of threat, hostility, fear, or mistrust.
4) Manifest behavior is the resulting action — aggression, competition, debate, or problem solving.
5) Conflict resolution or suppression has to do with bringing the conflict to an end either through agreement among all parties or the defeat of one.

---

[1]This section draws from the work of Pondy (1967, 1969); Corwin (1969); Walton and Dutton (1969); Fink (1968); and Schmidt (1973).

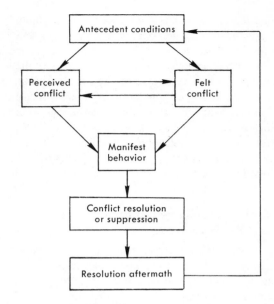

Figure 1. The conflict process.

6) Resolution aftermath comprises the consequences of the conflict.

We shall now consider each part of the conflict process in more detail. An understanding of the factors that lead to conflict is necessary if its occurrence is to be minimized.

THE ANTECEDENT CONDITIONS OF CONFLICT

Listed below are nine characteristics of social relationships that are associated with various kinds or degrees of conflictive behavior.

1) *Ambiguous jurisdictions.* Conflict will be greater when the limits of each party's jurisdiction are ambiguous. When two parties have related responsibilities for which actual boundaries are unclear, the potential for conflict between them increases. Conversely, when role definitions are clear, each party can expect a certain type of behavior from the other, and fewer opportunities for disagreement occur. For example, the argument of a married couple about who should make decisions relating to

household chores or the selection of evening entertainment was resolved by an agreement that on alternate days one of them would make all decisions and would be responsible for the success or failure of the decisions. On a more complex level, large organizations will define boundaries of individual responsibility through such tools as organization charts and job descriptions.

2) *Conflict of interest.* Conflict will be greater where a conflict of interest exists between the parties. One such situation is a competition for scarce resources. For example, one summer a married couple found themselves arguing about the use of the only air-conditioned room in their apartment, which also contained the television set. The woman was attending graduate school and the man was working; in the evening he wanted to watch the baseball games on television and she wanted to use the room for study, complaining that the noise of the television prevented her from concentrating. Another situation involves a case where the gain of one group is at the expense of another group. For example, Walton, Dutton, and Cafferty (1969) describe such an incident in which a maintenance department is evaluated on the basis of equipment performance. However, the equipment performance in a department served by maintenance is not part of the maintenance evaluation. The second department makes demands upon maintenance to increase its own performance record but in so doing reduces the rating of the maintenance department by interfering with the repair of other equipment.

3) *Communication barriers.* Conflict will be greater when barriers to communication exist. It appears that if parties are separated from each other physically or by time—for example, day shift versus night shift—the opportunity for conflict is increased. One explanation for this is the increased possibility of misunderstanding between the parties. Yet, as will be discussed shortly, the degree of knowledge which one party has about another is shown to be asso-

ciated with conflict (Walton, Dutton, and Cafferty, 1969). It seems more likely that space or time separations create natural groupings which promote separate group interests rather than advance a common effort toward joint goals.

4) *Dependence of one party.* Conflict will be greater where one party is dependent upon another. Where parties are dependent, they must rely on each other for performance of tasks or for the provision of resources. Thus, the opportunity for conflict to occur is increased. For example, a supervisor who depends upon the preparation of a cost effectiveness report by a subordinate in order to make a marketing decision may monitor the subordinate's progress. Closer supervision in itself contributes to the potential for conflict between the parties, as does their dependence upon each other.

5) *Differentiation in organization.* Conflict will be greater as the degree of differentiation in an organization increases. Where people work together in complex organizations, there is evidence (Corwin, 1969) that measures of conflict are related to the number of organizational levels, the number of distinct job specialties represented, and the degree to which labor is divided in the organization. The reasons may well relate to conditions already discussed. For example, the number of levels of authority may create difficulties of communication, conflicts of interest, difficult dependency situations, or jurisdictional disputes. In any case, the greater the degree of differentiation, the greater the potential for conflict.

6) *Association of the parties.* Conflict will be greater as the degree of association of the parties increases. *Degree of association,* as used here, refers both to the parties' participation in decision making and to informal relations between them. Where parties make decisions jointly, the opportunity for conflict is greater, which may explain the reluctance of some managers to involve others in decision

making. However, since groups often make superior decisions, the failure to utilize the potential of groups in decision making may be costly in terms of inferior judgments as well as in terms of employee dissatisfaction. An alternative logic would suggest that where participative decision making is used, the parties will need skills in conflict resolution. General conflict measures are positively associated with the degree of participation, although major incidents of conflict decrease as participation increases (Corwin, 1969).

The above holds true for informal association as well. Interaction and the degree of knowledge which parties have about each other are also related to rates of conflict.

7) *Need for consensus.* Conflict will be greater where consensus between the parties is necessary. When all parties must agree on a decision, at least to the point that no individual feels the decision is unacceptable, it is not surprising that disagreements will occur. Thus, it is possible to avoid conflict by having mechanisms such as voting, coin flipping, or adjudication to make decisions without the confrontation of consensus. As we shall see later, however, such mechanisms themselves are not without undesirable consequences.

8) *Behavior regulations.* Conflicts will be greater where behavior regulations are imposed. Regulating mechanisms include standardized procedures, rules, and policies. Regulating mechanisms seem to do two things at the same time. On the one hand, they reduce the likelihood of conflict since they serve to make relationships predictable and reduce the need to make arbitrary decisions. On the other hand, they increase the degree of control over parties, and this control may be resisted. If the adherence to or the imposition of rules becomes discretionary, further sources of disagreement are created. Furthermore, if the parties have high individual needs for autonomy and self-control, it is likely that the presence of regulating procedures will lead to conflict.

9) *Unresolved prior conflicts.* Conflicts will

be greater as the number of unresolved prior conflicts increases. As will be discussed later, the type of conflict resolution utilized will affect the resolution aftermath. Thus, prior experiences of the parties will themselves create antecedent conditions. Suppression of conflict by the use of power, or compromises to which the parties are uncommitted, create conditions and expectations which may lead to behavior conducive to further conflict.

The antecedent conditions need not lead directly to conflict, but they are certainly conditions which create opportunities for conflict to arise. Further development of overt conflict depends upon the perception of conditions which exist and the attitudinal characteristics of the parties.

PERCEIVED CONFLICT

Perceptions of the conditions which exist between the parties may enhance the likelihood of conflict or may reduce it. The failure to identify potentially conflictive conditions may prevent conflicts from developing. In many cases, however, it is the inaccurate or illogical perception of the situation which leads to overt conflict between the parties. Perceptual processes contribute to conflict in two ways. First, they provide an accurate or inaccurate assessment of the conditions which exist. This occurs when, for example, clear jurisdictions are perceived as ambiguous or when similar interests are perceived as conflicting. Second, they affect the extent to which the parties see the situation as one threatening a potential loss. The latter occurs when each party fails to recognize the availability of solutions which will satisfy the needs or requirements of both parties.

In the case of the couple in conflict about the use of the air-conditioned room containing the television set, the perceptions of one air-conditioned room and one television set were accurate. In fact, overt conflict resulted from this perception of the situation, and the conditions of dissimilar interests and scarce resources led to fighting behavior, as would be expected. Yet the perception of the problem could be and, in fact, was changed to suggest that the common interest was to find a way so that the wife could study in a quiet air-conditioned room and the husband could hear and watch the ball game in the air-conditioned room. Solutions to the conflict could be interpreted as unlimited when one considers not just the actual materials involved but the available combinations of these materials. In this particular case, the changed perceptions led to overt problem-solving behavior rather than conflict. The husband watched the game on television with the sound off and listened to the game through earphones. The wife then studied with her back to the television set.

Conflicts may also be perceived when antecedent conditions do not exist (Pondy, 1967). Such situations occur when the parties do not understand each other's actual positions or when either of the positions taken is based upon a limited knowledge of the facts. Both cases lend themselves to resolution by discussion between the parties to clarify the facts. In such situations, the difficulty lies not so much in the perceptual process and its clarification as it does in the attitudinal issues which arise when the parties become angry, mistrustful, or defensive. If these negative attitudes can be controlled, the eventual resolution is facilitated by discussion and clarification.

For example, if two arts administrators are planning a summer concert for a community and both agree that the objective is maximum entertainment value for the greatest number of people in the community, then the selection between two alternatives can be made easily by obtaining facts about the appeal of each to various client groups and by choosing the alternatives with the most appeal. Or, when two fishermen state potentially conflictive preferences for fishing deep or fishing shallow, the logical process is one of asking why each prefers his strategy and of determining more facts, in hope of finding a goal compatible to both fishermen and to their mutual goal of catching fish.

Finally, initial perceptions of conflict may result in conflict-avoiding processes. Two important methods which lead to this outcome are the suppression mechanism and the attention-focus mechanism (Pondy, 1967). The former occurs when individuals ignore conflictive situations that involve low potential loss or are viewed as minimally threatening (Blake, Mouton, and Shepard, 1964). The attention-focus mechanism occurs because parties can selectively perceive conflictive conditions and make choices about those to which they wish to attend.

It is likely that individuals attend more readily to those conflictive conditions which are perceived to have readily accessible processes for resolution or for which readily accessible outcomes are available. There also seems to be a preference for attending to those conflictive situations involving relatively fewer negative attitudes. Thus, the parties in a labor-management disagreement may focus on issues which lend themselves to established grievance systems or arbitration procedures and effectively ignore fundamental differences which cannot be handled routinely in the usual way. They may also be reluctant to deal with issues provoking anger and hostility and instead restrict attention to matters which do not create such feelings.

From the above discussion it may be seen that perceptual processes can act to create conflict or to avoid existing conflictive situations. The third important ingredient in the development of overt conflict or problem-solving behavior consists of the feelings or attitudes of the parties.

FELT CONFLICT

Feelings and attitudes, like perceptions, may create conflict where rational elements would not suggest that it might arise; feelings and attitudes also play a part in avoiding conflict where it might be expected to occur. The most important consideration in determining the outcome of the conflict is whether the situation is personalized or depersonalized. Personalized situations are those in which the whole being of the other party is threatened or judged negatively. Depersonalized situations are those in which the behavior of the other party, or the characteristics of the relationship, are *described* as creating a problem, rather than judged as being responsible.

To illustrate, feelings or expressions of feelings which say "You are bad" are personalized; feelings or their expression which say "What you believe is different from what I believe" are depersonalized. Similarly, the statement "You threaten me" is personal, while "Your behavior leads to fear on my part" is depersonalized. Personalized situations create tension and anxiety; depersonalized situations lend themselves to problem solving. We shall see later how much the language that parties use with each other can affect the personalized or depersonalized nature of the situation.

Feelings and attitudes which set the stage for overt behavior also arise out of characteristics of the individual personality. There is not as much likelihood of overt conflict when parties who are yielding or anxious to please are dealing with parties who are dominant or self-seeking, as there is when the parties are both of the dominant type. A married couple in which one partner is dominant and the other is submissive will experience less overt conflict than one in which both are dominant or both are submissive.

The feelings and attitudes about the mutuality of the relationship will further affect eventual behavior. Where the parties value cooperation and believe that success in their relationship involves the attainment of the needs of both, the situation is less conflictive than when the parties value competition and believe that one can win only at the other's expense. Such attitudes not only affect their perceptions of the situation but also determine the way in which they will judge the availability of solutions.

Again, mutuality of interests and scarcity of resources relate in part to the initial feelings and attitudes of the parties.

Finally, trust between the parties can strongly affect the outcome of a potentially conflictive situation. Trusting attitudes elicit recognition of the mutual vulnerability of the parties, which occurs in part through the sharing of information between them. Vulnerability is also exhibited through the sharing of control by the parties. In the absence of such trust, a party is more likely to withhold information against him. If a party does give information, however, he is likely to distort it in order to maintain his own advantage. Similarly, each nontrusting party will try to maximize his control over the other and to minimize the control of the other over himself. Thus, the presence of trust may prevent potentially conflictive situations from arising, while its absence may create conflict where actual conditions do not seem to warrant it.

No attempt is made here to determine the origins of the attitudes and feelings held by the parties. Undoubtedly some are cultural, while others have their origin in developmental experiences, perceptual processes, or personal experiences. Whatever the source, these feelings become important determinants of the development and resolution of overt conflict between the parties.

MANIFEST BEHAVIOR

The actual overt behavior of the parties, based upon antecedent conditions, perceptions, and attitudes, may be exhibited as conflictive or problem solving. Where there is a conscious (though not necessarily deliberate) attempt by one party to block the goal achievement of another party, the behavior may be considered conflictive (Pondy, 1967). Thus, when one party accidentally blocks the goal attainment of another, it is a chance occurrence in a social system. But when one party knowingly interferes with another, conflict is said to occur.

On the other hand, when the parties make

conscious attempts to achieve the goals of both by supportive efforts, the behavior is that of problem solving. As with conflict behavior, the accidental achievement of both sets of goals is a chance occurrence; the deliberate effort to achieve them is overt problem-solving behavior. Parenthetically, it may be noted that the methodology of conflict is learned early in life and is well practiced. Competition, dominance, aggression, and defense are part of an established process unconsciously learned in the family, in the school, and in other social institutions. Problem solving, on the other hand, appears to be learned less frequently through developmental experiences. Conscious effort is generally required to develop and practice problem solving skills.

Manifest conflict-resolution or problem-solving behavior may be described according to the degree to which it is programmed or unprogrammed. Programmed behavior follows specified or anticipated patterns in order to achieve outcomes readily identifiable by the parties. Its effectiveness is determined by the breadth of alternative behaviors available for utilization by the parties. For example, the skill of a chess player depends upon his ability to choose appropriately from among a wide variety of strategic moves. Similarly, the simulation of war through war games is designed to increase the variety of strategies and tactics available to the participants and to anticipate action-reaction sequences. Thus, programmed behavior is rational behavior.

Unprogrammed behavior in conflict resolution or in problem solving does not follow known patterns and is governed more by emotion. The appearance of anger, aggression, apathy, or rigidity in conflictive situations reduces each party's effectiveness in gaining a relative advantage and makes it difficult for both to terminate the interaction. For that reason, it is useful to program the conditions surrounding the relationship when it is not possible to program the actual action-reaction sequences. For example, where the boundaries

between the parties cannot be made unambiguous, it is more useful to provide mechanisms for resolving boundary issues than it is to leave such resolution to chance. Such is the case when two departments with overlapping responsibilities establish a coordinating committee to deal with unanticipated issues that could potentially lead to conflict between them.

In like manner, problem solving may be handled on an unprogrammed emotional basis or it may be handled rationally. Communal or cooperative groups, united by strong emotional ties, often attempt to use consensual methods in their interactions. While the problem resolutions may be acceptable, the lack of programming and the scarcity of consciously identified alternative behaviors make such processes lengthy and susceptible to failure (Filley, 1973).

Finally, manifest behavior may be identified as that of an individual or that of a group. In this book we shall not distinguish between the two as parties in overt conflict unless making specific references to one or the other. Behavior between groups rather than individuals does not alter the basic pattern in the conflict process itself.

CONFLICT RESOLUTION OR SUPPRESSION

The next step in the conflict process is that of conflict resolution or suppression. Although the activity here is directed at ending the manifest conflict, in many cases it may resemble a continuation of the manifest conflict or problem-solving activity. It is distinguishable from such manifest behavior by the processes of conflict reduction rather than conflict elevation. In competition, the resolution process is simple and programmed: Rules specify the outcome. In less programmed and more disruptive conflicts, resolution involves the imposition of a deliberate strategy of conflict reduction.

In the next chapter we shall identify a number of conflict resolution mechanisms. These involve three types or classes according to results: (1) a win for some parties and a loss for others; (2) a partial gain and a partial loss for all parties; and (3) an acceptable gain for all parties. We are chiefly concerned in this book with the third type, generally referred to as problem solving and identified specifically as (a) consensus and (b) integrative decision making (IDM).

RESOLUTION AFTERMATH

Usually the resolution of conflict leaves a legacy which will affect the future relations of the parties and their attitudes about each other. Perhaps the most neutral in its effects is the end of a simple competitive situation viewed impersonally as an event. In such cases the value of the competitive process probably outweighs the attitudes about the final victory or defeat. More often, however, the outcome of a conflict leaves the parties with positive or negative changes in resources and with attendant feelings which are also positive or negative.

As pointed out earlier in this chapter, a clear defeat may leave a party with antagonistic or self-destructive feelings that merely set the stage for further conflict. Losers intend to win on the next encounter and such determination necessarily is accompanied by less cooperation, less trust, more personalization of the role of both parties, and distorted communication between the parties.

Where the resolution is one of compromise, the agreement often involves some form of future reciprocity. The parties become bound together by some kind of antagonistic cooperation. Often both parties will judge that they have given more than they have received; and, although neither party loses all, they both may have feelings of defeat (Burke, 1970). Parties will prepare themselves for a better bargain in the next encounter and, as in the previous case, will exhibit less trust, more personalization, and more frequent distortions in communication. Perhaps most important, they will often tend to manifest a low level of commitment to the compromise agreement (Blake, Mouton, and Shepard, 1964).

Finally, where problem solving results in an integrative outcome which is viewed as a win by both sides, the parties are brought closer together. Cooperation increases, future issues are depersonalized, trust is enhanced, and communication is accurate and complete. Problem solving is likely to leave the parties with a high level of commitment to the agreement.

To summarize, we have outlined the sequence associated with the development and resolution of conflict. Antecedent conditions, plus perceptions and attitudes, generate manifest behavior of a conflictive or problem-solving nature which is followed by some mechanism for ending the overt behavior. The resolution may be one which increases the likelihood of future conflicts or one which contributes to future harmony and cooperation.

References

Blake, R. R., and J. S. Mouton. "Comprehension of own and outgroup positions under intergroup competition." *Journal of Conflict Resolution* 5 (1961a): 304-10.

Blake, R. R., and J. S. Mouton. "Loyalty of representatives to ingroup positions during intergroup competition." *Sociometry* 24 (1961b): 177-83.

Blake, R. R., and J. S. Mouton. "Reactions to intergroup competition under win-lose conditions." *Management Science* 7 (1961c): 420-35.

Blake, R. R., J. S. Mouton, and H. A. Shepard. *Managing Intergroup Conflict in Industry.* Gulf, 1964.

Boulding, K. B. "A pure theory of conflict applied to organizations." In *The Frontiers of Management Psychology,* G. Fish, ed., Harper & Row, 1964.

Burke, R. J. "Methods of resolving superior-subordinate conflict: The constructive use of subordinate differences and disagreements." *Organizational Behavior and Human Performance* 5 (1970): 393-411.

Corwin, R. G. "Patterns of organizational conflict." *Administrative Science Quarterly* 14 (1969): 507-21.

Filley, A. C. "Organization invention: A study of utopian organizations." Wisconsin Business Papers No. 3. Bureau of Business Research and Service, University of Wisconsin-Madison, 1973.

Fink, C. F. "Some conceptual difficulties in the theory of social conflict." *Journal of Conflict Resolution* 13 (1968): 413-58.

Lott, A., and B. E. Lott. "Group cohesiveness as interpersonal attraction: A review of relationships with antecedent and consequent variables." *Psychological Bulletin* 64 (1965): 259-309.

Pondy, L. R. "Organizational conflict: Concepts and models." *Administrative Science Quarterly* 12 (1967): 296-320.

Pondy, L. R. "Variances of organizational conflict." *Administrative Science Quarterly* 14 (1969): 449-506.

Rapoport, A. *Fights, Games, and Debates.* University of Michigan, 1960.

Schmidt, S. M. "Lateral conflict within employment service district offices." Unpublished doctoral dissertation, University of Wisconsin-Madison, 1973.

Walton, R. E., and J. M. Dutton. "The management of interdepartmental conflict: A model and review." *Administrative Science Quarterly* 14 (1969): 73-84.

Walton, R. E., J. M. Dutton, and T. P. Cafferty. "Organizational context and interdepartmental conflict." *Administrative Science Quarterly* 14 (1969): 522-43.

Confrontation

GERARD EGAN, Ph.D.

"Confrontation" is a word that inspires fear in many people, and perhaps rightly so, for they have seen themselves or others devastated by irresponsible interpersonal attack. At any rate, confrontation in human-relations-training groups is certainly a controversial issue, and both helpers and human-relations-training specialists continue to argue its pros and cons, its effectiveness and its risks. Confrontation has been the topic of a certain minimal amount of research (see Berenson & Mitchell, 1974, for a summary), and most of this research is related to helping rather than to human-relations training. Lieberman, Yalom, and Miles (1973), in studying a variety of approaches to sensitivity-training and encounter groups, found that confrontation in groups with low structure and low support led to a number of "casualties." To add to the confusion, there is no standard definition of confrontation and no agreement in the literature on what results it is supposed to have. Berenson and Mitchell (1974, p. 111) describe five different kinds of confrontation, but

they warn the reader so stridently about the possible abuse of confrontation that they seem almost to discourage its use altogether. Their thesis is that relatively few people are living effectively enough and are skilled enough to merit the "right" to confront others. Be that as it may, interpersonal life abounds in confrontations—for better or for worse. Confrontation has been a fact of everyday life throughout history. Kanter (1972, pp. 14ff, 37ff), for instance, in a study of different kinds of communes, found that both confrontation and self-criticism have characterized a wide variety of successful utopian communities. It is senseless, then, to suppose that confrontations can be eliminated from interpersonal transactions.

Given this confusion, you may well ask yourself: should I confront the members of my group or not? The answer is that it depends. Confrontation, if used skillfully by a caring person (and Berenson and Mitchell certainly recognize this), can serve the interests of both parties in an interpersonal transaction. No more definitive answer can be given, however, without a more concrete explanation and description of confrontation—its nature, its goals, its potency, its limitations, and the conditions under which it can be used constructively. The purpose of this section, then, is to help you understand the nature and the technique of confrontation so that you can decide what place it should have in your interpersonal repertoire. In these pages I would like to give confrontation a "better name" and describe a process that, if carefully handled, can enrich interpersonal transactions and relationships.

THE ANATOMY OF CONFRONTATION
Inadvertent confrontation

The process to be described in the following pages is *intentional* confrontation, or confrontation as a specific skill. However, confrontation is also "in the eye of the beholder"—that is, any transaction that is perceived by a person as confrontational. In this sense, even accurate empathic understanding can be seen as confrontation. Let me explain. If you attend carefully to another person, listen to what he has to say (both verbally and nonverbally), and communicate to him in a nonjudgmental way understanding of his feelings, experiences, and behaviors, you do two things. First, your communication is an act of intimacy, at least broadly defined. And, if the other person is fearful of intimacy, your getting close to him through an act of accurate empathy may well frighten him—that is, confront him with his own fears. Second, accurate empathy, if it is really on the mark, has a way of encouraging the other person to disclose or explore himself even further. In other words, there is a social-influence dimension even to primary-level accurate empathy. High-level accurate empathy is both supportive and demanding. Therefore, if for one reason or another the other person is reluctant to take a deeper look at himself, accurate empathy may appear confrontational to him, even if confrontation is not the intention of the speaker.

Advanced accurate empathy, insofar as it "digs deeper" and expresses what is only implied, is confrontational in itself, for it invites the other person to look at himself from a different perspective or in a new way, thus challenging him.

Confrontation as invitation

"Confrontation," as used here, is anything that you do that invites a person to examine his behavior and its consequences more carefully. Confrontation as invitation may be indirect. For instance, if you act patiently and caringly with a group member with whom I have been quite impatient, I may well experience your behavior as confrontational in that it invites me to assess my own (in this case, ineffective) behavior. In these pages we will stress the invitational character of confrontation and focus on direct verbal confrontations. Let's look at an example of direct verbal confrontation.

Group Member A: Mark, I wonder whether you are aware that, with some frequency, you change the topic or focus of a conversation when you respond to others. At least it strikes me that way. For instance, a little earlier Jim was talking about his fear of being controlled by people here whom he sees as stronger than himself. You responded to him, I think, with understanding; but somehow, as you talked about your own fears, *you* became the focus. And I'm not sure that Jim got a chance to explore his own fears. I hope I'm not distorting what actually happened.

Mark: Now that you mention it, that's just what happened. I'm not too aware that I do this as part of my style, but I'd like some help in monitoring that. I wonder whether anyone else here has noticed that.

Member A invites Mark to take a look at a possibly nonfacilitative dimension of his interpersonal style, and Mark responds by accepting his invitation. Maintaining the invitational character of confrontation is important. Otherwise, confrontation degenerates into parental (rather than adult-to-adult), accusatory, punitive, and/or recriminatory behavior, and the mutuality necessary for good interpersonal transactions is lost. It is usually not necessary to hit someone in the head in order to get him to examine his behavior. The invitational character of confrontation is part of the tentativeness that should characterize the use of all challenging skills.

Types of confrontation

Berenson and Mitchell (1974) describe five types of confrontation. Let's examine these as a way of getting into *how* and *what* to confront.

1. *Didactic confrontation.* This type of confrontation deals basically with information or misinformation. If you give one of your fellow group members information he doesn't have, or correct misinformation he has about relatively objective aspects of the world, including the "world" of the training group, then you are dealing in didactic confrontation. This type, too, can be invitational. It need not focus on the "ignorance" of the other.

Group Member C: Rita, there's one aspect of the group contract under which we're working that I'm not sure that you're aware of. At least I'd like to check it out. You refer fairly frequently to what happens in your interpersonal life outside the group. For instance, you've talked a great deal about dependency problems with your mother and father. But often enough we deal with them as problems "out there," and not much is done to relate what you say to your relationships within the group. And it turns into a kind of counseling session. This isn't bad in itself, but our contract asks us to relate there-and-then happenings to the here and now of our own group. Does this make any sense to you?

Rita: Now that you bring it up, I remember reading that in our contract, and I know I've let it slide. Yes, and I do end up in a counseling session—all of you become my counselors. I think two things are happening. First, I didn't read that part of the contract carefully enough. Second, my problems with my parents are sometimes so pressing on my mind when I come in here that I guess I'm just looking for help.

Member C is trying to find out whether Rita has some mistaken notion about the contract. His "invitation," therefore, centers around an information/misinformation issue. His hypothesis is that Rita's lack of information is getting in the way of her effective involvement with her fellow group members; and, as Rita's nondefensive reply indicates, to a degree he is correct. In this case a didactic confrontation helps clear the air and give sharper focus to Rita's problem of immediacy of involvement in the group.

2. *Experiential confrontation.* As you involve yourself more deeply with your fellow group members, you will notice that at times your experience differs from that of another group member: the other *experiences* himself, what is happening in the group, another group member, or you *differently* from the way you do. While avoiding making your own experience normative, you can still invite the other to examine these differences with you and the others. Let's take a look at a few examples.

Group Member E: Joan, you say that you're unattractive, and yet I know that you get asked out a lot. And, if I'm not mistaken, I see that people often react to you here with ways of saying "I like you." I can't seem to put this together with your being "unattractive."

Joan: Okay. What you say is true, and it helps me clarify what I mean. First of all, I'm certainly no raving beauty, and when others find me attractive, I think they mean personality—the fact that I'm a rather caring person and things like that. I think at times I wish I were more physically attractive, though I hate to admit it. But, more important, most of the time I *feel* unattractive. And sometimes I feel *most* unattractive at the very moment people are telling me directly or indirectly that they find me attractive.

Since Member's E's experience of Joan seems to be different from Joan's experience of herself, he invites Joan to explore that difference in the group. Joan's self-exploration clarifies the issue greatly.

Group Member F: Jim, I'll bet I'm not far wrong if I say that you see yourself as a person who appreciates humor and is fairly witty. I've often seen you be genuinely witty, but sometimes I think what you see as wit I see as perhaps cynicism or even, at times, sarcasm. It could be that I'm over sensitive, and I think it would be good to get feedback from others here.

Jim: Yeah, I think I'd like to hear what others have to say.

Here Jim does not say how he experiences himself, but he is willing to hear how others experience him.

Group Member G: Nancy, you say that you see Cheryl as "pushy," making demands of you. I might have another perspective. I guess I see Cheryl as gutsy. She's committed to the goals of this group, and she does make demands of you, me, herself, all of us. But I see these demands as falling within the scope of the group contract. Cheryl makes me uncomfortable at times, but I need to be made uncomfortable.

Nancy is invited to review her experiencing of Cheryl. This does not necessarily mean that G's view of Cheryl is correct. It *is* different from Nancy's, however, and worth exploring.

What are the sources of differences in experiencing? Discrepancies, distortions, evasions, games, tricks, and smoke screens, to name a few—and all of us are guilty of some of these at one time or another.

a. *Discrepancies*. In all of us there are various discrepancies—between what we think and feel and what we say, what we say and what we do, our views of ourselves and others' views of us, what we are and what we wish to be, and what we really are and what we experience ourselves to be. And, of course, discrepancies are common between our verbal and nonverbal expressions of ourselves. For instance:

- I'm confused and angry, but I say that I feel fine.
- I see myself as witty, whereas others see me as biting.
- I experience myself as ugly, when in reality my looks are somewhat above average.
- I say "yes" with my words, but my body language says "no."
- I say that I'm interested in others, but I don't attend to them or try to understand them.

- I say that I want to improve my interpersonal style, but I'm lazy and listless and don't put much effort into this group experience.

In this lab experience we are interested principally in discrepancies that affect interpersonal style and group participation.

b. *Distortions*. If we can't face things as they really are, we tend to distort them. The way we see the world, including our interpersonal world, is often an indication of our needs rather than a true picture of what the world is like. For instance:

- I'm afraid of you and therefore I see you as aloof, although in reality you are a caring person.
- I see the group leader in some kind of divine role, and therefore I make unwarranted demands on him.
- I see my own stubbornness as commitment.
- I see your talking about yourself in generalities as adequate self-disclosure because I am afraid of disclosing myself.

One way group members can help one another is to suggest to one another alternative frames of reference for viewing self, others, and interpersonal living. For instance, it is confronting to suggest that

- living more intensively in the group can be seen as challenge rather than as just pain;
- what seems like heroic forbearance in the face of painful learnings about oneself might be just self-pity;
- a person might be something of a seducer rather than merely a victim;
- a person might be afraid to act rather than unable to act;
- caring for another might be smothering rather than nurturing; or
- intimacy is rewarding rather than just demanding.

Seeing alternative frames of reference helps us break out of self-defeating views of self, others, and the world of relating.

c. *Games, tricks, and smoke screens.* If I am comfortable with my delusions and profit by them, I will obviously try to keep them. If I'm rewarded for playing games—that is, if I get others to meet my needs by playing games—then I will continue a game approach to life (see Berne, 1964; Harris, 1969; James & Jongeward, 1971). For instance, I'll play "Yes, but. . . ." That is, I get others to give me feedback on my interpersonal style and then proceed to show how invalid that feedback is. Or I make myself appear helpless and needy in the group (or to my friends outside the group), and when they come to my aid I get angry at them for treating me like a child. Or I seduce others in one way or another and then become indignant when they accept my covert invitations. The number of games we can play in order to avoid intimacy and other forms of effective interpersonal living is seemingly endless. When we are fearful of changing elements of our interpersonal behavior, we often attempt to lay down smoke screens to hide from one another the ways in which we fail to seize life. We use communication in order *not* to communicate (see Beier, 1966).

The best defense against game-playing in your training group is to create an atmosphere in which it is almost impossible to play games. Effective group participants don't get "hooked" into games. For instance, if you refuse to play the role of "helper" in your group, others are prevented from playing the "Yes, but . . ." game. However, if someone in the group does try to play any of the innumerable games available, he should be challenged in a caring and responsible way.

Group Member A: Maureen, you are the one in here that I can really talk to. You listen to me, and I'm sure you care about me. When I need feedback, I know I'm going to get it straight from you. You seem to know me so well. Your feedback is so accurate.

Maureen: I appreciate your trust very much. But I'm also uncomfortable being singled out like this. I'm

not sure whether you're implying that you can't develop other relationships in here similar to ours.

Member A involves himself in a game of "pairing," linking himself closely to another group member in seeming opposition to another or others. Maureen, however, doesn't let herself get hooked into "pairing." She challenges A to begin thinking about developing other strong relationships in the group.

3. *Strength confrontation.* Confrontation of strengths means pointing out to another the strengths, assets, and resources he is failing to use or is not using fully.

Group Member B: Rick, I'd like to make a comment on the *quality* of your interactions here. The times you've interacted with me, I've really listened, because you are totally present. You attend, listen, understand very well. I guess I'm not sure why you're not available to more people here in that way consistently. Your interactions with me are so rewarding that, when you "retire" for an extended period, I miss you. But, overall, a certain lack of *quantity* of interactions on your part seems in the long run to affect even the quality of your presence here. I'm just not sure why you tend to hold back.

Here B places a demand on Rick that he deploy unused resources. If, as many social scientists have told us, we tend to use less than a quarter of our human potential (including interpersonal potential) as we make our way through life, then strength confrontations should be the most widely used kind of confrontation. Such confrontations are obviously *experiential,* for they must be realistic—that is, based on observation of real strengths, assets, and resources that have been developed or are not being used. In their research studies, Berenson and Mitchell (1974) have demonstrated that high-level communicators do indeed use strength confrontations more frequently than low-level communicators do, and they use them instinctively. In the group, then, you and your fellow group members are asked to demand the best from one another in terms of interpersonal transactions. There is a negative element even in strength confrontations, for it means pointing out possible strengths that are *not* being used. Overall, however, such confrontations are quite positive, for emphasis is placed on the strength, asset, or resource, and not on its nonuse.

4. *Weakness confrontation.* As the name implies, weakness confrontation dwells on the deficits of the person being confronted. Although it is impossible to avoid such confrontations entirely in the realistic interchange that takes place in a training group or in everyday life, weakness confrontations become the preferred mode of confrontation only of low-level communicators.

Group Member C: Sheila, your silence here is beginning to drive me up the wall. It makes you seem so passive. When you're silent like that, I wonder what you're thinking; I begin to think that you're judging the rest of us. Your silence just doesn't get you anywhere. It makes you appear sullen and disinterested. And I want to block you out entirely.

Such confrontation may well reveal the impact that the silent member is having on many of the group members, but since it dwells merely on a weakness it probably does little good by itself. The person being confronted feels under attack and becomes defensive. My experience in groups tells me that the usual periodic weakness confrontation administered to a relatively silent member does practically nothing to increase such a member's participation. Nevertheless, group members continue to employ weakness confrontation in an almost ritualistic way.

Group Member D: Sheila, you've mentioned that part of the problem you have with silence here is a fear of barging into conversations, interrupting others, and the like. Well, you can call it "barging in" if you like, but I *welcome* your interruptions. I guess I just don't see them as interruptions. I see them as your thinking enough of me to want to make contact with me. And I like that very much.

Here D tries to understand Sheila's feelings, but the focus is on a strength—Sheila's presence as

an act of contact, an act of interest. Whenever you are about to challenge someone in the group, pause a moment and see whether you are emphasizing his strengths or his weaknesses. If a weakness is the primary focus, the odds are that your confrontation will be less effective than it could be.

5. *Encouragement to action.* As we take a look at this final type of confrontation, you will probably begin to notice that most confrontations are "mixed"; that is, they are combinations of elements from more than one type. Encouragement to action, as Berenson and Mitchell note, is my pressing you to act upon your world in some reasonable, appropriate manner and my discouraging in you a passive attitude toward life. High-level communicators are agents, doers, initiators; they are not afraid to make an impact on the lives of others. They are reasonably assertive and active, and they are unafraid to call others to action, especially when others say they want to act but fail to do so.

Group Member D: Ken, you and I have both admitted that we're not so assertive as we want to be in the group. I'm wondering whether you and I might enter into a little side contract with each other. Let's increase the frequency of our interactions. For instance, we can determine before a group meeting how often we would like to contact others, and then increase our contacts in a reasonable way. We could both help each other plan before the meetings and monitor each other's behavior during the meetings.

Not only does D confront Ken by encouraging him to act, but he suggests a way of going about it that emphasizes *mutuality*. Helping is going to take place, but it is *mutual* helping that doesn't cast either person in the role of "helper" or "helpee."

THE MANNER OF CONFRONTING

If confrontation is to be for better rather than for worse, the manner of confrontation is as important as the type of confrontation. First we will discuss some principles and then proceed to some practical applications of these principles. How should confrontation take place?

1. *In the spirit of accurate empathy.* We have already noted that even primary-level accurate empathy can be confrontational in itself. Advanced accurate empathy is in and of itself challenging and is therefore included among the challenging skills. However, the principle is that *all* interactions that take place among you and your fellow group members should be based on accurate understanding. If confrontation does not stem from understanding, it will almost inevitably be either ineffective or destructive.

Group Member E: If I can put together what you're saying, Mary, there seem to be two themes. You're attracted to George here and feel a good deal of respect for him, and you show this respect by making an effort to contact him, by working at understanding him, by giving him feedback on his style as he interacts with others. On the other hand, you haven't gotten over the fact that he ripped into you in a punitive, confronting way at the very first meeting we had. So you also still feel uneasy with him—and there's still some distrust, alienation, and perhaps at times dislike. It seems to me that these negative elements choke off free-flowing communication between the two of you. I'm just wondering whether you both feel that it might be time to face these issues directly with each other. I think a number of us have taken on the role of intermediary between you two.

If E's assessment is accurate, it is likely to be constructively confrontational.

2. *Tentatively.* As is the case with all challenging skills, confrontation should take place tentatively, especially in the earlier stages of the lab experience, when you and your fellow group members are working at building initial rapport with one another.

Group Member A: Jerry, you say that you swallow your anger a lot. Could it be that the anger you "swallow" here doesn't always "stay down"? From the feedback you're getting, it seems to dribble out somewhat in cynical remarks or periods of aloofness or uncooperative behavior. I'm wonder-

ing if you see some of this. I know you can deal with strong emotion directly. I've seen you do it here.

The fact that A's statement is filled with qualifications can help Jerry listen to and explore what is being said more easily. If you dump a ton of bricks on one of your fellow participants, you arouse his defensiveness, and he will have to pour his energy into recovering from the blow rather than into trying to assimilate and work with the confrontation. See how different the following confrontation sounds from the preceding one.

Group Member B: Face up to it. You don't "swallow" your anger. It's dribbling out unproductively all the time. I don't think you're fooling anyone but yourself.

This is confrontation, but it is unnecessarily accusatory. Perhaps the word "balance" would be good to use here. Although good confrontations are not accusatory, neither are they so qualified and tentative as to lose their force. There is a message in the overly tentative confrontation: it says to the person being confronted "You probably don't have the resources to hear this." Such confrontations are demeaning because they turn the other group member into a "helpee." Likewise, the overly tentative confrontation may say something about the confronter: that he is afraid to face another person directly.

3. *With care.* Basic respect demands that group members confront one another with care. Let's try to operationalize the expression "with care."

INVOLVEMENT. Confrontation should be a way of getting involved with the other person. If in the act of confronting you find yourself standing off from the other, you are probably not confronting with care. All interactions in a human-relations-training lab should heighten mutuality. If confrontation is alienating, it runs counter to the basic goals of the lab.

MOTIVATION. Your motive in confronting should be mutual help in understanding interpersonal style and behavior. Other motives—to show that you are right, to punish, to get back at someone, or to put someone in his place—are dysfunctional. If your confrontation is not a way of showing others that you are "for" them, you will be seen as untrustworthy in the group.

THE STRENGTH OF THE RELATIONSHIP. Confrontation should be proportioned to the relationship between yourself and the person you are confronting. We all know that we are more willing to hear strong words from some than from others. If you do little to establish rapport with your fellow participants, you should avoid the "strong medicine" interaction of confrontation. Caring confrontation presupposes some kind of intimacy between confronter and confronted.

THE STATE OF THE PERSON BEING CONFRONTED. Social intelligence demands that you be able to judge the *present* ability of your fellow group member to assimilate what you are saying. If the other person is disorganized and confused at the moment, it does little good to add to his disorganization by challenging him further.

Group Member A: I'm just getting in touch with the fact that I practically never do give support here. I had no idea that I could be so selfish, but as I look at my style "outside," it's much the same. I get my own way. I take little or no time to understand others. I'm embarrassed. I'm almost speechless. It's like being groggy. I don't want to look at it for a while.

Group Member B: I think you should see one more thing, while you're at it. Even though you don't give support, you demand it of us here. And that's infuriating!

Group Member C: What has just dawned on you is pretty painful and confusing. It seems that you'd like a little time to let it all sink in, to settle down, to get your bearings.

C recognizes A's disorganization and tries to give him support by understanding what is going on (primary-level accurate empathy). B, on the other hand, moves in for the kill. His confrontation is not a sign of caring but a way of

satisfying his own immediate need to express his pent-up emotionality and, possibly, to punish.

4. *Using successive approximation.* In many cases, confrontation will be more effective if it is gradual. The other person has to assimilate what is being said to him; he has to make it his own, or it won't last. If you are trying to change your own interpersonal behavior, it is usually not good to demand everything from yourself all at once. Space the demands you make on yourself; give yourself time to get a sense of success. This movement in small steps toward a behavioral goal, each of which is rewarded in some way, is called the method of "successive approximation." Therefore, if you are using encouragement-to-action confrontation, you will probably be more helpful if you start with simpler, concrete behavioral units that are relatively easy to change. Let's take a look at an example of what *not* to do.

Group Member A: Jim, if you want to get rid of your feelings of loneliness, you have to get out there *today* and start interacting effectively with other people.

Member A is unrealistic: he is not concrete, and he asks for everything at once. Asking for everything at once is a good way of getting nothing. Let's look at another example, in which the group member is much more aware of the method of successive approximation. Bill is worried over the fact that he makes, or at least thinks he makes, a poor impression on others. The group has been meeting long enough for the members to have established a fairly solid degree of rapport with one another.

Group Member B: Bill, you've said a few times here that you're pretty sure that you make a poor impression on people—that you seem, almost invariably, to start off on the wrong foot. First of all, it might be good to check that out with the people right here. I can give you some of my impressions. For instance, when we're together here, your posture frequently seems to say that you'd rather be someplace else. It could be that others would see you as being interested in them if you simply attended to them more carefully. At least that's my impression.

Although B may think that it is not just a case of poor attending that makes for Bill's poor impression on others, he starts there is his encouragement-to-action confrontation. Attending is a behavior that is relatively easy to change, and he challenges Bill to change his behavior here and now, in the group. Let's consider another example. In this case, a group member is too passive and ends up being ignored by the others.

Group Member C: You're too passive, Ted. You have to go out and seize life if you expect others to pay any attention to you.

The concept "passive" is too general, and the solution offered is too vague. Moreover, C has assumed a "helper" or parental role; he no longer seems to be "with" Ted but is standing off from him.

Group Member D: Ted, I have to admit that I ignore you here at times. When I ask myself why, I come up with a couple of things. I think enough has been said about your silence. But even when you do speak, your voice is so soft and quiet that sometimes it's hard to hear you. It's almost as if you don't want to touch me too strongly, even with your voice. I would feel better if you spoke up to me more.

D is involved and concrete, and he avoids the parental tones of C. He doesn't make wide-ranging demands but starts with something that may well be within Ted's control.

Some practical hints concerning the manner of confrontation

If the effect of your confrontation is to set up a barrier between you and the other person, this confrontation is useless. Here are some ways to avoid erecting barriers.

KEEP CURRENT. If another person's behavior is of some concern to you, don't keep your concern locked up inside yourself by bottling up your feelings, withholding feedback, ignoring the person, or engaging in other substitutes for directness. Try to stay current within the group; as issues come up, face them directly with the other person. This doesn't mean that you should become picky or specialize in challenging others. However, if you notice in another a behaviorial theme that seems unproductive, don't hesitate to deal with it directly. For instance, if it becomes clear that another person is habitually passive or domineering in the group, don't wait until these patterns solidify and become part of the group culture. By that time it will be difficult to do much about them. Or, if you identify a resource or a strength that another uses only abortively, feel free to use a strength confrontation. In my experience, the majority of participants in human-relations-training groups (although there are disastrous exceptions) err by delaying confrontation too long—until it is useless or hostile—rather than by engaging in premature confrontation.

NONVERBAL BEHAVIOR IS INSUFFICIENT. Nonverbal hints about what you are thinking or feeling in the group are not enough. If you fall silent, refuse to look at someone else, exclude another, smile, slouch in boredom, or bite your lips, you are indeed sending messages—some of which may well be confrontational—but these messages must be backed up by words if they are to be direct and unambiguous.

USE DESCRIBING BEHAVIOR. Perhaps the most important practical hint for confronting others is one suggested by Wallen (1973): *describe* what you see as counterproductive behavior in another, and *describe* the impact you think it has on the person himself, yourself, and the other members of the group. There is a strong tendency, as Wallen notes, to substitute less useful forms of verbal behavior for descriptions. What are some of these?

Commanding rather than describing

- *Commanding:* John, don't keep asking Mary how she feels. That's become a cliché with you. Tell her how *you* feel and what impact she has on you. Then she might do the same.

- *Describing:* John, unless I'm mistaken, almost every time you ask Mary how she feels—and you seem to do so often enough—I see her wince. You ask her to share her feelings with you, but I'm not sure I see you sharing yours with her.

Judging, labeling, or name-calling instead of describing

- *Judging:* Peter, you're selfish!
- *Describing:* You're very verbal, Peter, and very assertive. At almost every group meeting you begin with your own agenda. We've almost developed a ritual here—we wait for you to start. I don't think that you or any of the rest of us is doing anything to change this pattern.

Accusing instead of describing

- *Accusing:* Gene, you have it in for Kay. You don't like her. You haven't accepted her from the start.
- *Describing:* Gene, I know that Kay has to work out her own relationship with you—but I see her sitting there and taking things that would drive me up the wall. You don't initiate conversations with her. When she contacts you, your part of the dialogue seems very brief. Even your voice strikes me as very matter-of-fact. I've noticed this kind of behavior from the very beginning of the group. I'm in the dark. I don't know what's going on between you two.

Questioning instead of describing

- *Questioning:* Jim, is it safe or productive for you to reveal so much about yourself so quickly?
- *Describing:* Jim, you have revealed yourself more than anyone else in this group. And now this evening you have begun to explore your sexuality—and it's only the third meeting! Frankly, it scares me when someone moves that fast.

Sarcasm or cynicism rather than describing

- *Sarcasm:* Boy, you really know how to put people at ease!
- *Description:* Paul, now that Craig has stormed out of here, I'll bet you're wondering what angered him so. I don't want to talk about him, since he's not here, but this is my view of what you did. You told him point-blank that he's not the kind of per-

son you usually make friends with, but you did it with such cool deliberation and lack of feeling in your voice. I shuddered a bit inside and began wondering what was happening inside Craig. Your expression hasn't changed since he's left, and I'm not sure what's happening inside you.

Describing behavior has a kind of objectivity to it that helps the person being confronted avoid the kind of natural defensiveness that arises with confrontation.

THE RIGHT TO CONFRONT

Does anyone and everyone in the training group have the right to confront fellow participants? It depends. By subscribing to the laboratory contract, you say in effect to your fellow group members "I want to place on myself the demands outlined in the contract. However, although I want to make these demands on myself, nevertheless I am a member of a learning community, and I expect my fellow group members to help me place these demands on myself without their becoming role "helpers" or casting me in the role of "helpee." Confrontation, then, is a legitimate form of interaction in the group, because it is one of the ways in which you and your fellow group members help one another live up to the legitimate demands of the training experience.

Does this mean that everyone in the group has an automatic right to confront? I think not. You must earn the right to confront others, and in general you can do so by living up to the contract yourself. Only active group members really earn the right to confront. Let's examine what this statement means more concretely. Berenson and Mitchell (1974) name certain qualities that must characterize a helper before he has the right to confront.

1. *Relationship-building.* In order to earn the right to confront, you must actively engage in the process of relationship-building as it has been described so far in this book. If you do not have a solid relationship with someone, don't confront him, for mere acquaintance does not

supply a solid enough foundation for confrontation. Leave confrontation to someone who has a
more solid relationship with the person. In
order to confront, you must be "in" the group
and not just a peripheral member.

2. *Understanding at a deep level.* Do not
confront anyone until you have spent a good
deal of time trying to understand him. Effective
confrontation is built on understanding and
flows from it. Without understanding, the confrontation is usually hollow. Moreover, unless
the other person feels that you understand him,
he will probably not listen to your confrontations anyway. Therefore, before confronting
ask yourself whether you have spent sufficient
time understanding the person.

3. *Being able to disclose oneself.* Do not confront others unless you are active in revealing
yourself appropriately in the group. When you
make yourself "visible" through self-disclosure, you too open yourself up to confrontation.
The mutuality that should characterize transactions in the group demands that you disclose
yourself. Don't expect to deal with the vulner-
abilities of others without at the same time making yourself vulnerable.

4. *Being in touch with oneself.* The person
who confronts should be in touch with his own
emotionality, should have a feeling for the
strength of the relationship between himself and
the person to be confronted, and should know
why he is confronting. If I am out of touch with
my own experience, I may be confronting in
order to "get even," in order to compete, in
order to express my counterdependency, or for
a variety of other counterproductive reasons. If
your reasons for confronting are foggy to you,
delay your confrontation unless you can work
out your motivation with the help of the rest of
the group.

5. *Having a dynamic relationship with the
confronted.* Confront only those with whom
your relationship is growing. If you and another
person are on a kind of interpersonal plateau,
delay confrontation and find out why nothing is

happening between you. Unless you have a
sense of the interpersonal movement of the
other, your confrontation may well be stale or
ill-timed. Confront only those with whom you
have a currently active relationship.

6. *Living fully.* Berenson and Mitchell (1974)
claim that only a person who is striving to live
fully according to his value system has the right
to confront another, for only such persons are
potential sources of human nourishment for
others. In other words, don't confront others
unless you are the kind of person who challenges yourself.

7. *Not allowing your virtues to be exploited.*
Don't allow your virtues to be turned against
you in the process of confrontation. For example, if you are an understanding person, don't
let the other be self-servingly selective in what
he will listen to from you. If the other person is
willing to be understood as fully as possible by
you, he is also opening himself up to be confronted by you. Don't let yourself become the
victim of the "MUM effect," which refers to
people's tendency to withhold bad news from
others (Rosen & Tesser, 1970, 1971; Tesser &
Rosen, 1972; Tesser, Rosen, & Batchelor,
1972; Tesser, Rosen, & Tesser, 1971). In ancient times the bearer of bad news was often
killed. In modern times he may not fear death,
but he does fear something. Research has
shown that, even when the bearer of bad news
is assured that the one receiving the news will
take it well, he is still as reluctant as the bearer
who knows that the receiver will take it hard.
Bad news—and, by extension, the "bad news"
involved in any kind of confrontation—arouses
negative feelings in the sender (the confronter),
no matter what the reaction on the part of the receiver. If you are uncomfortable with human-
relations training as a social-influence process,
you may well fall victim to the MUM effect,
and your communication with others will become watered-down and safe. Conversely, if
you are the kind of person who earns the right
to confront, you will probably engage in con-

frontation—not as a specialty, but naturally. Never confronting may be a sign that the quality of your other interactions is poor or weak.

8. *Responding well to confrontation*. Finally, confront only if you yourself have learned how to respond well to confrontations. What constitutes effective response to confrontation? Let's try to answer that question now.

RESPONDING GROWTHFULLY TO CONFRONTATION

Confrontation, even when it is executed with care by someone who has our interests at heart, has the tendency to pull us up short. It isn't always easy to be challenged. Therefore, we all have the tendency to respond defensively to confrontation. Since we are such resourceful creatures, this defensiveness can take many forms.

Defensive response to confrontation

Confrontation usually precipitates some degree of disorganization in the person being confronted. It can leave us feeling inadequate. One way of looking at confrontation and response to it is from the point of view of the cognitive-dissonance theory. Confrontation induces dissonance. For instance, I have always seen myself as a witty, humorous person, and now the suggestion is made that my humor is often biting or sarcastic, that it is a way of avoiding intimacy, and that it ignores the needs of others. All of a sudden I am forced to think of myself in a different way, and this shifting of gears is not easy. I am somewhat taken aback, pulled up short, and confused. This is dissonance. Since dissonance is an uncomfortable state, my immediate tendency is to try to get rid of it. But I can try to get rid of it in ways that don't allow me the opportunity of examining the confrontation in order to see if there is something to it. They simply protect me. What are some of these? (See Egan, 1975; Harvey, Kelley, & Shapiro, 1957; King, 1975.)

1. *Don't think about it*. I can listen, say "I see," and then proceed to file what has been said in the deepest recesses of my mind. This seems to happen all too often in groups, and no one does much about it.

2. *Distort the evaluation*. Someone tells me that I am an attractive person and that my verbal skills are good, but that I don't use them assertively enough. I hear the part about my attractiveness and my verbal skills, but the rest is lost. In this case I distort the evaluation by not hearing the whole message.

3. *Discredit the confronter*. Another ploy to reduce dissonance is to destroy the credibility of the confronter. Counterattack becomes a strong defense.

Group Member A: It's easy for you to ask me to become more involved here. You're attractive and skillful and can do easily what demands a great deal of effort from me. If you would stand in my shoes a little while, I don't think you'd be so quick in telling me what I'm doing wrong. Not only that, there are two people here whom you practically ignore. I think you should tend to your own garden first.

Obviously, you need not discredit the confronter so vocally. You can also do it silently, and just let him whistle in the wind.

4. *Persuade the confronter to change his views*. Win him over by persuasion or rationalization. Defuse the confrontation by linking up with the confronter.

Group Member B: I know I don't express much feeling here, John, but I'm not sure that it's called for—not as much as you ask for, at any rate. After all, there *is* something artificial about these groups. I don't want to manufacture emotion; in fact, that's part of our contract. I want to let what comes flow naturally.

B's "reasonableness" here prevents him from facing up to the issue.

5. *Devaluate the importance of the topic in question*. This is another form of rationalization. For instance, if one of the group members is being confronted about his sarcasm, he may

point out that he doesn't really mean it, that he is rarely sarcastic, that "poking fun at others" is a very minor part of his interpersonal style and not worth spending time on. The person being confronted has a right to devaluate a topic if it really isn't important. This fact emphasizes the necessity of your attending carefully to his behavior and understanding him before you confront him.

6. *Deny, reject the confrontation.* One defense is merely to deny what the confronter has to say. This approach, however, lacks subtlety, and more indirect defenses are usually preferred.

7. *Seek support elsewhere.* I can probably always find people in the group who are "on my side." Then, if I don't like what someone is saying to me, I can seek support for what I do from "my friends" or from those who find it difficult to say anything confrontational at all.

8. *Agree with the confronter.* I can readily agree with what the confronter has to say. But this too can be a game. It gets the confronter off my back, and my "honesty" wins approval from other group members. I find that, if I readily agree with the confrontation, that is the end of it. It is difficult for the confronter to confront me again, because I have already admitted what he has to say. The point is that I do little or nothing about it.

Obviously, there are many more defenses against confrontation, some blatant and some subtle. Use your imagination and list some further dodges.

Creative response to confrontation

If someone takes the risk of confronting you and does so reasonably and responsibly, then mutuality demands that your response be just as open and direct. What are the implications of this demand?

First, make sure you *understand* what the other person is saying. Use primary-level accurate empathy. Very often the confronter finds it difficult to say what he feels he should say.

Respect for him demands that you get what he is saying straight, and that you understand how he feels as he says it. Obviously, your own emotions come into play. Since you don't like what you are hearing, it is easy for you to distort and misunderstand the message. You may have to fight your own emotions in order to understand. Confrontation, even when it is reasonable, can *feel* like an attack, and attack calls for instinctive defense and/or counterattack. Therefore, it may *sound* simple and easy to understand what the confronter has to say and make sure you get the message straight, but in practice it is not that easy.

Second, you are in a group, so use the resources of the group. If you are confused, or if you don't understand, deal with your confusion in the group. A good confronter often throws the question open to the entire group.

Group Member A: Peter, you are a very active person in this group. Perhaps even overactive. Because you are so active, in both initiating conversations and responding when others talk about themselves, in some sense you end up controlling a lot of what goes on here. I wonder sometimes whether you possibly avoid some of your own interpersonal issues by being so active. What I'm saying is a hunch. I'd like to check it out with the others here.

Peter: You're saying that anyone as active as I am has a kind of advantage. He can control his own agenda and thus, to a degree, he can control what is going to be said to him. You know, I may well be avoiding some interpersonal issues. I'd like to find out from the rest of you what some of these issues are—I mean the ones that pertain to this group.

Peter understands A and follows his suggestion by calling on the resources of the group. There is a big difference between calling on the other group members for one's defense and calling on them in order to explore the confrontation as carefully as possible. I have often been in groups in which both confronter and willing confrontee have tried unsuccessfully to get to the heart of the confrontation. But they didn't call on the resources of the wider group, and apparently no one else wanted to "interrupt.". . .

Third, respond to the confrontation, once you understand what is being said, by using the resources of the group in order to explore it as concretely as possible. For instance, if someone challenges you because you are a low-level initiator in the group, find out whether others see you in this way, find out how they feel about it, and explore how you yourself feel about it. Examine your own values related to being an initiator in interpersonal situations. You may find that you want to increase your level of initiation because your present level is so low that it interferes with the overall quality of your presence. However, you may also come to realize that you don't want to be an extremely assertive person. For instance, you may not want to be so assertive as the person who challenged you in the first place. Within the group you want to live up to the demands of the contract, but you also want to be yourself. In brief, whereas defensiveness is almost always counterproductive, mere compliance to the expressed or implied demands of the confronter is hardly ideal. If you are to actively choose the elements of your own interpersonal style, you certainly should listen to the challenges presented to you by others; but you should also adapt these challenges to your own needs, wants, and values. If you determine that a given confrontation has merit, your ultimate response will be some kind of *change of behavior*. Often enough it takes time for a particular confrontation to sink in and take effect. Good response to confrontation doesn't mean leaping into action. Giving yourself time is useful, providing it is not just your way of sidestepping the issue.

CONFRONTATION AND MUTUALITY

Confrontation can be a very beneficial transaction when it is used reasonably and in a context of mutuality. Its obvious drawback is that the confronter becomes the "more knowing"

person and the confrontee becomes the "less knowing" person, and mutuality is thus lost. Once a group is divided into "those who confront" and "those who are confronted," the group is no longer a learning community but a group of "helpers" and "helpees." Finally, as research has shown (see Berenson & Mitchell, 1974), anyone who makes confrontation his *specialty* does all things poorly, even his specialty.

Gordon (1970), in teaching parents ways of being effective in their relationships with their children, speaks of the "dirty dozen"—twelve categories of ineffective parental behaviors. Seen in the context of adult-adult relationships and human-relations training, these dozen sets of behaviors are caricatures or perversions of confrontation. As you read what follows, it may strike you that Gordon is overstating his case—that some of the behaviors he discusses are quite legitimate and do not destroy mutuality. Let's first go through the "dirty dozen" and then return to this issue.

- *Commanding, ordering, directing:* "John, talk to Jane. Your last remark hurt her." This set of behaviors constitutes an attempt to *control* the other. They suggest that the other person doesn't have enough social intelligence to be in control of his own interpersonal behavior. The implication is nonacceptance of the other.
- *Warning, admonishing, threatening:* "Jane, you know it's not good to pout like that. You'll just end up ostracizing yourself from the group." This remark certainly assumes that the other person is a child. These behaviors promote fear and submissiveness and usually evoke resentment and hostility.
- *Exhorting, moralizing, preaching:* "Peter, the contract is not an obstacle. It's here for our growth and protection. Following it actually frees us." Unfortunately, the temptation to preach in human-relations-training groups is sometimes quite strong. Sterile preaching effects little or nothing in religious contexts, so we should expect little from it in training groups.
- *Advising, giving suggestions, offering solutions:*

"Sarah, why don't you relax and count slowly to five before responding to anyone who confronts you? I'll bet that will take the edge out of your voice." Again, this is helping behavior, with the inevitable "helper-helpee" role-casting.

- *Lecturing, giving logical arguments:* "Tony, first of all, you disclose little about yourself. Second, your attempts at accurate empathy are too widely separated. Therefore, you can't expect others to listen when you complain about their 'selfish' behavior." Teaching turns the other into a student, and, in most educational contexts, lecturing does not imply mutuality.
- *Judging, criticizing, disagreeing, blaming:* "Alice, it's your fault that Connie left in tears. You're too blunt and harsh. That behavior of yours is one of the reasons for the low level of trust in here." Judicial functions have no place in the training group. Perhaps more than other "parental" behaviors, they elicit feelings of inadequacy, inferiority, stupidity, and worthlessness. They provoke defensiveness, anger, and even hatred.
- *Approval behaviors such as praising, agreeing:* "Rich, you're the most understanding person in this group. You put yourself out for others, and that's great. More of us should do that." Such behavior usually makes the person being praised squirm in his chair and arouses resentment in others because of the expressed or implied comparisons. Praise can also be ingratiating and manipulative.
- *Name-calling, ridiculing, shaming:* "Dorothy, you really say stupid things at times. You act like such a little child." It goes without saying that such behavior seldom evokes beneficial change.
- *Interpreting, analyzing, diagnosing:* "Tom, from what you've said, I'd say that your fearfulness in groups stems from your childhood. You were too protected and sheltered by your parents. I think you still look for parent substitutes in this group." Playing psychologist is, again, a strong temptation. And it is endless, for when will we ever discover our "real" motives for doing things? The pursuit of insight too often leads nowhere, at least in terms of constructive behavioral change.
- *Reassuring, consoling, supporting, sympathizing:* "Cindy, don't let this get you down. I know we're making demands on you, but we care about you. We even respect your tears." Such behaviors make

the other a "weak child" and usually cut off communication. They are distortions of accurate empathy and in no way encourage mutuality.
- *Probing, questioning, interrogating:* "Carl, how do you feel right now? Did Mark's comment embarrass you?" Questions usually beget little but more questions. Such cross-examination is demeaning. Questions imply that information is more important than understanding, that you are gathering data in order to "solve" a problem, and that *you* must solve the problem rather than let the other solve it. Questions limit the freedom of the other to talk about what *he* wants to talk about.
- *Withdrawing from, humoring, distracting:* "Kathy, let's put the issue of your relationship to Andy on the shelf for a while. Too many cooks here are spoiling your broth!" Humor too often implies a lack of interest and/or respect.

I don't mean to suggest that none of the behaviors above is ever useful in human interactions. I do suggest that parentalness is no substitute for mutuality. Some of these behaviors may be used beneficially once a certain degree of mutuality is established. The stronger a relationship the stronger the interactions can be—including strong confrontation. I include the "dirty dozen" here as a way of asking you to be careful in confronting. If you do use some of the "dirty dozen," it may help the interaction to consider your motivation for doing so. It may also help if you identify *what* you are doing, so that the person being confronted does not feel attacked. Finally, any kind of confrontation is suspect when it is used as a substitute for understanding.

SELF-CONFRONTATION

Challenging one another in the group has been emphasized up to this point. However, mutuality is well served if you and your fellow group members learn how to challenge yourselves. Put crudely, you should "get yourself before others get you." This statement is crude, because responsible confrontation is not a "getting." But there is a great deal of value in this idea. If I learn how to confront myself, I will be less defensive in dealing with the issues I bring up, will not force others into the position of constantly challenging me, and will put the responsibility for change directly where it belongs—on myself. If I challenge myself, I can then call upon the resources of the other members of the group to help me monitor my behavior, to give me feedback, and to provide some of the encouragement and support I need to work through a change-of-behavior program. Ideally, then, self-confrontation should be more frequent than confrontation by others (or at least should grow in frequency). For most of us this means that we must adopt new behavior. The laboratory is precisely what we need—a place where we can experiment with new behavior under controlled and supportive conditions.

Further readings

Carkhuff, R. R., & Berenson, B. G. In search of an honest experience: Confrontation in counseling and life. Chapter 11 in *Beyond counseling and therapy*. New York: Holt, Rinehart and Winston, 1967, Pp. 170-179. Chapter 11 is a collaborative effort under the direction of John Douds and with assistance from Richard Pierce.

Egan, G. Confrontation in laboratory training. Chapter 9 in *Encounter: Group processes for interpersonal growth*. Monterey, Calif.: Brooks/Cole, 1970, Pp. 287-335.

References

Beier, E. *The silent language of psychotherapy*. Chicago: Aldine, 1966.

Berenson, X. G., & Mitchell, K. M. *Confrontation: For better or worse*. Amherst, Mass.: Human Resource Development Press, 1974.

Berne, E. *Games people play*. New York: Grove Press, 1964.

Egan, G. *The skilled helper*. Monterey, Calif.: Brooks/Cole, 1975.

Gordon, T. *Parent effectiveness training*. New York: Wyden, 1970.

Harris, T. *I'm OK–you're OK: A practical guide to transactional analysis*. New York: Harper & Row, 1969.

Harvey, O. J., Kelley, H. H., & Shapiro, M. M. Reactions to unfavorable evaluations of the self made by other persons. *Journal of Personality*, 1957, *25*, 383-411.

James, M., & Jongeward, D. *Born to win: Transactional analysis with Gestalt experiments*. Reading, Mass.: Addison-Wesley, 1971.

Kanter, R. M. *Commitment and community*. Cambridge, Mass.: Harvard University Press, 1972.

King, S. W. *Communication and social influence*. Reading, Mass.: Addison-Wesley, 1975.

Lieberman, M. A., Yalom, I. D., & Miles, M. B. *Encounter groups: First facts*. New York: Basic Books, 1973.

Rosen, S., & Tesser, A. On reluctance to communicate undesirable information: The MUM effect. *Sociometry*, 1970, *33*, 253-263.

Rosen, S., & Tesser, A. Fear of negative evaluation and the reluctance to transmit bad news. *Proceedings of the 79th Annual Convention of the American Psychological Association*, 1971, *6*, 301-302.

Tesser, A., & Rosen, S. Similarity of objective fate as a determinant of the reluctance to transmit unpleasant information: The MUM effect. *Journal of Personality and Social Psychology*, 1972, *23*, 46-53.

Tesser, A., Rosen, S., & Batchelor, T. On the reluctance to communicate bad news (the MUM effect): A role play extension. *Journal of Personality*, 1972, *40*, 88-103.

Tesser, A., Rosen, S., & Tesser, M. On the reluctance to communicate undesirable messages (the MUM effect): A field study. *Psychological Reports*, 1971, *29*, 651-654.

Wallen, J. L. Developing effective interpersonal communication. In R. W. Pace, B. D. Peterson, & T. R. Radcliffe (Eds.), *Communicating interpersonally*. Columbus, Ohio: Charles E. Merrill, 1973, Pp. 218-233.

Chapter 9

PERFORMANCE EVALUATION

An uneasy look at performance appraisal

DOUGLAS McGREGOR, Ph.D.

Performance appraisal within management ranks has become standard practice in many companies during the past 20 years and is currently being adopted by many others, often as an important feature of management development programs. The more the method is used, the more uneasy I grow over the unstated assumptions which lie behind it. Moreover, with some searching, I find that a number of people both in education and industry share my misgivings. This article, therefore, has two purposes:

1. To examine the conventional performance appraisal plan which requires the manager to pass judgment on the personal worth of subordinates.

2. To describe an alternative which places on the subordinate the primary responsibility for establishing performance goals and appraising progress toward them.

CURRENT PROGRAMS

Formal performance appraisal plans are designed to meet three needs, one for the organization and two for the individual:

1. They provide systematic judgments to back up salary increases, promotions, transfers, and sometimes demotions or terminations.

Douglas McGregor, ''An Uneasy Look at Performance Appraisal,'' *Harvard Business Review*, September-October, 1972. Copyright 1957 by the President and Fellows of Harvard College; all rights reserved.

2. They are a means of telling a subordinate how he is doing, and suggesting needed changes in his behavior, attitudes, skills, or job knowledge; they let him know ''where he stands'' with the boss.

3. They also are being increasingly used as a basis for the coaching and counseling of the individual by the superior.

Problem of resistance

Personnel administrators are aware that appraisal programs tend to run into resistance from the managers who are expected to administer them. Even managers who admit the necessity of such programs frequently balk at the process—especially the interview part. As a result, some companies do not communicate appraisal results to the individual, despite the general conviction that the subordinate has a right to know his superior's opinion so he can correct his weaknesses.

The boss's resistance is usually attributed to the following causes:

• A normal dislike of criticizing a subordinate (and perhaps having to argue about it).

• Lack of skill needed to handle the interviews.

• Dislike of a new procedure with its accompanying changes in ways of operating.

• Mistrust of the validity of the appraisal instrument.

To meet this problem, formal controls—scheduling, reminders, and so on—are often instituted. It is common experience that without them fewer than half the appraisal interviews are actually held. But even controls do not necessarily work. Thus:

In one company with a well-planned and carefully administered appraisal program, an opinion poll included two questions regarding appraisals. More than 90% of those answering the questionnaire approved the idea of appraisals. They wanted to know how they stood. Some 40% went on to say that they had never had the experience of being told—yet the files showed that over four fifths of them had signed a form testifying that they had been through an appraisal interview, some of them several times!

The respondents had no reason to lie, nor was there the slightest supposition that their superiors had committed forgery. The probable explanation is that the superiors, being basically resistant to the plan, had conducted the interviews in such a perfunctory manner that many subordinates did not realize what was going on. Training programs designed to teach the skills of appraising and interviewing do help, but they seldom eliminate managerial resistance entirely. The difficulties connected with ''negative appraisals'' remain a source of genuine concern. There is always some discomfort involved in telling a subordinate he is not doing well. The individual who is ''coasting'' during the few years prior to retirement after serving his company competently for many years presents a special dilemma to the boss who is preparing to interview him.

Nor does a shift to a form of group appraisal solve the problem. Though the group method tends to have a greater validity and, properly administered, can equalize varying standards of judgment, it does not ease the difficulty inherent in the interview. In fact, the superior's discomfort is often intensified when he must base his interview on the results of a *group* discussion of the subordinate's worth. Even if the

final judgments have been his, he is not free to discuss the things said by others which may have influenced him.

The underlying cause

What should we think about a method—however valuable for meeting organizational needs—which produces such results in a wide range of companies with a variety of appraisal plans? The problem is one that cannot be dismissed lightly.

Perhaps this intitutive managerial reaction to conventional performance appraisal plans shows a deep but unrecognized wisdom. In my view, it does not reflect anything so simple as resistance to change, or dislike for personnel technique, or lack of skill, or mistrust for rating scales. Rather, managers seem to be expressing real misgivings, which they find difficult to put into words. This could be the underlying cause.

The conventional approach, unless handled with consummate skill and delicacy, constitutes something dangerously close to a violation of the integrity of the personality. Managers are uncomfortable when they are put in the position of ''playing God.'' The respect we hold for the inherent value of the individual leaves us distressed when we must take responsibility for judging the personal worth of a fellow man. Yet the conventional approach to performance appraisal forces us not only to make such judgments and to see them acted upon but also to communicate them to those we have judged. Small wonder we resist!

The modern emphasis upon the manager as a leader who strives to *help* his subordinates achieve both their own and the company's objectives is hardly consistent with the judicial role demanded by most appraisal plans. If the manager must put on his judicial hat occasionally, he does it reluctantly and with understandable qualms. Under such conditions, it is unlikely that the subordinate will be any happier with the results than will the boss. It will not be surprising, either, if he fails to recognize that he has been told where he stands.

Of course, managers cannot escape making judgments about subordinates. Without such evaluations, salary and promotion policies cannot be administered sensibly. But are subordinates like products on an assembly line, to be accepted or rejected as a result of an inspection process? The inspection process may be made more objective or more accurate through research on the appraisal instrument, through training of the "inspectors," or through introducing group appraisal; the subordinate may be "reworked" by coaching or counseling before the final decision to accept or reject him; but as far as the assumptions of the conventional appraisal process are concerned, we still have what is practically identical with a program for product inspection.

On this interpretation, then, resistance to conventional appraisal programs is eminently sound. It reflects an unwillingness to treat human beings like physical objects. The needs of the organization are obviously important, but when they come into conflict with our convictions about the worth and the dignity of the human personality, one or the other must give.

Indeed, by the fact of their resistance managers are saying that the organization must yield in the face of this fundamental human value. And they are thus being more sensitive than are personnel administrators and social scientists whose business it is to be concerned with the human problems of industry!

A NEW APPROACH

If this analysis is correct, the task before us is clear. We must find a new plan—not a compromise to hide the dilemma, but a bold move to resolve the issue.

A number of writers are beginning to approach the whole subject of management from the point of view of basic social values. Peter Drucker's concept of "management by objectives"[1] offers an unusally promising framework within which we can seek a solution. Several companies, notably General Mills, Incorporated, and General Electric Company, have been exploring different methods of appraisal which rest upon assumptions consistent with Drucker's philosophy.

Responsibility on subordinate

This approach calls on the subordinate to establish short-term performance goals *for himself*. The superior enters the process actively only *after* the subordinate has (a) done a good deal of thinking about his job, (b) made a careful assessment of his own strengths and weaknesses, and (c) formulated some specific plans to accomplish his goals. The superior's role is to help the man relate his self-appraisal, his "targets," and his plans for the ensuing period to the realities of the organization.

The first step in this process is to arrive at a clear statement of the major features of the job. Rather than a formal job description, this is a document drawn up *by the subordinate* after studying the company-approved statement. It defines the broad areas of his responsibility as they actually work out in practice. The boss and employee discuss the draft jointly and modify it as may be necessary until both of them agree that it is adequate.

Working from this statement of responsibilities, the subordinate then establishes his goals or "targets" for a period of, say, six months. These targets are *specific* actions which the man proposes to take, i.e., setting up regular staff meetings to improve communication, reorganizing the office, completing or undertaking a certain study. Thus they are explicitly stated and accompanied by a detailed account of the actions he proposes to take to reach them. This

---

[1] See *The Practice of Management* (New York, Harper & Brothers, 1954).

document is, in turn, discussed with the superior and modified until both are satisfied with it.

At the conclusion of the six-month period, the subordinate makes *his own* appraisal of what he has accomplished relative to the targets he had set earlier. He substantiates it with factual data wherever possible. The "interview" is an examination by superior and subordinate together of the subordinate's self-appraisal, and it culminates in a resetting of targets for the next six months.

Of course, the superior has veto power at each step of this process; in an organizational hierarchy anything else would be unacceptable. However, in practice he rarely needs to exercise it. Most subordinates tend to underestimate both their potentialities and their achievements. Moreover, subordinates normally have an understandable wish to satisfy their boss, and are quite willing to adjust their targets or appraisals if the superior feels they are unrealistic. Actually, a much more common problem is to resist the subordinates' tendency to want the boss to tell them what to write down.

Analysis vs. appraisal

This approach to performance appraisal differs profoundly from the conventional one, for it shifts the emphasis from *appraisal* to *analysis*. This implies a more positive approach. No longer is the subordinate being examined by the superior so that his weaknesses may be determined; rather, he is examining himself, in order to define not only his weaknesses but also his strengths and potentials. The importance of this shift of emphasis should not be underestimated. It is basic to each of the specific differences which distinguish this approach from the conventional one.

The first of these differences arises from the subordinate's new role in the process. He becomes an active agent, not a passive "object." He is no longer a pawn in a chess game called management development.

Effective development of managers does not include coercing them (no matter how benevolently) into acceptance of the goals of the enterprise, nor does it mean manipulating their behavior to suit organizational needs. Rather, it calls for creating a relationship within which a man can take responsibility for developing his own potentialities, plan for himself, and learn from putting his plans into action. In the process, he can gain a genuine sense of satisfaction, for he is utilizing his own capabilities to achieve simultaneously both his objectives and those of the organization. Unless this is the nature of the relationship, "development" becomes a euphemism.

Who knows best?

One of the main differences of this approach is that it rests on the assumption that the individual knows—or can learn—more than anyone else about his own capabilities, needs, strengths and weaknesses, and goals. In the end, only he can determine what is best for his development. The conventional approach, on the other hand, makes the assumption that the superior can know enough about the subordinate to decide what is best for him.

No available methods can provide the superior with the knowledge he needs to make such decisions. Ratings, aptitude and personality tests, and the superior's necessarily limited knowledge of the man's performance yield at best an imperfect picture. Even the most extensive psychological counseling (assuming the superior possesses the competence for it) would not solve the problem because the product of counseling is self-insight on the part of the *counselee*.

(Psychological tests are not being condemned by this statement. On the contrary, they have genuine value in competent hands. Their use by professionals as part of the process of screening applicants for employment does not raise the same questions as their use to "diagnose" the personal worth of accepted members of a management team. Even in the latter instance, the problem under discussion would not arise if test results and interpretations were given to the *individual himself,* to be shared with superiors at his discretion.)

The proper role for the superior, then, is the one that falls naturally to him under the suggested plan: helping the subordinate relate his career planning to the needs and realities of the organization. In the discussions, the boss can use his knowledge of the organization to help the subordinate establish targets and methods for achieving them which will (a) lead to increased knowledge and skill, (b) contribute to organizational objectives, and (c) test the subordinate's appraisal of himself.

This is help which the subordinate wants. He knows well that the rewards and satisfactions he seeks from his career as a manager depend on his contribution to organizational objectives. He is also aware that the superior knows more completely than he what is required for success in this organization and *under this boss.* The superior, then, is the person who can help him test the soundness of his goals and his plans for achieving them. Quite clearly the knowledge and active participation of *both* superior and subordinate are necessary components of this approach.

If the superior accepts this role, he need not become a judge of the subordinate's personal worth. He is not telling, deciding, criticizing, or praising—not "playing God." He finds himself listening, using his own knowledge of the organization as a basis for advising, guiding, encouraging his subordinates to develop their own potentialities. Incidentally, this often leads the superior to important insights about himself and his impact on others.

Looking to the future

Another significant difference is that the emphasis is on the future rather than the past. The purpose of the plan is to establish realistic targets and to seek the most effective ways of reaching them. Appraisal thus becomes a means

to a *constructive* end. The 60-year-old "coaster" can be encouraged to set performance goals for himself and to make a fair appraisal of his progress toward them. Even the subordinate who has failed can be helped to consider what moves will be best for himself. The superior rarely finds himself facing the uncomfortable prospect of denying a subordinate's personal worth. A transfer or even a demotion can be worked out without the connotation of a "sentence by the judge."

Performance vs. personality

Finally, the accent is on *performance,* on actions relative to goals. There is less tendency for the personality of the subordinate to become an issue. The superior, instead of finding himself in the position of a psychologist or a therapist, can become a coach helping the subordinate to reach his own decisions on the specific steps that will enable him to reach his targets. Such counseling as may be required demands no deep analysis of the personal motivations or basic adjustment of the subordinate. To illustrate:

Consider a subordinate who is hostile, short-tempered, uncooperative, insecure. The superior need not make any psychological diagnosis. The "target setting" approach naturally directs the subordinate's attention to ways and means of obtaining better interdepartmental collaboration, reducing complaints, winning the confidence of the men under him. Rather than facing the troublesome prospect of forcing his own psychological diagnosis on the subordinate, the superior can, for example, help the individual plan ways of getting "feedback" concerning his impact on his associates and subordinates as a basis for self-appraisal and self-improvement.

There is little chance that a man who is involved in a process like this will be in the dark about where he stands, or that he will forget he is the principal participant in his own development and responsible for it.

A NEW ATTITUDE

As a consequence of these differences we may expect the growth of a different attitude toward appraisal on the part of superior and subordinate alike.

The superior will gain real satisfaction as he learns to help his subordinates integrate their personal goals with the needs of the organization so that both are served. Once the subordinate has worked out a mutually satisfactory plan of action, the superior can delegate to him the responsibility for putting it into effect. He will see himself in a consistent managerial role rather than being forced to adopt the basically incompatible role of either the judge or the psychologist.

Unless there is a basic personal antagonism between the two men (in which case the relationship should be terminated), the superior can conduct these interviews so that both are actively involved in seeking the right basis for constructive action. The organization, the boss, and the subordinate all stand to gain. Under such circumstances the opportunities for learning and for genuine development of both parties are maximal.

The particular mechanics are of secondary importance. The needs of the organization in the administration of salary and promotion policies can easily be met within the framework of the analysis process. The machinery of the program can be adjusted to the situation. No universal list of rating categories is required. The complications of subjective or prejudiced judgment, of varying standards, of attempts to quantify qualitative data, all can be minimized. In fact, *no* formal machinery is required.

Problems of judgment

I have deliberately slighted the many problems of judgment involved in administering promotions and salaries. These are by no means minor, and this approach will not automatically solve them. However, I believe that if we are prepared to recognize the fundamental problem inherent in the conventional approach, ways can be found to temper our present administrative methods.

And if this approach is accepted, the traditional ingenuity of management will lead to the invention of a variety of methods for its implementation. The mechanics of some conventional plans can be adjusted to be consistent with this point of view. Obviously, a program utilizing ratings of the personal characteristics of subordinates would not be suitable, but one which emphasizes *behavior* might be.

Of course, managerial skill is required. No method will eliminate that. This method can fail as readily as any other in the clumsy hands of insensitive or indifferent or power-seeking managers. But even the limited experience of a few companies with this approach indicates that managerial *resistance* is substantially reduced. As a consequence, it is easier to gain the collaboration of managers in developing the necessary skills.

Cost in time

There is one unavoidable cost: the manager must spend considerably more time in implementing a program of this kind. It is not unusual to take a couple of days to work through the initial establishment of responsibilities and goals with each individual. And a periodic appraisal may require several hours rather than the typical 20 minutes.

Reaction to this cost will undoubtedly vary. The management that considers the development of its human resources to be the primary means of achieving the economic objectives of the organization will not be disturbed. It will regard the necessary guidance and coaching as among the most important functions of every superior.

CONCLUSION

I have sought to show that the conventional approach to performance appraisal stands condemned as a personnel method. It places the manager in the untenable position of judging the personal worth of his subordinates, and of acting on these judgments. No manager possesses, nor could he acquire, the skill necessary to carry out this responsibility effectively. Few would even be willing to accept it if they were fully aware of the implications involved.

It is this unrecognized aspect of conventional appraisal programs which produces the widespread uneasiness and even open resistance of management to appraisals and especially to the appraisal interview.

A sounder approach, which places the major responsibility on the subordinate for establishing performance goals and appraising progress toward them, avoids the major weakness of the old plan and benefits the organization by stimulating the development of the subordinate. It is true that more managerial skill and the investment of a considerable amount of time are required, but the greater motivation and the more effective development of subordinates can justify these added costs.

A systems approach to evaluation of nursing performance

CHRISTINE BENSON, R.N., M.S.N., PEGGY SCHMELING, R.N., M.S.N., and GARY BRUINS, R.N., B.S.N.

The problem of accurately and objectively evaluating the performance of nurses in a hospital has been extremely difficult for nursing administration. In designing an evaluation system for nursing, it is essential to consider the concept that evaluation is an emotionally-charged area, and that its interpretation by the nurses being evaluated can have a strong impact on their self-esteem and subsequent performance of patient care.[1] The design of an evaluation system, then, must be carefully selected and detailed to both conserve the integrity of the individual practitioner and to provide for competent care delivery.

Our interest in evaluation systems evolved from personal involvement with a 300-bed acute care teaching hospital in urban Milwaukee. The special care units include a six-bed intensive care unit, a six-bed coronary care unit, and a 25-bed intermediate care unit. They

Reprinted with permission from *Nursing Administration Quarterly*, 1978

will be collectively referred to as the critical care areas.

At the time this project was undertaken, the staff in the critical care areas, in response to multi-faceted problems, lacked their usual motivation and interest. Administration, concerned about the rapid turnover and wishing to improve the quality of patient care, had promised the staff a wage increase based on the clinical ladder concept. The rationale for this concept, in which clinical expertise is rewarded via a promotional system, has been described by Marie Zimmer.[2] Emphasis was placed on the fact that nurses are responsible and accountable for their own practice. In accordance with this concept, a job description for critical care staff nurses had been developed by an ad hoc committee. The original plan was to base the evaluation on percent accomplishment of the criteria defined in the job description. No immediate plans had been made for the development of a formal evaluation tool for implementation of the program. This situation presented itself to us as an interesting and challenging problem to approach within the framework of administrative theory.

THE SYSTEMS APPROACH TO PROBLEM SOLVING

In order to organize a method for developing a tool for evaluation based on the ladder concept we decided to utilize the systems approach to problem-solving. The process we used was devised by Janet M. Kraegel et al.[3] In selecting the best system we followed the steps outlined below:

    I. *Statement of purpose.* The purpose was to plan an evaluation system for critical care nurses based on the ladder concept.

    II. *Expanded purposes.* Through the process of expanding our purposes we deduced that the ultimate goal was to provide quality patient care.

    III. *Restrictions.* The most imposing restriction was that we were required to remain within the confines of the job description developed for critical care staff nurses.

    IV. *Criteria.* We wanted the evaluation system to be applicable to evaluation of critical care nurses as a pilot study, to be objective and account for bias, halo effect and central tendency,[4] to allow for interchange between nurses and their evaluators, and to reward self-motivation and quality of patient care with status and wage increase.

    V. *Unit of regularity.* The tool would basically be designed for the purpose of regular evaluation of staff nurses at predetermined intervals by their immediate supervisors.

    VI. *Ideal system.* We conducted a thorough search of the literature to gather all available ideas that would fulfill our defined purpose.

    VII. *Selecting the best system.* In selecting the best possible system from our long list of alternatives, we decided to use Maslow's hierarchy of needs as a theoretical base in devising the evaluation tool. This is a conceptual framework that most nurses relate to well and could be easily adapted for our purposes. The major responsibility for evaluation lies with head nurses who may choose to delegate their authority to assistant head nurses in charge of various shifts. In order to eliminate bias, input is contributed by head nurses, assistant head nurses, nursing supervisors, clinical specialists, and assistant directors of nursing. This administrative evaluation would be compared with a self-evaluation by nurses in a goal-setting conference in which their performance can be contrasted with their own pre-determined objectives and own prior performance. In this manner nurses and evaluators would determine the nurses' placement on the ladder and direction of planned progress. A conceptual model offers a complete explanation of the evaluation process and how it fits into the total system. (See Figure 1).

UTILIZATION OF MASLOW'S HIERARCHY OF NEEDS

In designing the best ideal system we devised three categories which implied progression for vertical advancement, titled Clinician I, Clinician II, and Clinician III. Within the existing job description for critical care staff nurses, there are five major categories on which the nursing staff should be evaluated. These are 1) direct patient care; 2) teaching/learning; 3) coordination/leadership; 4) professional development; and 5) research.[5] Also within the job description were generalized criteria that staff nurses were expected to attain. Thus, a major task for our project became establishment of measurable criteria for each clinician level. Maslow's theory of individual human motivation served as a frame of reference for this task.

Maslow's hierarchy consists of a continuum

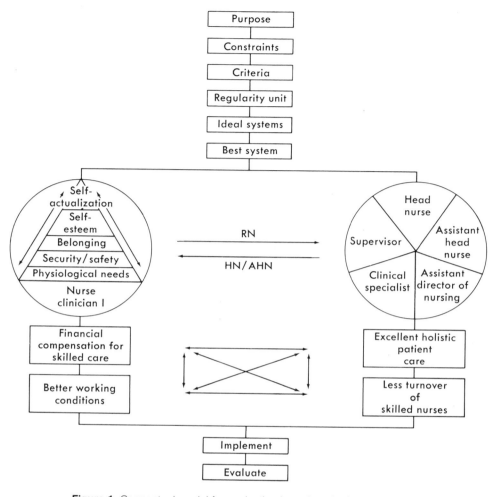

Figure 1. Conceptual model for evaluation based on the ladder concept.

or sequence of needs ranging from the most basic physiologic need to survive through the various psycho-social needs to the point of self-actualization. Maslow referred to the fact that prior to accomplishing higher level needs, one must first accomplish the lower level needs. Therefore, inherent in this theory is a ladder concept.

In relating staff nurse performance to Maslow's theory, the following assumptions were made:

1. In order to meet survival needs in one's job, one must meet the basic qualifications for the position.
2. In order to meet the security needs in one's job, one must display a sense of awareness of trust and self-confidence.
3. In order to meet the belonging needs in one's job, one must communicate effectively.
4. In order to meet the self-esteem needs in

one's job, one must be totally committed and display involvement.

5. In order to meet the self-actualization needs in one's job, one must take responsibilities and display autonomy.

Having established this parallel to Maslow's theory, it became necessary to consolidate the basic process so that three behaviors remained:

1. Display of awareness of the rationale for actions and self-confidence in performance.
2. Display of ability to communicate effectively.
3. Display of autonomy and responsibility for action.

These behaviors of nurses become the main threads in devising the performance criteria expected for the three levels of clinical practice. When applying our three threads to this criteria, the expected behavior for the three various clinicians became:

Clinician I: Gives pertinent information regarding patient's problems, unit activities and personal needs when asked.

Clinician II: Gleans insights into patient problems, unit problems and personal needs and initiates communication to proper authority.

Clinician III: Identifies problems, gathers pertinent data regarding problems and communicates appropriately in suggesting solutions to appropriate authority.

Devising the evaluative criteria became a realistic task only after we had conceptualized Maslow's theory and made assumptions based on his theory.

DETAILING THE SYSTEM

The final aspect of detailing the system evolved around the presentation of the tool to administration, the ad hoc committee, and the staff. The tool was first presented to the assistant director of nursing for critical care. With her acceptance and approval, she in turn presented it to the assistant administrator of nurs-

ing. In the interim, the evaluation system was presented to the staff for questions, comments, and further input. After the director's approval, the tool was presented to the ad hoc committee for final approval. With the approval of the ad hoc committee, the tool was presented to the staff in its final form for use in the pilot study.

RECOMMENDATIONS FOR IMPLEMENTATION

The following recommendations were suggested for successful implementation of the evaluation system.

1. Each of the five evaluators maintain anecdotal notes.
2. Utilize sources for further evaluation and observation:
   a. Periodically review care plans
   b. Audit nurses' documentations in chart
3. Individual nurses keep track of the team conferences they have given through a card file kept in the unit where they work.
4. Record daily observed factual data regarding effective and ineffective performance. This is designed for the nurses' benefit to discuss strengths and weaknesses.
5. Hold summary conferences after evaluation is given whereby aspects of the evaluation can be discussed and mutual goal-setting can take place. Goal-setting, not criticism, should be used to improve performance.
6. Coaching conferences between formal evaluations should be ongoing, help according to the needs of the individual nurse.
7. Keep conferences open and future-oriented.

IMPLEMENTATION OF THE SYSTEM

The evaluation system was implemented as a pilot project in the critical care areas in January 1976. Twenty-one registered nurses were admitted onto the ladder, nineteen as Clinician I and two as Clinician II. All nurses prepared a self-evaluation and participated in a goal-setting conference with the head nurse to determine initial placement. Further information on the systems process was given, emphasizing specifics of each individual's nursing practice within the confines of the system.

ASSESSMENT OF IMPLEMENTATION PHASE

In assessing the implementation phase, the assistant director of nursing, personnel director, both head nurses and two staff nurses were interviewed. A major problem was the lack of sufficient orientation of the evaluators to the evaluation tool itself. Both head nurses felt that some categories were subject to varied interpretation and that some of the language used was cumbersome and abstract. One head nurse complained that the evaluation form did not allow her to delve into personality problems and their effect on nursing performance.

Problems were encountered in the attempt to apply the evaluation to the part-time nurse and the administrative personnel themselves, as neither were free to devote most of their time to development of clinical expertise. It also seemed difficult, in some areas, to use identical criteria to evaluate both nurses from the intensive-coronary care unit and the intermediate care unit. Another difficulty expressed was the lack of time to document critical events, and the absence of administrative personnel to record events on PM or night rotations.

In comparing administrative evaluations with staff evaluations, most categories were rated closely, with staff nurses generally ranking themselves lower on the scale than their head nurse evaluators ranked them! Both head nurses stated that the goal-planning conferences allowed them to communicate on a new, more in-depth level with their professional staff. One head nurse also expressed the feeling that since

her staff members had goals, she felt more confident in her own ability to direct them. She also felt that the evaluation focused primarily on patient-centered care and the nursing process, giving the entire group a common direction.

Staff nurses expressed pleasure with the goal-setting conferences. One nurse maintained that she noted an initial difference in staff performance, but that the effect was only temporary. Another nurse maintained that she had more initiative due to the positive and personalized nature of the conferences. All expressed the idea that the evaluation form itself, while being comprehensive in nature, was not concise in many categories and needed some change.

The personnel director stated that the evaluation system was a good attempt to describe and quantify the position of the professional nurse, and that it was an excellent start in the recognition and rewarding of both education and performance. He did question the training of the nurse evaluators and their ability to be objective, stating that money does have an effect on evaluation and that the tendency is to lean toward reward and positive evaluation. Therefore, if the evaluators are being given the authority to spend hospital dollars, they must be in control of the system. Since both nurses and evaluators have expressed some difficulty with consistent interpretation of all items, he recommends evaluation and revision of the tool to provide for a more objective evaluation based on measurable behaviors.

EVALUATION OF THE SYSTEM

As projected by the system, evaluation of the project began in January 1977, after the one year pilot study had been completed. The two major goals of the evaluation study now underway are; 1) to test the reliability and practicality of the evaluation tool, and 2) to determine whether the basic objectives of the system are being accomplished.

The tool developed to determine the reliability and practicality of the system had to answer the following questions:

1. Is this evaluation form one which can produce reliable ratings when used by the same rater on the same individual for two successive intervals and also when used by two different raters for the same individual concurrently?[6]
2. Should administrative personnel be included in the ladder system at all?
3. Can the same form be utilized for full-time and part-time personnel? Intensive care/coronary care and intermediate care personnel?
4. Is the evaluation form too complex or abstract? Are all items objectively measurable?

Information derived from these answers will guide the committee in finalization of the evaluation form.

Each of the objectives defined by the system has a separate focus and can be tested by its own criteria.

1. *Objective:* Excellent holistic patient care.
   Criteria: Are nurse-defined goals patient-oriented? Are nurses meeting their goals?
2. *Objective:* Financial compensation for skilled care.
   Criteria: Percentage of eligible nurses being compensated.
3. *Objective:* Better working conditions.
   Criteria: Attitude-testing for job satisfaction.
4. *Objective:* Less turnover of skilled nurses.
   Criteria: Statistical comparison of turnover before and after implementation of the evaluation system.

The integration of results of the evaluation study will ensure that the intent is being accomplished, that the needs of the hospital and the nurses are being met, and that the revisions will be responsive to changing organizational goals.

WORKING CONCEPTUAL MODEL

Utilization of the systems approach in our task of developing a ladder system of evaluation and promotion provided us with an organized framework and led us to the development of a conceptual model. The result was a theory-based process of evaluation with a built-in design to integrate it into the philosophy and objectives of nursing. Even though the evaluation form itself will need revision, the model will offer guidance to assessment and re-evaluation of the system and its goals as it is expanded into the total hospital system to form the basis of a comprehensive career ladder.

The system defined is one way to support the trend of professional nursing in today's society. The ladder concept defines levels of competence and recognizes nurses, who are directly involved in providing care to patients and families, as being responsible for their practice and accountable for the quality of nursing care provided to the consumers. Recognition of performance in nursing practice and provision of an environment which enables nurses to grow in competence should result in a higher rate of retention of nurses with motivation to achieve an advanced level of competence in practice and to pursue careers at the bedside.

An organized, high level approach to management tasks such as evaluation of personnel could aid nursing administration in directing the nurse to the development of a patient-oriented practice and make the evaluation process itself meaningful and constructive.

References

1. Thompson, P. H. and Dalton, G. W., "Performance Appraisal: Managers Beware." *Harvard Business Review* (January-February 1970) p. 150.
2. Zimmer, Marie J. "Rationale for A Ladder for Clinical Advancement in Nursing Practice." *Journal of Nursing Administration* (November-December 1972) p. 18-24.
3. Kraegel, J. M. *et al. Patient Care Systems* (Philadelphia: J. B. Lippincott Co. 1974).
4. Nash, A. N. and Carroll, S. J. "Individual-Wage Determination." Chapter 6. *The Management of Compen-*

sation (Monterey, California: Brooks/Cole Publishing Company, Inc., 1975) p. 177-89.

5. Anderson, M. I. and Denyes, M. J. "A Ladder for Clinical Advancement in Nursing Practice: Implementation." *Journal of Nursing Administration* (February 1975) p. 11.

6. Tate, B. L. *Test of a Nursing Performance Evaluation Instrument,* (New York: Research and Studies Service National League for Nursing 1964) p. 10.

Suggested readings

Chopra, A. "Motivation in Task-Oriented Groups." *Journal of Nursing Administration,* (January-February 1973) p. 16-22..

Colavecchio, R., Tescher, B., and Scalzi, C. "A Clinical Ladder for Nursing Practice." *Journal of Nursing Administration:* (September-October 1974) p. 54-8.

Conforti, M. F., Ed. D. "Understanding and Motivating Employees." *Occupational Health Nurse Nursing* (January 1972) p. 14, 20, 47.

Jehring, J. J. "Motivational Problems in the Modern Hospital." *Journal of Nursing Administration* (September-December 1972) p. 35-41.

Lysaught, J. P. "No Carrots, No Sticks: Motivation in Nursing." *Journal of Nursing Administration:* (September-October 1972) p. 43-50.

Evaluation as an Objective Approach. National League for Nursing 1972) Report of the 1971 Workshops of the Council of Diploma Programs.

Is the position description obsolete?

CHARLES GEROLD, Consultant

Is the position description obsolete? A growing number of behaviorists say it is, but personnel technicians, searching for an adequate replacement, claim that there is no substitute for it. Operations personnel in the middle, trying to do their jobs, ask just to be left alone. Despite the disparity of opinions, many in each group agree that, as presently used, the position description is too often a waste of time.

However, proponents of the position description ask whether this need be the case. Does the manager who misuses or permits abuse of the position description deprive himself of one of his most useful tools? Advocates of the position description argue that when it is used in conjunction with management by objectives (MBO) and appraisal by results (ABR), it can be a key to planning, staffing, work organization, scheduling, productivity control, review, and reporting. Its advocates claim that when MBO and ABR are built into the position description—as they easily can be—it becomes a working tool of unsurpassed value.

Not so in reality, say critics, who see the position description as an anachronism from the outmoded scientific management movement, as repugnant as the stopwatch. And they marshall impressive arguments to support their opinion.

A typical discussion between a proponent and opponent of the position description might follow the direction of the following conversation.

Con: *My job is different. It's too dynamic and complex to reduce to writing.*

Pro: What you really mean is that no one has clarified what you're supposed to do or achieve, so of course you feel threatened by any attempt to plan or measure the objectives or performance standards of your non-job.

Con: *It's too time-consuming. I would have to spend hours every month updating details of goals, tasks, and schedules. New performance standards would have to be devised for every new assignment, and the domino impact of this effort would require endless toil. I don't have time.*

Pro: In this era of permissive play-work, it may

Reprinted by permission from *Hospital Progress,* May, 1971, and the author.

seem bizarre to ask a manager to plan, direct, and review performance. But what higher priority functions are you paid to perform? A participative approach to developing the position description is not prohibited; in fact, it is recommended. But keep in mind that you are ultimately responsible for the use of material-human-cash resources in your unit and that a significant percentage of work being done this minute should probably not have been undertaken in the first place. (Consult Parkinson, Drucker, and Townsend, plus your own experience.) There is a larger multiplier of reward in productivity and savings for every minute you spend planning and controlling work.

Con: *The best laid plans. . . . When unforeseeable circumstances crop up, all my planning effort goes down the tubes anyway.*

Pro: The truth is that imaginative planning can anticipate emergencies. Even interruptions that can't be anticipated can be better fielded by an organized team able to shift ordered priorities and assignments in order to cope with new factors. The ability of a champion quarterback to call effective audibles under stress is founded upon prearranged targets and tasks, well drilled into each team member. Are you a team leader or just padding?

Con: *Don't fence me in! Staked-out assignments kill initiative, promote lethargy, reinforce resistance to change, and destroy the will to progress.*

Pro: Creative chaos may be appropriate in a few truly breakthrough assignments. But the vast majority of work is best accomplished by organization and ordered performance. Indeed, many highly creative people require a structured environment to free them from routine detail. Disorganization inevitably results in costly gaps and overlaps. Any manager who permits apathy to develop in an organized work situation is certainly likely to tolerate unproductive anarchy.

Con: *All this paperwork is a putdown. Overplanning stultifies the self-actualizing enthusiasm essential to high morale, effective teamwork, and unique individual performance. Who wants to take a trip if every milestone along the way has been pre-identified and pre-examined in numbing detail? Interest palls.*

Pro: Are you conducting a country club gambol

or being paid to reach a target by doing only what is necessary, in an acceptable manner, within budget, on schedule? Is the pleasure and pride that comes from completing a given task no longer worthy of consideration?

Con: *Position descriptions are fundamentally phony, anyway, insofar as influencing management to give equal pay for equal work. Even if a position description is honestly written, words have multiple meanings, so that, strung out in paragraphs, the ambiguities and generalizations are overwhelming. Subjective interpretation is inevitable. When the chips are passed out, favoritism, politics, even honest misunderstanding will still decide who gets what and when.*

Pro: Not if objectives, tasks required to achieve each, and standards of performance are built in and enforced by use in performance review. Combined with the strategic performance budget, the position description is a tactical tool that is very difficult to "fix."

ARE THERE ALTERNATIVES?

Having identified some pros and cons, let's briefly explore the alternatives to the position description to see if there are other means of achieving the functions that it performs. The objective of this task is to find a tool that is free from the major defects of the position description, which even its champions admit. These include heavy investment of time, rapid obsolescence, subjectivity, some inflexibility, and generalization. At the same time, keep in mind that we are searching for a tool that can perform all the functions which the position description performs when properly and fully used. A brief list of these might include:

1. Planning:
   a. Specify goals per job, pyramiding into goals for the unit and for the organization.
   b. Specify management's expectations.
   c. Specify performance constraints: Time, cost, and error. Prescribe productivity standards.

Job title:	State the title of the position being described.		Info: Information
			Rec: Recommendations
Grade:	Enter its grade (41 through 90, or "executive").		Dec: Decisions
			Svc: Services
Shift:	A.M., P.M.. or Night.	Substance of contact:	What the contact is all about: Products, subjects, kinds of services, organizational meetings, etc.
Days:	Number of days worked per week, if irregular; otherwise, "Mon-Fri," "Sat-Sun," etc.		Examples: Report XYZ
Immediate supervisor:	Name of first level supervisor.		Inhalation therapy treatments
Grade:	His (her) grade.		Maintenance work orders
Qualifications required:	The minimum background needed to perform this job at the level of responsibility indicated by its grade.		Nursing schedules
			Policies ABC
			Purchase of medicines
Education:	Level of schooling believed to be required. Formal education is not to be equated with either intelligence or ability.	Item No.	Numerical identification of objectives and tasks: One to infinity.
License/certificate required:	If any. Example: RN, engineer, CRNA, MD.	Objectives:	List the broad goals or basic objectives which this position exists to achieve within the next time period (6-month minimum; 12-month maximum). Basically, objectives are not actions, so use nouns here in declarative sentences.
Experience:	How many months or years; specify general or specific requirements, i.e., five years in general office work, two years as therapist, etc.	Related tasks:	Tasks required to achieve each objective. There may be few or many. Try to start each task statement with a verb. The key to easy identification of units per measure and standards of performance later on is to break the tasks down to a level of detail small enough to produce visibility on desired results. At first, you may find it easier to start by identifying the standards of performance now used to judge whether a job has been well or poorly done. Then, specify the task to which those standards apply, singly or as a group.
Equipment used:	Machinery or devices which employe must operate.		
Special skills required:	Languages, interpersonal competence, etc., not specified elsewhere.		
Unusual environmental factors:	Examples: Laundry room heat; frequent entry/exit to cold storage lockers; other unusual factors affecting physical or psychological comfort.	Volume/frequency:	The volume and frequency of work involved in a task.
			Examples: Meetings per week
Time required to reach proficiency:	How many months of practice needed to do this job at the required level:		Reports per month
	A. Generally: Starting with the education specified above.		Applicants per hour
	B. In this hospital: Starting with the education and experience specified above.		Forms to be processed per day
Person(s) dealt with:	Enter in descending order according to hours spent per month. If list is long, group classes of persons according to reason for contact. Be complete, but avoid duplicate statements.		For tasks that are not of a recurring nature, it may be difficult to specify frequency. Also, where intangibles are concerned, the volume may be difficult to measure. However, it is surprising how many tasks can be identified in terms of product volume and frequency, if the task is stated at a low enough level of detail.
Individual or class:	If numbers of nurses, clerks, maintenance personnel, etc., are dealt with, do not list individual names, but note the general class. If individual contact outside general classes takes more than five per cent of total time per average month, name the individual dealt with.		
Title:	Position held by person(s) referred to.	Unit of measure:	In evaluating performance, how do you measure? Normally, measures are made in terms of counts: Time deadlines to be met; number of units to be processed, produced, or affected; number or percentage of permissible defects.
Grade:	Grade held by person(s) referred to. This may be a range.		
Hours spent per month:	One hundred and seventy-two hours constitute a standard work month based on 4.3 40-hr. weeks. Therefore, the total of all entries in this column should not exceed 172 hours. For each entry, estimate hours per average month.	Performance of standard:	How many units per time period? How many errors per count? What percentage of errors is acceptable? What time slippage is permissible? How do you tell that the job has been well done? More often than may be supposed, specific standards are already known. The labor comes in trying to reduce them to writing. Once done, however, performance evaluation standards are also complete.
Type of contact:	How the relationship is maintained:		
	Tel: By telephone		
	Per: In person		
	Grp: In group meetings		
Reasons for contact:	Purposes served by contacts. Basically, these dealings entail supplying or obtaining:		

Figure 1. Suggested content: position description reflecting MBO/ABR.

d. Basis for task assignment recurring daily/weekly/monthly/quarterly/annually.

2. Staffing:
   a. Forecast manpower resources and development needs.
   b. Personal services.
   c. Identify skills needed for specific advertising, interviewing, training, transfer, and promotion actions.
   d. Clarify organizational boundaries by function analysis.
   e. Structure for assigning newly-hired employes.
   f. Basis for classification and pay structure, yielding internal consistency and rational relation to the external labor market.
   g. Orientation tool: Tasks and standards.

3. Organizing work:
   a. Pre-slice the activity pie.
   b. Tailor the job to the man or train the man to the job.
   c. Stimulate self-assessment and development.

4. Directing Work: A compass pointing through task squalls to objectives in the light of standards.

5. Performance Evaluation: Position description contains the forecast and standards to compare with actuals.

6. Reporting: A unit manager's responsibilities comprise the sum of each position description reporting to him, plus those functions which he alone performs. Reports up, out, and down will properly evolve from objective- and task-planning reflected at the start of a cycle. Breakouts of the data, of course, are possible.

Figure 1 gives some samples of position descriptions.

Alternative tools available to supplant the position description include: Salary surveys, ranking, collective bargaining, individual exploitation of the marketplace, factored performance evaluation, job enlargement, and rank in person. These related methods are well-known and are discussed in standard texts, so they need not be elaborated upon here.

Using different arguments to skew the material presented in Figure 1 in the direction of any prejudice, it is still obvious that no tool exists that can do as many things as well as the position description. The real superiority of the position description as a management tool is best realized, however, when MBO and ABR are built in.

SUMMARY

Although the position description is still a far from perfect tool, a workable substitute has not yet been developed. In fact, many other supervisory management tools and techniques are so dependent upon sound position analysis, that many management weaknesses can be traced to inadequate position descriptions. No other tool can so readily identify recruitment needs, orientation, requirements, training problems, performance standards, results criteria, etc. The position description "puts it all together."

Chapter 10

CHANGE PROCESS

Theoretical considerations involved in the process of change

JANET A. RODGERS, R.N., Ph.D.

In an age in which the single constant is radical and rapid change, we all suffer in varying degrees from what Toffler calls ''future shock.'' If we are to steer a course between disorganizing cognitive dissonance and reactive psychic and social inertia we need to increase our understanding of the nature and dynamics of change.

WHO IS THE CLIENT?

When examining the principles and strategies for changing social behavior, we frequently encounter the debate over who is the appropriate client: the individual or the social system? Schein reminds us that the issue is reminiscent of Koestler's distinction between the Yogi and the Commissar—between those who turn inward for insight and nirvana and those who turn outward for social salvation. (1:202) Put another way, it is the difference between those who look to self-actualization for ultimate social improvement and those who believe in the manipulation of external forces, such as legal, technological, economic, and political. Sometimes the debate takes the guise of theoretical preferences—Freud versus Skinner, or individualism versus statism.

The target of change is both the individual

Reprinted with permission from *Nursing Forum*, Vol. XII, No. 2, 1973.

and the social system, usually a formal organization or some subdivision of it. The dynamics inherent in the change process are the same; the strategic differences lie in the complexity.

I am reminded of Ujhely's excellent paper '' 'And' Instead of 'Either-or' or the 'Fallacy of False Opposition,' '' (2:10-13) for certainly this is not an either-or phenomenon. Ujhely speaks on the seeming dichotomy of ''social action'' versus ''working with individuals.'' After empathizing with the nurse's utter frustration at the multiplicity of problems in which patients are ensnared, and recognizing that nurses frequently would rather be active in other endeavors than witness the patient's plight, day in and day out, she says:

. . . I am not sure at all that we have to either be with the patient or in the social arena. Is there any reason why we cannot do both? Is there any reason why, in the innumerable intolerable hospital situations we cannot help the patient by giving what little support we can . . . by aiding him . . . to survive in the system, while at the same time trying to alter his surrounding atmosphere by working with the staff and while also seeking power so that we can participate in top decision making with respect to his welfare? . . . Of course, it is much more difficult to keep involved in the patient's present situation while at the same time attempting to chip away at the walls that hold him bound. . . . It is not enough for him to know that you are trying to hoe a future exit out of his prison; he also needs someone who can be with him and help him bear the life he must lead now. (2:12)

MODELS OF CHANGE

Let me review the assumptions of three analytic models of change described by Chin: the system model, the developmental model, and the model for changing. (3:201-214)

The primary emphasis in a *system model* is on the manner in which stability is achieved. Change is derived from the structure and evolves out of the incompatabilities and conflicts in the system. The assumption is made that in an organization interdependency and integration exist among its parts, and that change is dependent upon how well the parts of the system fit together—or upon how well the system fits with other surrounding and interacting systems. The source of change is primarily structural stress, either externally induced or internally created. The process of change is one of tension reduction. The goals of change can be either internally or externally imposed and are set by vested interest groups. Stresses, strains, and tensions are the presenting symptoms, and adjustment and adaptation are the goals of intervention. Feedback mechanisms offer important inputs in restoring balance to the system. The change-agent's role is that of diagnostician and action initiator, and his position is, by necessity, external to the client system.

This "apartness" of the change-agent requires an expansion of the system model into an intersystems model to account for the internal system of the change-agent. The connectives between the two interacting open systems may be either cohesive or divisive, and these relational issues are, as we all know, crucial factors in the promotion of, or resistance to, change. The intersystems model seems especially useful as a tool for studying problems of leadership, power, communication, organizational conflict, and intergroup relations of all sorts.

Underlying the *developmental model* is the assumption that there is constant change and development, and growth and decay of a system over time. The stability is that of a living organism, a progression—one stage giving way to another stage. Change is seen as "natural," rooted in the nature of the organism (social or biological), end-related and purposeful. Difficulties develop when a major blockage results in a gross discrepancy between potentiality and actuality. The change-agent's role in the developmental model is that of diagnostician, obstacle remover, and promoter of growth. His position is external to the client-system.

The change-agent in the developmental model has been compared to a horticulturist or midwife. A teacher, for example, may be seen as tending and cultivating the individual mind—feeding, watering, and weeding the student's intellectual garden to promote growth to full bloom or maturity. The psychotherapist aids the individual as he passes through various developmental phases, helping him to break loose and move forward if he has become "fixated" at a given stage. The midwife guides the delivery, removes any blockage, and aids the individual in giving "birth."

The third model—*a model for changing*—incorporates elements of the system model along with ideas from the developmental model into a framework in which the emphasis is on the forces producing change. In this model, stability is studied in order to unfreeze and move parts of the system. Change is induced and controlled, and built on rational choice. Goals are not fixed but instead are arrived at through a collaborative process. The change-agent is an active participant in the situation, playing the role of helper to the client-system.

PACE OF CHANGE

In examining the process of change we need to pause briefly to consider the pace of change. Lewin defines "no change" as a quasi-stationary equilibrium, ". . . a state comparable to that of a river which flows with a given velocity in a given direction during a certain time interval.'' (4:208) He describes a social change as comparable to a change in the velocity or direction of that river.

Earlier I referred to Toffler's concept of future shock, ''the shattering stress and disorientation that we induce in individuals by subjecting them to too much change in too short a time.'' (5:4) Toffler's point is that the rate of change has implications quite apart from, and sometimes more important than, the direction of change. Physical and psychological distress arise from an overload of man's physical adaptive systems and his decision-making processes. Thomas Holmes and Richard Rahe have shown that change itself—not a specific change but the rate of change in one's life—is intimately related to physical health. Together they developed a life-change units scale for measuring the amount of change an individual had experienced in a given span of time and have found a positive correlation between high life-change scores and the frequency and severity of subsequent illness. (5:291-6).

The *psycho-physiological responses to novelty* are well known: pupils dilate, hearing becomes momentarily more acute, general muscle tone increases, brain wave patterns are altered. ACTH secretion is increased, peripheral blood vessels constrict, and respiratory and heart rates are altered. These changes are part of what is known as an alarm or orientation response. This response is one of man's key adaptive mechanisms, but it does exact a price in bodily wear and tear.

Change is essential to life but there are limits on one's adaptability. Just as environmental overstimulation causes physical damage, so does it affect one's ability to think and behave rationally. The combat soldier, the disaster victim, and the culturally dislocated traveler respond to overstimulation in strikingly parallel ways. With sensory overload comes confusion, disorientation, or a blurring of the lines between illusion and reality.

James Miller, Director of Mental Health Research Institute at the University of Michigan, suggests that information overload, like environmental overload, may be related to mental illness. He speculates that ''. . . schizophrenia (by some as-yet unknown process, perhaps a metabolic fault which increases neural 'noise') lowers the capacities of channels involved in cognitive information processing. Schizophrenics consequently . . . have difficulties in coping with information inputs at standard rates like the difficulties experienced by normals at rapid rates. As a result, schizophrenics make errors at standard rates like those made by normals under fast, forced-input rates.'' (5:315)

Decision stress is another form of overstimulation. With the increasing tempo and complexity in our lives comes a great increase in the need for private and public decision making. The question becomes one of a delicate balance between ''programmed'' and ''nonprogrammed decisions.'' As Toffler points out, each of us needs a blend of the two.

If this blend is too high in programmed decisions, we are not challenged; we find life boring and stultifying. We search for ways, even unconsciously, to introduce novelty into our lives, thereby altering the decision ''mix.'' But if this mix is too high in nonprogrammed decisions, if we are hit by so many novel situations that programming becomes impossible, life becomes painfully disorganized, exhausting and anxiety-filled. Pushed to its extreme, the end-point is psychosis. (5:317)

RESISTANCE TO CHANGE

In looking at the change process it is important that we examine the issue of resistance. Many people, perhaps most people, including the well-educated, find the idea of change so threatening they attempt to deny its necessity if not its existence. Because no one can change all his beliefs and still retain his sanity, people frequently prefer problems that are familiar to solutions that are not. (6:8) In a society in which every area of life is subject to change, we should not be surprised to find individuals, consciously or unconsciously, digging in and hanging on to that which is familiar.

Stability in one area of life often enables a person to feel comfortable enough to risk or even seek change in other areas. It should come as no surprise that frequently the area of stability so tenaciously clung to is the work area. It is essential that a would-be change-agent recognize and take into account this likely possibility.

All psychiatric nurses are familiar with the phenomenon of resistance. When in the course of therapy a patient feels threatened by a painful awareness he balks, becomes silent, changes the subject, fills the interview with irrelevant chitchat, misses or comes late for appointments, or becomes angry with the therapist—all an effort to resist change and maintain the status quo. Similar resistance occurs when the target of change is a group or organization. Hostility, either overtly or covertly expressed, is a common defense against real or implied threats to an individual or group's self-image.

There are a number of conditions conducive to resistance to organizational change. For example, if the persons to be influenced by a proposed change are not given adequate information regarding the nature of the change, resistance can be expected. Moreover, personal idiosyncrasies and life experiences cause people to read different meanings into a proposed change. Adequate explanation, however, does not always assure that there will be no resistance to change. Explanations can be distorted, and information is not a panacea for the problem of implied threat to one's personal status or power position. Resistance may be expected when one feels pressured to make a change and will be decreased when one has a "say" in the nature or direction of the change. Resistance is also likely if a change is made on personal grounds rather than on impersonal require-

ments. And lastly, if the change ignores existing alliances within a group, resistance by the individuals in the group is a certainty. (7:543-8)

I do not want to leave the issue of resistance without commenting on its paradoxical form, namely, resistance to stability and order. Some people are so deeply attracted to an ever-changing, accelerated pace of life they feel tense, bored, and depressed when the pace is slow and the system relatively stable. They long to be "where the action is," without regard for whether the action is goal directed or not. For them, the goal is excitement, not constructive change. The hysterical personality and the fixated adolescent are classical examples.

They need a storm about them as a distraction from the essential emptiness or storm within. Though ostensibly dedicated to external change, these people are implacably resistant to internal change and are frequently an obstacle to external change because of the counter-transference resistance they evoke in others.

Another obstacle to change, although not resistance *per se,* is relative satisfaction with the existing system. It is commonly agreed that most hospital personnel work very hard, are usually dedicated to their jobs, and are kept so busy within the present system they do not feel any particular pressure to make changes. If it doesn't hurt, that is, if a person is not dissatisfied, there is no motivation for changing the status quo: "if it doesn't itch, don't scratch." The important point to keep in mind here, however, is that though the hospital personnel may not itch, the patient may have a fulminating rash.

PROCESS OF CHANGING

The actual process of changing is described by Lewin as a three-step procedure: unfreezing, moving, and refreezing. (4:210-11) The first two stages are necessary conditions of change. The third, refreezing, ensures the stability of whatever change occurs. Unfreezing involves "breaking the habit"—disturbing the equilibrium. To break open a shell of complacency it is often necessary to deliberately cause an emotional disturbance. An analogy that comes to mind is the act of giving up smoking. (I am tempted to refer to the process as an art rather than an act.) The point here is that breaking the habit (the step of unfreezing) is frequently accomplished only when there is a severe threat to the self-system. That shell of complacency is disturbed only when the threat is seen as a very real and present danger—not a problem that one might have to cope with at some vague point in the future.

In the unfreezing process the information which is introduced leaves the person feeling uncomfortable. It creates a sense of uneasiness, a disequilibrium. He feels frightened and sometimes guilty. As suggested earlier, he frequently reacts with anger, a defense against the loss of a previous form of stability. (The process of change has many parallels with the process of mourning.)

That the person not become too defensive or rigid, some type of psychological safety must be built into the situation, either by reducing the threat or removing some of the barriers to change. As the individual begins to feel safe, he will begin to seek new information about himself or his relationship to others. He may look for relevant cues from others around him or he may identify with some particular person whose beliefs seem to be viable. In other words, the changee may start to view himself from the perspective of another person or several other persons. As his frame of reference shifts, he will develop new beliefs which will lead to new feelings and responses. When these new feelings and responses become comfortable for the individual and are confirmed or reinforced by others, a kind of consolidation or freezing takes place. Thus, a degree of permanency is acquired. (1:275-76)

In essence, what I have been describing is the process of attitude change. An individual's core personality is deeply rooted in his formative

years. However, the peripheral aspects of personality emerge at later developmental levels. When we attempt to introduce change, we are attempting to change the peripheral aspects of a person's personality. Thus, in order to initiate change it is important that we assess the attitudes and beliefs of those involved in the change. The characteristics that need to be looked at are the extremes of attitudes, the multiplicity of attitudes, their degree of consistency, the needs served, and the centrality of their related values. We also need to look at such general characteristics of the participants as level of intelligence, cognitive needs and style, personal ability, and group affiliations.

NEED FOR A THEORETICAL FRAMEWORK

In providing leadership in change it is essential that we move away from considering personal characteristics of the change-agent and toward a conceptual and operational framework. That is, although personal charisma may help some people effect change, knowledge is more reliable. Change theory must be derived from learning theory, communications theory, systems theory, and interpersonal theory.

In whatever type of work or community situation we find ourselves, once established, it is a system rather than a random collection of individuals. Thus, we need to understand the components of a system, the repetitive patterns of a system, our own part as a system representative, and the fact that any change attacks vested interests of system members and frequently changes their economic and social status. The issue of prestige allotments immediately points up the major, and at times seemingly insurmountable, difficulties in system change.

THE PROBLEM-SOLVING PROCESS

The phases of the change process have been identified by such writers as Greiner, (8:487-492) Foote and Cottrell, (9:175-208) and Kolb and Frohman. (10:51-66) Intrinsic to each of these phase models is the concept of the problem-solving technique. That is, one needs to:

1. *Identify the problem.* Enough pressure is exerted on the power structure to make it aware of the existence of a problem and of the possibility of change.
2. *Collect sufficient data to accurately diagnose the problem.* This involves examining the components of the system and assessing the attitudes and beliefs of the system members.
3. *Make inferences and judgments.* Look at for whom the present structure works and for whom it doesn't work. Assess the system's goals, one's own motivations and one's resources.
4. *Plan intervention on the basis of the above inferences and judgments.* Formulate imaginative and creative proposals. Prepare alternatives. After developing effective solutions obtain commitment for implementing them. Select an appropriate place to start and the appropriate role of the change-agent.
5. *Intervene.* Maximize the participation of personnel by involving people in the system in the change-making process. Give people adequate opportunity to express themselves. Use the leaders in the traditional setup and deal with resistances at all levels.
6. *Evaluate the change process and the solution.* Throughout the process the criteria of change should be clear, verbalized, and shared. Emphasis should be on growth as opposed to success or failure.

THE FUNCTION OF POWER

Implicit throughout this discussion is the differentiation between planned change and other forms of change, since obviously not all change is planned. A major distinguishing feature involves the concept of power, or, "Who's in control of the change?" A primary feature of planned change is equal power distribution, that is, shared deliberations and goal setting. (11:154) Both indoctrinations (as practiced in many schools, prisons, and mental hospitals) and coercive change (thought control and brainwashing) are examples of an imbalanced power ratio, although indoctrinational change involves shared goal setting whereas coercive change does not. (11:154-55)

In the world of medicine and health-care delivery, power is generally sufficient to maintain things as they are. The role of the change-agent is to reorganize the distribution of power, either by encouraging the development of new sources of influence or by making old power centers more responsive to, and representative of, the structure as a whole. Both fragmentation of power and competitiveness, two related characteristics, profoundly affect the change process. A crucial task of the change-agent is to turn intergroup competition into intergroup collaboration. Successful change depends on a redistribution of power within the group system; usually, in the direction of greater shared power. The change-agent's power or influence within a system is derived from a combination of two sources: expert power and line power (1:208-9); that is, the change-agent is seen as possessing expert skills and competencies or as occupying a certain position or holding a certain status in the system which legitimizes his influence.

Power is the means of access to all other values. However, as Deloughery points out, "Nurses, as a group, seem poorly equipped to recognize power, label it as such, and utilize it effectively, either in themselves or others." (12:127) It seems difficult for nurses to view power as other than a negative concept. The reasons for this are fairly obvious. Nurses have historically been a relatively powerless group. We have more frequently been the victims of power than the wielders of power. This is true in our roles as professionals and as women. Nursing is still a "feminine profession" and is likely to remain so within the foreseeable future. However, this fact in no way condemns nurses to traditional powerless and statusless roles.

CONCLUSIONS

There are a number of characteristics basic to the change-agent role. The change-agent is a professional who relies heavily on a body of knowledge to realize his aims. He is frequently a marginal individual without formal membership in the system. The role of the change agent, a somewhat ambiguous one, involves certain risks, frequently drawing suspicion and hostility because of its ambiguity. At the same time, to be effective, any person intimately concerned with change needs to possess a tolerance for ambiguity. The role of the change agent is both insecure and risky. He may frequently be viewed as the most expendable person, and with the complexity of organizational change, unanticipated consequences of his actions can lead to totally undesirable outcomes. (1:217-8)

Probably the most singular skill of the successful change agent is that of *interpersonal competence*. Competence implies the capacity to meet and deal with a changing world, to formulate ends and to implement them. The interpersonally competent individual is healthy, intelligent, empathetic, autonomous, sound in his judgments and innovative. (9:36-60) He is the kind of individual who can size up a situation, maintain an awareness of the human factors involved, and develop a diagnostic sensitivity as well as behavioral flexibility in dealing with human problems.

References

1. Schein, Edgar H. and Bennis, Warren G., *Personal and Organizational Change through Group Methods: The Laboratory Approach,* New York: John Wiley & Sons, Inc., 1965, p. 202.

2. Ujhely, Gertrud, " 'And' Instead of 'Either Or' of 'The Fallacy of False Opposition,' " *Image* (Sigma Theta Tau), 4(3):10-13, 1970-71.

3. Chin, Robert, "The Utility of System Models and Developmental Models for Practitioners," in *The Planning of Change: Readings in the Applied Behavioral Sciences,* (edited by Warren G. Bennis, Kenneth D. Benne and Robert Chin). New York: Holt, Rinehart and Winston, Inc., 1961, pp. 201-214.

4. Lewin, Kurt, "Group Decision and Social Change," in *Readings in Social Psychology* (edited by Eleanor E. Maccoby, Theodore M. Newcomb, and Eugene L. Hartley), New York: Holt, Rinehart and Winston, Inc., 1958, p. 208

5. Toffler, Alvin, *Future Shock,* New York: Random House, 1970, p. 4

6. Postman, Neil and Weingartner, Charles, *The Soft Revolution,* New York: Dell Publishing Company, Inc., 1971, p. 8

7. Zander, Alvin, "Resistance to Change—Its Analysis and Prevention," in *The Planning of Change: Readings in the Applied Behavioral Sciences,* (edited by Warren G. Bennis, Kenneth D. Benne, and Robert Chin). New York: Holt, Rinehart and Winston, Inc.; 1961, pp. 543-548.

8. Greiner, Larry E., "Patterns of Organization Change," in *Interpersonal Behavior and Administration,* (edited by Arthur N. Turner and George F. Lombard), New York: The Free Press, 1969, pp. 477-493.

9. Foote, Nelson N., and Cottrell, Leonard S., Jr., *Identity and Interpersonal Competence: A New Direction in Family Research,* Chicago: The University of Chicago Press, 1965.

10. Kolb, D., and Frohman, A., "An Organization Development Approach to Consulting," *Sloan Management Review* 12:51-66 (Fall) 1970.

11. Bennis, Warren G., "A Topology of Change Processes," in *The Planning of Change: Readings in the Applied Behavioral Sciences,* (edited by Warren G. Bennis, Kenneth D. Benne, and Robert Chin), New York, Holt, Rinehart and Winston, Inc., 1961, p. 154.

12. Delougbery, Grace W., Gebbie, Kristine M., and Neuman, Betty M., *Consultation and Community Organization in Community Mental Health Nursing,* Baltimore: The Williams & Wilkins Company, 1971, p. 127.

Unit two □ STUDY GUIDE

1. Defining the characteristics of a leader can be difficult.
   a. Identify the person that you consider the most effective leader you have ever known. List the five characteristics that you believe make this person an outstanding leader. Compare your list of characteristics with others in your group who have done the same thing. Tally and group the characteristics to find the five selected most often. Discuss the implications of your findings.
   b. Repeat this exercise, looking at the most ineffective leader you have known.
2. Applying Tannenbaum and Schmidt's model, classify the style of leadership utilized by the most effective leader you identified above. Repeat for the ineffective leader. Discuss.
3. Identify your own leadership style.
4. After forming discussion groups of nine to twelve people, the instructor distributes copies of Controversial Statements Sheet. Select a statement from the sheet and discuss. When the discussion is concluded, the instructor reassembles large groups and asks students to describe any new learnings they have experienced from the activity in terms of increased knowledge, insights into others, and insights into themselves. Implications of these new learnings for management are discussed. Suggested controversial statements:
   a. The equal opportunity program has wiped out discrimination in federal employment.

   b. Full compliance with the equal employment opportunity program requires that the organization relax character and suitability standards.
   c. The performance of white and black employees should be judged by the same standards.
   d. Blacks ought to get equal treatment, but it is not fair to give them preference over whites for jobs and promotion.
5. Do an observational study in an agency to collect data from which you can identify and list:
   a. the extrinsic motivating factors for employees
   b. the intrinsic motivating factors for employees
6. Use the topic of motivation as a subject for a staff conference. Identify motivating factors the group can influence and those they cannot. Which factors might you as an individual be able to influence if you were in a different position of power?
7. What is the format for evaluation used in your clinical situation? How do the ideas McGregor put forth fit in with the process being used? Are they compatible? Could they be combined?
8. a. List factors that contribute to resistance to change.
   b. Identify in your clinical area some change that has been or is being initiated.
   c. Using the list of behaviors identified in *a*, carry out a study to see if indeed resistance is involved in that change.

d. Do you see these behaviors as positive or negative?

9. Make a change in your clinical situation. Select your model for change from Rodgers' article and examine the situation, using as much of her theoretical material as possible. Evaluate the outcomes. What did you learn from making this change that you could apply in another situation?

Economic or extrinsic factors and their influence on efficient organizational functioning

☐ This unit deals with three areas of functioning relatively new to the nurse-leader's management activities: budgeting, affirmative action, and labor relations.

Health care as a major national industry is currently confronted with inflationary costs that have escalated beyond predicted levels. Cost containment has become a national, state, and local priority, creating a greater emphasis on sound fiscal management as part of organizational responsibility. Decentralization of authority and accountability in health care delivery systems have resulted in increased responsibility for administrative decisions at every level of nursing practice. For example, nurse-leaders are being required to make decisions about operational and program planning, budgeting, utilization of staff, participation in affirmative action policies, and political negotiations for which they often feel inadequately prepared. Expansion of the nurse-leader's knowledge base in these areas and the use of skilled problem-solving can contribute to organizational effectiveness.

Until recently, only nursing administrators in hospitals, nursing homes, and community agencies were involved in budget preparation. Today, nurse-leaders at all management levels are being asked to prepare unit or departmental budgets and to participate in the overall agency budget, forecasting, and program planning. One of the most keenly felt knowledge deficits for many nurses is that necessity for budget preparation. Nurse-managers need to know about the beginning points for budget preparation and how to estimate expenses for budget purposes. The budget can be a device to communicate departmental objectives by describing programs to be pursued to achieve those objects. It may also serve as a device to allocate resources and a method to monitor programs.

Nurse-managers familiar with the concepts of budgeting and financial planning can use this information in the management of their daily operation. These concepts are essentially concerned with expenses and revenue. Some examples related to expenses are:

Concept of variable expenses: these vary proportionately to changes in volume such as salaries, benefits, supplies, and contracted services

Concept of fixed expenses: these remain reasonably stable during changes in volume, such as insurance, interest, utilities, and depreciation.

Some examples related to the concept of revenue are:

Concept of the mix in a nursing unit: the type of patient and the amount of care required

207

Concept of volume: the quantity of work to be performed

Concept of the workload unit: the measurement of volume, that is, patient days, examinations, procedures, emergency room visits, hours of surgery, etc.

Concept of rate: revenue, expense, or profit per workload unit

Concept of capital expenditure: current outflow of cash that will cause an expense to occur during each period in the future

It must be recognized that there is a reciprocal relationship between budget and staffing in the delivery of health care. Staffing of nursing personnel has evolved into a complex activity. There are at least four influences that have stimulated this evolutionary process and have contributed to its complexity:

1. As recent educational goals have been refocused, student nurses have moved from a primarily hospital-based experience into a more academic setting. At the same time, many community facilities other than hospitals came into use for student learning experiences. This change took from some hospitals an important segment of their nursing staff.

2. When information from the behavioral sciences began to be used to evaluate how the goals of institutions could be met without violating the rights of the individual, new patterns of staffing had to be found that would satisfy both the personnel and the organization.

3. Until recently, increased power and status for nurses were awarded only by promotion to staff positions with greater administrative responsibility and less patient care responsibility. Nurses now are demanding recognition for clinical competence, and administrators have been expected to provide greater incentives for that competency.

4. As health care costs have escalated, nursing administrators have become increas-

ingly concerned with maximizing efficient use of equipment, facilities, and personnel. With nursing personnel comprising the largest single work force in most patient care facilities, nursing actions have fallen under the scrutiny of time and cost analysis.

Basically, then, the task of staffing health care agencies has led to the development of patterns of assignment that attempt to satisfy the variable needs of patients, personnel, and the supporting institutions.

Affirmative action or equal job opportunity programs are required both by law and by accrediting commissions for all health agencies employing fifteen or more persons. Nurse-managers must be knowledgeable about the law and about the institutional program and must use this knowledge astutely in recruiting, hiring, promoting, counseling, and dealing with personnel grievances.

The nurse-leader new to labor relations and collective bargaining activities may be faced with a conflict between personal and professional values and the demands of the labor management situation. The changes in traditional masculine-aggressive, feminine-passive roles occurring in our culture might also create confusion within the individual. The nurse may be uncomfortable with the expectation of increased aggressiveness, or the labor management group may be reluctant to accept a more assertive stance on the part of nurses.

As a group, nurses have been loathe to become involved in political maneuvering and power strategies. Consequently they have operated without knowledge about such matters; as nurse-leaders attempt to become competent in labor management activities, they find themselves without the necessary skills.

The chapters in this unit present information about each of the identified areas of functioning. In Chapter 11, Stevens discusses the necessity of understanding expenses and revenues and looks at methods to document the cost of nursing services. She maintains that once nursing care has been priced, then the kinds of services an agency can offer and the allocation of resources can be more realistically ascertained.

Nurse-managers need to become familiar with some of the common approaches to program planning in relation to building budgets. Among these approaches are the traditional historical budget base, management by objectives, program planning budgeting systems, critical path method, program evaluation review track, and zero-base methods. Anderson explains the essence of the zero-base approach, the fundamental steps for building "decision packages," and the highlights of the zero-base process. In addition, he points out the potential benefits for producing cost-effective results for management.

In the final article of this section, Kretschman gets down to the very basics of costs. He defines types of costs—that is, direct, indirect, real, or opportunity—and the various types of cost savings. A cost-saving measurement model is described as well as its usefulness for different decision-making processes in evaluating proposed or existing cost savings plans.

Ramey's article, in Chapter 12, presents a comprehensive eleven-step approach that systematized staffing for a specific hospital. Of particular importance is the implication that nurses must be involved in the early stages of problem identification and policy-making as well as the implementation phase of a staffing pattern.

Many articles are currently being written about primary nursing and how it is being implemented in many agencies on both a trial and a permanent basis. Ciske states that there is still confusion in primary nursing that relates to staffing and patient assignment. She discusses the responsibilities of the nurse leader in decision-making, delegating, and staff development for both professional and nonprofessional personnel. In addition, she identifies the primary patient population and some of the staffing situations that require problem-solving.

In Chapter 13, in an original article, Austinson presents a historical review of the development of the labor movement in nursing from the 1930's to the present. Grand traces the historical development of nursing from the ethic of service to the present-day orientation of "professional collectivism." Chamot cites the increasing numbers of employed professionals and white-collar workers who are turning to unions as a means of settling conflicts through collective bargaining. The special problems of discontent among professionals are emphasized, as are the needs for professionals to obtain a greater measure of dignity and a larger share of economic rewards. Obstacles to cooperative relationships in labor management activities lead to situations in which management and employee associations must deal with each other as adversaries. Werther and Lockhart suggest techniques and precautions for both parties. He stresses the need for those who provide health services to develop a reasonable philosophy of labor relations.

The article by Pati and Fahey presents an excellent synopsis of affirmative action programs and the impact of public policy in many functional areas of management. The legal requirements are well outlined. The implications for the nurse-manager in terms of recruitment, selection, staff development and training needs, manpower inventory audit, control, and record-keeping are clearly identified.

Chapter 11

BUDGET PLANNING

What is the executive's role in budgeting for her department?

BARBARA J. STEVENS, R.N., Ph.D.

What is the appropriate role of today's nurse executive in the financial management of her department and of her institution? At one time, nurses knew the answer to that question: the nurse executive has succeeded when she has been given the opportunity to plan, recommend, and defend her own budget. Unfortunately, this right, once it has been attained, often has been viewed as an end in itself rather than a means to achieving some further end.

One is reminded of the historial struggle of women for the vote. That right, once attained, was used by many merely to ratify the candidate of their husbands' or their fathers' choice. Nurse executives place themselves in a similar position if their budgetary input is an end in itself and if they merely ratify their institutions' present system of financial management.

Now that nurse executives have input into the budgeting and financial systems of their organizations, the question becomes, "How can they use those channels in the best interest of nursing and of the patient?" Input into the budgetary process certainly gives the nurse executive a needed opportunity to make others aware of nursing's contribution to the organization and to the patient's welfare.

Reprinted with permission, from *Hospitals, Journal of the American Hospital Association,* vol. 50, November 16, 1976, p. 83.

Why is it important that others recognize nursing's contribution? The plain fact is that those who are perceived as "pulling their own weight" are respected and rewarded. In the health care system, such rewards come in the form of added resources and, in nursing, added resources mean more or better patient care. All too often, however, the budgeting systems that others devise for nursing—either intentionally or unintentionally—place nursing at a great disadvantage.

When one looks at the typical budget system of most health care institutions, nursing appears on only one side of the ledger—the side marked "expenses." On the other side marked "revenues," nursing does not appear. Although a naive consumer may perceive nursing as one of the major services for which he is paying and nurses tend to agree with this perception, nursing does not appear to be a source of revenue according to the budget. Sources of revenue appear to be pharmacy, X ray, anesthesia, and so on. There also is a substantial figure called a "room rate"—a comprehensive item including maintenance costs such as meals, fresh linens, mopped floors, and nursing care. Consequently, other managers often view nursing as the department that brings in no money and that spends the most. Unfortunately, this distorted perspective exacts a toll from nurse executives; they often feel called upon to apologize for what others perceive to be a profligate operation.

Nursing's first priority in financial management must be to strive for realistic representation on both sides of the ledger. The nurse executive must be prepared to put a price tag on nursing as well as to document the cost of nursing services. Putting a price tag on nursing services and removing fees for nursing services from the room rate is the place to start. (Indeed the present system that forces patients who need less nursing care to subsidize the care received by others is inequitable and unfair.)

There are two ways to put a price tag on nursing. One approach involves billing patients for each separate nursing task; the second involves billing based upon a patient classification system. The accuracy of the first approach probably is not sufficiently advantageous to offset the administrative problems of such a multiple billing system. The second method, in which a patient's placement in a care classification system determines cost, is an alternative worth exploring. Pioneering in separate billing for nursing already has been done in some institutions. Although there is as yet no accepted formula or system, this is an area in which nursing must concentrate its energies.

In addition to billing patients based upon their varying needs for nursing services, it also is possible to specify more than one level of care. The level of care actually delivered might depend upon consumer preference or upon other constraints. For example, an institution might be unable, in spite of its financial status, to obtain enough nurses to deliver optimal care. Similarly, the consumer might choose an economy care package under one circumstance and a comprehensive nursing care plan at another time.

The nursing experience with quality control systems has provided practice in assessing care and care outcomes; quality control systems could be adapted to the task of putting price tags on different levels of care. Thus, by combining quality control systems and patient classification systems, it should be possible to set price schedules related to both patient needs and standards of care.

Nurse executives must begin to put realistic price tags on potential care packages. A nursing department on an economy budget cannot give deluxe care. Indeed, the attempt to deliver deluxe services will prevent the department from systematically determining what services are essential and therefore must be given priority in an environment of scarcity.

Putting a fair price tag on nursing services based on differences in patient care needs is only the start of an accurate billing system for nursing. The level of nursing care that a patient receives is influenced not only by his relative need for care but also by the total nursing resources available at any given time. Again, a look at typical budgeting procedures is illuminating.

"BUSINESS AS USUAL?"

The nurse executive spends many man-hours producing a budget that is adequate to supply those resources such as manpower, equipment, and supplies, that she needs to deliver nursing care. If she is very fortunate, the budget is approved, she gets the requisite rosources, and she delivers the nursing care as planned. More often, particularly in today's economic crunch, the nurse executive finds her budget cut by a sizeable percentage, and she does not get the requisite resources. However, she does deliver the nursing care as planned and, as a result nursing suffers a decline in the quality of care, directly related to the budget cuts. Clearly, the care received by a patient under these circumstances is different from the care received by a patient with similar needs in a resource-rich environment.

Just as other managers often fail to recognize nursing's contribution to the organization, they also may fail to appreciate the difficulties of nursing management under conditions of severe scarcity of resources. Other managers see no overt signs of deficiency. No patient unit is closed, no physician is told that there aren't enough nurses to carry out his orders, no patient sues for nursing malpractice.

Only a system that assigns costs (and fees) directly to nursing acts will allow nursing to make changes or potential changes in the quality of care evident to other managers. The nurse executive must accept this challenge to make nursing visible to others, visible in terms that they can understand. She must be a linguist, translating the meaning of nursing care from "nursese" into clear english. In addition, she then must convert clear English into a third language, the universal language of managers—money.

The nurse executive cannot realistically set a defined level of patient care and assume that it can and must be reached with whatever resources happen to fall nursing's way. What the nurse executive must do is to inform higher administration that for X amount of money, she can provide X type of care; and that for Y amount of money, she can provide Y type of care.

FIRST THINGS FIRST

The suggestion that services provided be matched with available resources usually is met by criticism from nurses. The counterargument runs that first the services are determined and then one sets about, somehow, to get the requisite resources. Indeed, when this is possible, it may be the desirable course of action. On the other hand, if those resources are not forthcoming, it is unreasonable to go on acting as if they had been supplied.

The nursing ethos runs counter to the notion of adapting care levels to available resources or to patient choices for care. Most nurses have in mind an idealized picture of the care that "every patient deserves." The educational system has ensured that this image is firmly in the mind of each nurse graduate; to profess to deliver less than this idealized nursing care is seen as heresy.

Putting a price tag on nursing will take a selling job among nurses. The typical nurse tends to see hospital costs from the perspective of the patient, not from the perspective of the nursing department or of the organization. Indeed, it is not uncommon to find nurses purposefully failing to process charges for patients known to be in financial difficulties. These nurses fail to see that such practices belittle the value of their own services. Educating staff to the worth of their services must be part of any program to account financially for nursing services.

In contradiction to the nurse's image of resource-rich care, many consumers do not want to invest ever larger proportions of their income in health care services—either in direct payments, insurance payments, or taxes. If we have reached or nearly reached a ceiling in terms of what people are willing to pay for health services, the logical question is not how to cajole them into paying more but how to get more and better health care for the amount they are willing to pay. Here the nurse executive has a responsibility for exerting leadership in organizational decisions regarding financial priorities and distribution of limited funds.

COST/BENEFIT ANALYSIS

In recent years, investments in nursing services consistently have lost out to the purchase of fancy equipment and to programs that will help a few patients in a dramatic way. An elaborate computerized diagnostic center or a new kidney dialysis unit will make news in a Sunday supplement; an addition in nursing manpower will not.

The nurse executive has a responsibility to her organization and to its administrators to keep cost/benefit issues at the forefront when major financial investments are being considered. The more precisely that she can document beneficial patient outcomes and relate them to both nursing actions and to costs, the more successful she will be in winning resources for nursing. A clear determination of the costs and benefits of a proposed program or project will give the nurse manager important input for decision making. Ultimately, however, determining whether a program's perceived benefits are worth the cost is a value determination. The section among different health objectives with different price tags cannot be solved with a quantitative, mathematical formula.

CONCLUSION

Once nursing has been realistically priced, then the nurse executive can face the issue of what kind of nursing care nurses, administrators, and patients want and what the alternatives for levels of care are. If a nurse executive and her institution opt for optimal, comprehensive care, then that price would be reflected in patient fees. If appropriate resources are not available in that institution, some patient units or nursing projects would be eliminated rather than offered at a lower care level. In contrast with the typical practice of "business as usual," the goal of optimal care, if decided upon, could realistically be achieved by having necessary services priced and patient fees set accordingly, thus making adequate resources available to achieve that goal.

If an institution chooses a lower level of care for an economic patient fee system, the nursing department in that institution would have to look at the realities of the situation and to set appropriate nursing priorities. The department would have to determine what services it would and could not offer to the patient. The sparcity of resources might cause this department to discriminate between nursing measures critical to the achievement of desired patient outcomes and those measured that are inessential. Again, the nursing department would be ahead, for it would have determined realistic work loads, eliminating both staff frustration and unrealistic patient expectations.

Yet another institution might opt for flexible levels of care related to the price the consumer wants to pay. In this case, nursing has accomplished something else; making the consumer look at what he is purchasing. This may make some nurse executives anxious, for the patient may start demanding his money's worth, wanting to know what he is getting for his dollar. However, the nurse executive may see the patient as a potential new ally. Putting a price tag on and merchandising nursing may help both the consumer and the nurse to know the profession's contribution—or potential contribution—to the nation's health.

Furthermore, the patient has a right to know the level of nursing care he will receive in any given institution. At present, the patient, seldom chooses a hospital on the basis of the level of nursing care it provides. Yet, he has a right to know that one hospital will give him "bare bones care," while another hospital will give good care plus amenities. Indeed, nothing has more potential for shifting resources to nursing in a well-informed public. If patients choose to avoid a hospital that puts its few resources into nursing, the empty bed count will soon make administrators see the need to reconsider priorities.

Zero-base budgeting: how to get rid of corporate crabgrass

DONALD N. ANDERSON

For companies in a budget squeeze, the obvious target for quick remedial action is that portion of the income statement most amenable to management control—controllable operation and maintenance expenses. But exercises in crash budget reductions too often yield only temporary improvements.

During the past two or three years, rising operating costs and declining growth rates have put companies in a profitability crunch that demands significant, innovative approaches to doing something about improving bottom-line results. And managers who have had to make agonizing decisions on budgets now realize that for favorable long-term results, you need budgetary reductions that will stick.

Administering operating budgets, however, is a lot like getting crabgrass out of your lawn. You can apply weed killers to eradicate it or pull it out by the roots, but despite expensive chemicals and backbreaking work, crabgrass usually creeps back—and the weekend gardener's job is never really done.

The parallel between ''managing'' crabgrass and administering a corporate budget is not so far fetched as it might seem. Corporations and their managers have crabgrass activities in their budgets that compete for the same dollars needed by essential, basic activities. We can mow budgets and take 5 to 10 percent off the top, but that doesn't affect the crabgrass. We can selectively pull out crabgrass activities, but if we don't get the roots out, it isn't long before

people and dollars are drawn into the same activities again. What's needed is a kind of selective treatment that can be applied to the entire budget to knock out the weeds and provide an overall net reduction—while keeping the desired activities functioning efficiently.

A technique that many companies are adapting and implementing to improve their budgetary front lawns is called Zero-Base Operational Planning and Budgeting (ZBOP). It's a formula we use at Southern California Edison, and we believe it does a good job of getting rid of budgetary crabgrass and keeping it out.

IMPROVING ON TRADITIONAL TECHNIQUES

Although the buzz words ''zero-base budgeting'' are relatively new to many managers, the underlying concept is nothing more than a systemization of tratitional operational planning and budgeting processes. In recent years, however, the traditional processes have not measured up to the tough decision making required because they assume that the projects and ongoing activities making up the historical budget base are (1) essential to the mission of the company and must be continued during the budget year; (2) are being performed in an optimal, cost-efficient manner; and (3) are projected to be cost-effective in the budget year, requiring budget dollar increases only for uncontrollables such as pay increases and materials costs.

Some projects and activities do, of course, meet these criteria, but it is unrealistic to assume that all do. It becomes a question, then, of which activities and projects are not really essential and what criteria should be used for making a judgment. The answers must come from a joint effort of each manager, his boss, and the members of senior management. This combination—which ensures that both corporate and individual organization needs are satisfied—is the essence of the ZBOP approach.

HOW ZBOP WORKS

The zero-base approach has two fundamental steps. The first requires preparation of a decision-oriented summary plan for each activity or project. Called a "decision package," this summary (operational plan) usually includes a statement of the expected business result or purpose of the activity, its costs, personnel required, measures of performance, alternative courses of action, and an evaluation—from a corporate or organizationwide perspective—of the *benefits of performance and consequences of nonperformance.* In developing the summary plan, each manager must evaluate two types of alternatives:

- Different ways of performing each activity (for example, in-house versus contracted maintenance services), and
- Different levels of effort and resources required for performing each activity.

Managers also must identify a minimum level of spending for each activity and then identify in separate decision packages the costs and benefits of incremental, additional levels of spending.

The second fundamental step in ZBOP requires that each decision package be ranked against packages for other current and proposed new activities and projects, thus allowing each manager to specify his priorities for new and old programs. The end result is a prioritized list of priced-out operational plans built from the ground up, or "zero base."

The list can be used in senior management to evaluate and compare relative needs and priorities in making crucial funding decisions. As the list of approved operational plans increase, the total cost also increases, and top

management can decide at what point the added costs outweigh the benefits.

Under this procedure, the entire budgeting process need not be recycled back through the operating organizations when expenditure levels must be changed; instead, the decision-package ranking identifies the activities, projects, and operations (as summarized in the decision packages) to be added or deleted to implement a budget change. As an additional benefit, managers at all organizational levels become involved in the process, and they develop a greater sense of responsibility for budgets and related accomplishments. The zero-base documents provide a convenient reference plan that they can use for controlling their activities during the operating year.

GETTING STARTED IN ZBOP

The prospect that 1974 earnings would fail to meet company objectives prompted Southern California Edison to begin experimenting with the ZBOP concept. The need for prompt, effective action of some kind had been foreseen in December 1973 during the wrapup of the 1974 budgeting process when fuel shortages, rising prices, and reduced sales resulting from a statewide energy conservation program pointed to projected earnings substantially below 1974 goals. As a result, department managers were directed to submit by mid-January 1974 their estimates of activities that could be reduced and the expected consequences of such action.

During an all-day meeting of the SCE Management Committee held early in February, each manager was given an opportunity to explain and defend his proposed budget revisions. The session, which provided senior managers with broad visibility over the operational aspects of the proposed budget changes, was the first time senior managers had an opportunity to participate actively in budgeting and concurrent activity-planning decisions on a companywide basis.

Subsequent discussions of senior managers focused on development of a strategy to be used in preparing budgets for 1975. The arbitrariness of "crash" reductions by either specifying a spending limit, as was done for the 1974 budget, or ordering an across-the-board percentage cut, was acknowledged. Rapid changes occurring in the 1974 business environment, however, made it clear that the planning and budgeting processes had to be made more flexible and responsive to unanticipated changes in costs, revenues, and operating conditions. The idea of developing contingency plans for each of a series of alternative assumptions concerning 1975 business conditions was tested briefly and discarded for two reasons: excessive paperwork would be required, and development of contingency plans to meet hypothetical future conditions is a concept that does not appeal to busy, pragmatic operating managers.

At this point, it became apparent that a zero-base planning and budgeting approach might be useful to Southern California Edison, and the Management Committee agreed to (1) a pilot test of the entire zero-base process in six small staff departments reporting to the finanical vice-president and (2) the use of portions of the process in all other departments.

The results of the 1974 pilot test were, of course, limited, but over all, it was an enlightening learning experience. Some of its key benefits and lessons were:

• The budget director's staff had an opportunity to begin counseling departments concerning the benefits of analytical operational planning aimed at achieving long-term cost savings through changes in operation, organization, work processes, and so forth, as opposed to remedial actions having only a short-run effect in improving earnings. Managers thus were encouraged to weigh alternatives and evaluate them in terms of the dollar consequences to the company as a whole even though some alternatives might require the addition of personnel to the company payroll. Evaluation of benefits from a companywide perspective also was encouraged.

• We found that budgeting activity in the company was viewed by many as a numbers-oriented clerical exercise that managers frequently delegated to staff personnel; also there was a continuing attitude that the burden of proof as to where and how much a proposed budget should be reduced rested with the budget staff (and the Management Committee).

• This inappropriate over-concern with the clerical aspects of filling in numbers on forms pointed to an apparent need for budgeting guidelines emphasizing the crucial managerial aspects of the process. Logically, the burden of justifying all components of a proposed budget rests with the responsible operating manager because he is in the best position to know where and how much budgets can be reduced without seriously jeopardizing the company.

HIGHLIGHTS OF THE ZBOP PROCESS

1. Under the traditional budgeting technique, you:
   • Fit a trend line to historical recorded data and extrapolate to the budget year.
   • Assume that the current "base" is made up of only necessary cost-efficient activities that should be perpetuated.
   • Concentrate on justifying the incremental increase only.
   In the chart [p. 218, top] each block represents dollars needed to perform a project or continuing assignment having a defined scope of work and time schedule.

2. In ZBOP, each project and each continuing work activity must be broken down into smaller elements for detailed analysis and planning (see chart [p. 218, bottom]). To avoid excessive detail, however, an element should comprise no less than one full person and all associated costs. If the element involves no employees (as in the case of contracted work), the dollar value should gen-

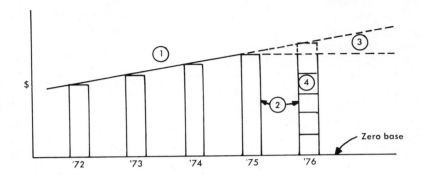

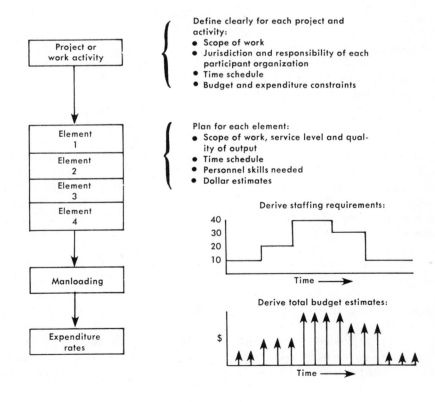

Objective no._____   DECISION PACKAGE   Date ___August 15, 1975___

Activity (or objective) name	Department	Prepared	Rank
PBX maintenance and subset installations	Communications	Ralph Schwartz	5
Level no. 2 of 3	Division Central	Approved B. Miller	

Purpose of activity	Resources required*	Current year (75)	Budget year (76)
Maintain company-owned PBX telephone switching equipment and related equipment to provide reliable intra-company communications and dependable linkages with the Bell System network.	Personnel	2	2
	Labor $	28	30
Description of activity	Outside services $	0	0
This level provides supervisors for both the day and swing shifts. This level plus 1 of 3 comprises the total 1975 staffing and workload. Maintains PBX equipment, call director, keyset and instrument equipment 2 shifts. Installs, moves, removes keysets and instruments 2 shifts.	Other $	2	2
	Total $	30	32

Alternative ways of performing work or program and costs

Because supervision and PBX maintenance capability are combined, no lower cost alternative is discernable. However, deleting swing shift maintenance and installation would require one less person for this package at a savings of $15,000 and increase average response time for working instrument and key equipment orders from 2 to 16 days.

Advantages of retaining activity

Permits maintenance of PBX equipment to hold average dial-tone delay to 5 seconds or less, minimizing caller inconvenience, and permits most instrument and key equipment install, move or remove orders to be worked during swing-shift hours with minimum inconvenience to office and professional employees.

Consequences if activity is eliminated

Total elimination of this activity would result in reduced maintenance leading to average dial tone delays of 30 seconds or more within 6 months and increased response time for key equipment and instrument orders from 2 to 20 working days. Orders could be worked only during day shift.

erally not be less than some meaningful minimum, say $10,000.

3. Analysis summaries—"decision packages" —for each level of effort are then prepared. A sample decision-package form is illustrated [above]. A fundamental step in the ZBOP process, the form summarizes a scope of work, cost, personnel, and implied time schedule, plus assessments of the benefits of performing the work and the expected consequences if it is not. The format makes it relatively easy for a manager to decide whether or not the work should be done and what its relative priority is.

4. The listing illustrated [p. 220, top] represents a priority ranking of decision packages at a divisional level.

5. The priority ranking continues with each higher level manager or officer merging and reranking lower priority packages for all organizations reporting to him [p. 220].

6. The objective is one companywide list of prioritized decision packages as illustrated in the chart [p. 221]. Thus the chief administrative officer or a management committee reviews the rankings of senior officers and managers in terms of corporate needs and establishes individual department and total company budget levels.

PRIORITY RANKING   Date August 15, 1975

Department	Division	Prepared	Ralph Schwartz	Page	1
Communications	Central	Approved	B. Miller	Of	1

Activity				Current year (75)		Budget year (76)		
Rank	Name and description	Level No.	of no.	Personnel	$ (000)	Personnel	$ (000)	Cumulative $ (000)
1	PBX maintenance and subset installations	1	3	4	60	4	63	63
2	Trunking maintenance	1	2	2	30	2	32	96
3	PBX operations	1	2	6	72	6	77	172
4	Directory and paging services	1	2	1	12	1	13	186
5	PBX maintenance and subset installations	2	3	2	30	2	32	217
6	Trunking maintenance	2	2	1	15	1	16	233
7	PBX operations	2	2	3	36	3	30	272
8	Equipment engineering	1	2	2	40	2	44	316
9	PBX maintenance and subset installations	3	3	0	0	2	16	332
10	Equipment engineering	2	2	1	20	1	22	354
11	Directory and paging services	2	2	1	12	1	13	367
	Totals			23	327	25	367	

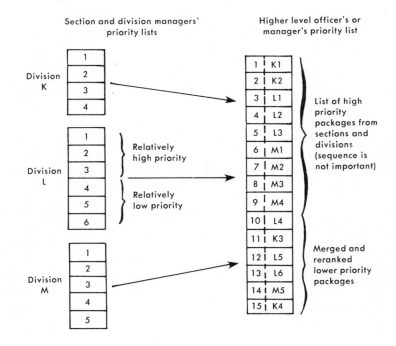

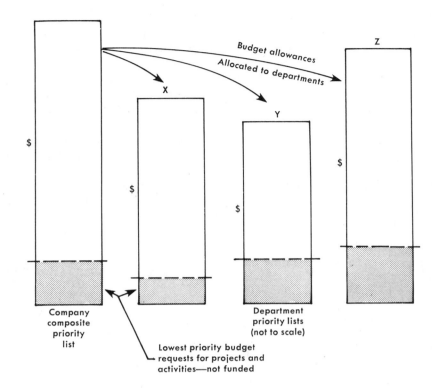

Budget allowances
Allocated to departments

Company composite priority list

Department priority lists (not to scale)

Lowest priority budget requests for projects and activities—not funded

AN ALL-OUT TEST

The 1974 experience with ZBOP demonstrated that only a full-scale implementation of ZBOP would highlight nonessential and discretionary crabgrass activities sufficiently to permit selective cultivation of the entire operations and maintenance budget. Accordingly, the ZBOP process was extended throughout the entire company during 1975, and managers used it with varying degrees of success. At least one more annual cycle will be required to achieve a uniform level of understanding of its usefulness and to attain a corresponding high level of achievement. We can point, however, to some examples of significant progress:

• In preparing their 1975 and 1976 programs, each manager reporting to an officer analyzed all of his proposed activities in terms of continued need, relative contributions to the corporation, consequences if not funded, personnel and dollars required, and priority. These decision packages were then prioritized and summarized on ranking forms.

• Each officer reviewed the packages and ranks of each of his managers and assured himself that they were reasonable. As a final step, he merged and reranked the lowest priority activities of all his managers and forwarded his documentation through the corporate budget staff (for screening and summarization) to the Management Committee. During a two-day working session last December, the Management Committee met with each officer and department head to review the zero-base documentation and set an authorized personnel and funding level for each in 1976.

• Although the Management Committee scanned summaries of all activities, discussion centered on the details of the lowest priority programs since these were the most likely candidates for deletion, postponement, or de-emphasis during budget year 1976.

• As a result of ZBOP and other on-going cost-reduction efforts during the latter part of 1974 and throughout 1975, we were able to achieve significant savings in the 1975 and 1976 budgets, including personnel reductions of approximately 9 percent from previously budgeted figures. Many of these reductions provided permanent dollar savings that will continue into future years—but only if the deleted crabgrass activities are not permitted to reseed and grow back in some other form.

• While many managers have come to appreciate the usefulness of ZBOP in planning and budgeting their own areas of responsibility, it appears the most significant utility of the process is at the middle and lower ranks of management. This is because the operating detail produced during the development of the zero-base data is a useful working guide during the budget year itself.

• Because they knew ZBOP documentation gives senior management an opportunity to scrutinize operations in more depth than ever before, a number of managers deleted or scaled down certain activities in their proprosed budget requests before submitting them to the Management Committee.

On the other hand, requiring managers to evaluate cost-effective alternatives has encouraged some to propose an increased level of spending for the budget year because they could demonstrate a compelling cost benefit or operational benefit in the near- or long-term. After candid discussion of the proposed increases, most were approved by the committee. In the absence of zero-base documentation, such proposed increases would have rarely survived senior management review in a period of fiscal restraint.

FUTURE EXPECTATIONS

Southern California Edison's use of the ZBOP process thus far has concentrated on

identifying potential areas for budget reductions because of the need for general fiscal holddowns. But this represents only a partial use of the power of the process; equally as valuable is the use of ZBOP as a flexible planning-budgeting tool that permits managers to respond quickly and effectively to improvements in the business climate.

Having pre-planned, costed, and prioritized activities at hand, a manager is equipped to proceed with additional cost-effective activities in support of company objectives should additional funds become available. We expect this aspect of the process to become increasingly useful as the company experiences an upturn in business activity.

GUIDELINES FOR GETTING STARTED IN ZBOP

For ZBOP to work, managers must be convinced there is something in it for them. After all, they will be asked to devote time to learning the concept—plus much additional time and effort in doing what is required to come up with an acceptable operating plan and budget. If they can't see some worthwhile benefits downstream, don't expect them to grasp ZBOP to their bosoms even if it does seem compellingly logical and appropriate to its advocates.

Long-range or strategic planning should precede the zero-base budgeting cycle. ZBOP concentrates on development of the operating budget, while long-range planning focuses on the general direction and development of the organization. Long-range planning should provide the goals, policy guidance, and assumptions for the zero-base process; zero-base should provide the first year's operating budget within the planning framework and should identify any conflicts between long-range goals and short-range growth and cost-reduction opportunities.

Most operating managers support a zero-base approach, especially during periods of severe budget reductions because ZBOP avoids a flat percentage reduction. But it also should be recognized that some managers will oppose any process that forces them to display their effectiveness and justify what they are doing. To overcome this problem, management support is needed.

It should be emphasized that ZBOP cannot be applied to an entire budget; it can be used for operations and programs over which management has some discretion. In the utility industry, for example, the zero-base approach can be used to develop budgets for administrative and general support, marketing, research, engineering, maintenance, construction and fabrication support, and some plant additions. It cannot be used for direct labor, direct material, and some direct overhead typically budgeted through ''standard costing'' procedures.

TAILORING PROCEDURES TO "MANAGEMENT STYLE"

The zero-base process encourages—indeed, it requires—a grassroots, bottoms-up approach to operations planning that necessitates the involvement of managers at all levels of the organization. If the process is followed faithfully and repeated each year, the positive benefits in terms of managerial effectiveness and organizational performance are impressive. The key to developing a tough-minded, professional spirit among managers lies in the simple fact that the zero-base process requires them to critically analyze, plan, adjust, and control their organizations in a way that brings their authority and responsibility into clear focus.

The process also requires an adjustment of the attitudes and perhaps even the managerial style of managers and their bosses. These adjustments are sometimes painful; not everyone can make the necessary transition successfully. But if the continued viability of a company is at stake, senior management is generally eager to make certain adjustments and sacrifices for themselves, to require the same of their subordinate managers, and through active,

visible leadership bring about the required shift in managerial thrust.

NO PANACEA, BUT WORTH A TRIAL RUN

ZBOP is not an optimal answer to every manager's prayer for a simple, effective operational planning and budget system, but it comes about as close as any. It is not for every organization or every manager in an organization, but it can produce cost-effective results in most segments of organizations. An added advantage is that the zero-base approach sometimes can highlight deeply rooted management problems not related to zero-base itself.

The SCE experience indicates it is best to make a trial run in a small, representative organization for one full budget cycle. You assess these results, then either drop the idea completely or make necessary fine-tuning adjustments and implement it throughout the remainder of the organization where, from the perspective of senior management, it has a high probability of success.

KEY TO SUCCESS: TOUGH-MINDED MANAGERS

The ZBOP process can be adopted by virtually any organization willing to aggressively eliminate its budgetary crabgrass, but only tough-minded managers intimately acquainted with the organization culture can make it work effectively. Although the process is ideally suited for cost-effective, planned growth, most managers probably will be initially interested in its enduring cost-reduction aspects and the capability it provides for responding flexibly to sudden shifts in an operating environment.

The final test of the net value of ZBOP is the way it is viewed by senior management. If, in spite of the time, cost, and anguish expressed by some managers, senior managers believe that on balance a lasting, significant benefit has been achieved, what more can be desired?

Know how to analyze costs in evaluating savings projects

CARL G. KRETSCHMAR

Most discussions of cost control in hospitals contain little documentation of expected or actual cost savings. However, in understanding cost savings measurement, it is necessary to understand the nature of costs and how the various types of costs are related to cost savings. The purposes of this article are to discuss some of the cost characteristics more relevant to cost savings and to suggest a model for cost savings measurement.*

TYPES OF COSTS

Each cost may exhibit characteristics that are not mutually exclusive. Therefore, in order to define cost savings, it is useful to elaborate on some of the more relevant characteristics that a cost may exhibit.

Costs may be direct or indirect costs. Direct costs are clearly identifiable with a good or a service. Indirect costs must be assigned or must be allocated to a good or a service.

Costs may be either real or opportunity costs. Real costs are reflected in actual flows of resources. Opportunity costs represent the potential benefits foregone or the costs avoided by the selection of a particular course of action. In some cases, opportunity costs can be quantified and can be included in the decision model. In other cases, opportunity costs must be identified and evaluated subjectively. The relevant opportunity costs always should be included in the final cost savings analysis.

Reprinted with permission from *Hospitals, Journal of the American Hospital Association*, vol. 50, September 16, 1976, p. 69.
*This article is based on work performed pursuant to Contract SSA-PMB-74-175 with the Social Security Administration, Department of Health, Education, and Welfare.

Some costs can be shifted to other areas but do not reduce total system costs and, thus, do not represent cost savings.

Most costs can be described as fixed, variable, or semivariable. Fixed costs do not change with changes in volume, whereas variable costs vary directly nad porportionately with changes in volume. Although all costs are variable in the long run, many costs incurred in hospitals are relatively fixed over short periods.

In differential cost analysis, alternative courses of action are judged by considering only the differences in costs among their alternatives rather than by evaluating each project's total costs. Any cost that does not vary among the alternatives is irrelevant to the decision-making process.

In measuring the cost of capital equipment, the problem is to assign a dollar value to the cost of capital. Direct real capital costs include historical cost depreciation and interest paid on the money borrowed to finance the capital acquisitions. The cost of capital also should include opportunity costs. When a hospital does not use debt financing, the interest that would have been earned had the money been invested should be calculated as an opportunity cost. In addition, the difference between historical cost and replacement cost depreciation should be caluclated as an opportunity cost.

TYPES OF COST SAVINGS

There are at least four types of cost savings: (1) direct savings resulting from a net reduction of resource flows; (2) opportunity cost savings, such as those associated with avoiding costs or securing intangible benefits; (3) improvements in the quality of services without an increase in costs; and (4) increased output of services without increases in costs.

Each of these types of cost savings can be divided into actual cost savings and potential cost savings. Actual cost savings have been experienced during a specific period; potential cost savings could be experienced when a plan is fully implemented. Potential cost savings should be estimated prior to implementing a cost containment program and, after the program has been put into operation, should be compared with actual cost savings in order to evaluate the success of the project.

The value of opportunity cost savings cannot always be measured accurately in monetary terms and, instead, must be described narratively. A positive opportunity cost represents a negative benefit and, therefore, can be described as a negative opportunity cost savings.

Hospitals have placed great emphasis on maintaining the quality of care through the influence of peer groups and federal legislation. Few monetary incentives currently exist to provide rewards for improving the quality of care. No agreement concerning how quality of care should be measured has been reached among authorities. Thus, the effects of cost savings programs on the quality of care could be considered opportunity cost savings and could be evaluated subjectively rather than as a part of a measurement model.

Reducing the average cost per unit by increasing output benefits payers of care but will not be reflected in most direct cost savings, because it may involve increased demands for services—a factor beyond the control of a hospital's administration.

MEASUREMENT MODEL

In order to evaluate cost savings projects, it is desirable to measure several of the types of cost savings. A proposed model for cost savings measurement is presented as a form that can be completed (table on [p. 226]).

Prior to the completion of a cost savings project, the potential and the opportunity cost savings can be estimated and should be entered in columns d and f of this form. Positive and negative opportunity cost savings should be entered in column f. The form provides space in column g to add opportunity cost savings to direct cost savings. However, it often is preferable to provide a narrative describing the characteristics of a particular opportunity cost savings rather than to estimate the dollar value of that cost savings; such characteristics could be considered subjectively.

When the project has been implemented, the form can be used to evaluate the success of the project by dividing all costs into the categories of labor, material, and capital. The annual direct costs that would have been incurred had the project not been implemented should be entered in column a; the annual direct costs that actually are experienced, in column b; and the annual direct costs that are expected when the plan is fully implemented, in column c. Subtracting column c from column a provides an estimate of potential direct cost savings. Subtracting column b from column a provides a measure of actual direct cost savings. Few cost savings programs achieve their entire potential in their first year, if at all.

The following discussion is intended to help clarify the process of implementing the cost savings measurement model.

Direct cost savings can be defined as the net decrease in cash flows throughout the hospital, caused by changes in programs or activities. The method of measuring these cost savings is best described as differential cost tracing— tracing the costs associated with a project, an activity, or a department and measuring the cost savings as the difference between what the costs actually were and what they would have been had no activities been changed. Differences in cost must be measured in terms of their impact on total hospital costs in order to eliminate the possibility of including shifted costs as cost savings. Differential cost tracing also should be used to measure actual and potential direct cost savings.

COST SAVINGS MEASUREMENT MODEL WITH EXAMPLE PROJECT ANALYSIS
Effects of cost savings plan
Year end _____

Hospital _____ Department _____

Prepared by_____

Date _____ Project _____

Approved by _____

	a	b	c	d	e	f	g
Costs	Prior costs	New costs, actual	New costs, annually expected	Potential direct cost savings (a-c)	Actual direct cost savings (a-b)	Opportunity cost savings	Total cost savings (d+f)
Direct labor							
Salaries	$48,730	$ 0	$ 0	$48,730	$48,730		
Engineering time		3,600			(3,600)		
Transfers to non-vacancies		6,820			(6,820)	$ 3,500	
Direct materials							
Supplies	3,200	0	0	3,200	3,200		
Operating costs		15,500	10,500	(10,500)	(15,500)	120 sq. ft. floor space freed	
Equipment amortization	2,235	12,100	12,100	(9,865)	(9,865)	(11,040)	
TOTAL	$54,165	$38,020	$22,600	$31,565	$16,145	($7,540)	

The cost of operating a hospital includes salaries, supplies and other expenses, and capital costs. The differential cost of salaries is measured as follows: (budgeted manhours × budgeted wage rate)—(actual man-hours × actual wage rate). This measurement includes the effects on cost savings of changes in the mix of employees. The measurement also must be adjusted for the effects that reduced payroll has on fringe benefits and for the effects that employees who are transferred rather than discharged have. The value of the services performed by an employee who is transferred to a position that previously was not defined as vacant does not reduce resource flows within the hospital; it is an opportunity cost savings rather than a direct cost savings.

Direct actual supply cost savings are measured as follows: (actual cost of supplies)—(budgeted cost of supplies). Potential supply cost savings are measured as follows: (unit price prior to the cost saving project × quantity used per year)—(new unit price × new quantity used per year).

Capital costs can be measured using straight line depreciation plus the interest on borrowed capital. Depreciation is best measured by using replacement cost. When replacement cost is not readily available, price level depreciation can be used as an approximation. In addition, some administrators prefer to use historical cost depreciation in order to be consistent with the capital cost measure used for rate setting and for third-party reimbursement. Although historical cost depreciation is conceptually inferior to replacement cost depreciation, its use can be considered satisfactory. When the relevant depreciation charge for a cost savings project is based on the current cost of obtaining capital equipment, replacement cost, price level, and historical cost depreciation all are the same. Depreciation will increase as a result of implementing many individual projects and, thus, often will be a negative factor when measuring project cost savings.

When a hospital borrows the money necessary to finance a project, the interest paid is a direct cost. When a hospital finances a project using funds on hand, there is no actual interest expense. The interest that would have been earned had these funds been invested, however, is an opportunity cost.

It is necessary to consider the effects of opportunity cost savings in order to correctly evaluate a cost savings program. For example, reducing the average inventory level from $50,000 to $30,000 may not save a hospital any direct cost, but it does free $20,000 in working capital. If this $20,000 is invested, it will produce interest income, which is a direct cost savings; otherwise, freeing this capital is an opportunity cost savings. In this case, the effects of the opportunity cost savings can be measured by assuming some reasonable cost of capital.

Another type of opportunity cost savings occurs when the work load in a department is reduced but no employees are fired or transferred. No direct cost savings occur, but the hospital may be in the position to benefit by having these employees take on new tasks and assignments. In this case, the administrator may choose to make a monetary estimate of the value of the new activities. However, because such estimates are quite subjective, it may be preferable to provide a written description of such benefits.

An important factor in cost savings measurement is the cost of the engineering and other time necessary to initiate and to implement a cost savings project. Some of these costs, such as the time of an outside consultant, are direct. Other costs, such as a hospital employee's applying his time to the project rather than to his normal duties, are opportunity costs. However, any employee costs that would not have been incurred had the employee not participated in the project, such as overtime costs, should be included among direct costs rather than among opportunity costs.

EXAMPLE OF USE OF MODEL

An approach to cost savings that frequently is suggested in the literature—replacing personnel with equipment through automation—illustrates how the cost savings measurement model and form can be used.

The wage cost savings from reducing the staff will affect the annual cash flow. The costs of automation include an initial outlay and annual operating costs. The annual outlay in capital costs must be derived from a lump sum; it is suggested that straight line depreciation on estimated replacement cost be used to determine the annual effect on costs of capital expenditures. Replacement cost will equal historical cost during the year that capital equipment is acquired. When a previously acquired asset is retired, the cash value received for it is an immediate, one-time cash flow. To determine the annual effects of this cash flow, the cash received should be deducted from the cost of the new asset before depreciation is calculated. When an asset that is retired from use in one project is converted for use in another, the value of the asset to the department that will be using it should be deducted from the cost of the new equipment before depreciation is calculated. If the asset is diverted to a new use in a way that prevents an additional cash outlay, the cost savings is direct. If the asset is used in a way that may benefit the hospital but that does not prevent a cash outflow, the diversion of the asset represents an opportunity cost savings.

Assume that a project eliminates a department within a hospital and substitutes some automated equipment costing $150,000, with an estimated 10-year life and a $17,000 salvage value. Operating cost would be $15,500 for the first year but were expected to drop to $10,500 in future years.

Prior to automation, the departmental costs were as follows: salaries—$44,300; supplies—$3,200; movable equipment—$1,450; building space—$785; total—$49,735.

When the department was disbanded, one of its employees was transferred to another department but did not fill a position that previously was defined as vacant. The salary paid to that employee was $6,200 for the first year, and his actual value to the new department was estimated to be $3,500. The old equipment was sold for $12,000. The floor space previously used was converted to a storeroom that was useful but not necessary to the operation of the hospital. Fringe benefits for employees amounted to an average of 10 percent of wages and were not allocated in the ledger. The hospital paid $3,600 to an outside consulting firm to develop and to implement the project.

Cost savings for this project are shown in the table on [p. 226]. The department's total costs would have been $54,165 ($49,735 plus 10 percent of $44,300 for fringe benefits) if the department had not been eliminated. These figures are encountered in column *a*.

New salaries and supply cost potentially could be reduced to zero; therefore, zero is entered in column *c*. Because one employee was transferred to an unnecessary position, the actual salaries cost of $6,820 ($6,200 plus 10 percent for fringe benefits) must be entered in column *b*, and the value of this time ($3,500) must be entered in column *f* as an opportunity cost savings. The cost of the consulting engineer's time devoted to the project ($3,600) is a direct actual cost and is entered in column *b*. No actual supply costs were incurred during the first year, so zero is entered in columns *b* and *c*.

Equipment amortization of $12,100 ([$150,000 cost −$17,000 salvage value −$12,000 cash proceeds from equipment sales] ÷ 10 years) and operating costs of $15,500 were experienced in the first year that the department was automated and are entered in column *c*. Because the floor space that was converted to a storeroom did not prevent a cash outflow, it is an opportunity cost savings and is noted in narrative form in column *f*. The hospital used existing funds to purchase the automated equipment. Assuming an eight percent cost of capital, an opportunity cost of $11,400 ([$150,000 cost −$12,000 sale of existing equipment] × .08) is derived and is shown in column *f* as a negative opportunity cost savings.

Thus, the model shows direct actual cost savings to be $16,145; direct potential cost savings to be $31,565; and opportunity cost savings to be −$7,450 and the positive benefits of the use of additional storage space.

CONCLUSION

The model for measurement of cost savings that is recommended in this article is best described as differential cost tracing applied to direct actual cost savings. The model is intended to produce at least three cost savings measurements, each useful for different decision-making processes in evaluating proposed or existing cost savings plans.

Chapter 12

STAFFING PATTERNS

Eleven steps to proper staffing

IRENE G. RAMEY, R.N., Ph.D.

Pressures to trim hospital costs and to increase the productivity of employees point to a need for nursing service departments to utilize a rigorous methodology for developing staffing patterns for patient units. The development of a staffing pattern is not an easy procedure. Much preliminary work should precede it to provide a framework. First, a statement of philosophy should be developed that spells out the values and beliefs of the nursing service department regarding its contribution toward the care provided by the total institution. General objectives for the department as a whole and specific objectives for the individual patient units should state in operational terms what the nurses hope to accomplish.

Two other prerequisites to the development of an appropriate staffing pattern are the delineation of a table of organization that shows the line and staff relationships of the personnel in the department and the development of job descriptions that list the functions of the various types and levels of personnel.

The success of any staffing pattern rests upon having the correct number of appropriately prepared personnel to meet the needs of patients. Therefore, in order to determine a staffing pattern, it is first necessary to conduct a careful survey of patients' needs.

The methodology proposed here is different from methodologies in which determinations are made of activities staff members currently are performing. Obviously, there may be a great difference between what a patient is having done for him and what he needs to have done for him. It is absolutely essential, therefore, that the data be collected by highly skilled and knowledgeable professional nurses who are capable of determining the kind and amount of care that the patients ought to have.

Other important factors that must be taken into account in planning staffing include the type of equipment that is available to facilitate the work of the staff, the physical design of the unit and its proximity to other departments, and the availability of specialists from other disciplines.

ELEVEN STEPS TO PROPER STAFFING

1. Survey each patient unit on 10 to 15 nonconsecutive days (with several days between each survey so that the same patients are not counted repeatedly) to determine the number of patients requiring intensive, moderate and minimal care. An example of criteria for classifying patients may be found in the article, ''Predicting change in nursing values,'' by Thomas.*

Reprinted, with permission, from *Hospitals, Journal of the American Hospital Association*, **47**(6), March 16, 1973, p. 98+.

*Thomas, L. A. Predicting change in nursing values. *J. Nursing Admin.* 1:50, May-June 1971.

Such a survey should be conducted several times a year to determine seasonal trends. Record the data on the *classification of patients form* (Figure 1).

2. Develop a *patient data collection form* (Figure 2) listing the various direct and indirect nursing activities that are carried out in a patient unit. The form will be used to indicate the number of times in a 24-hour period each procedure

is to be performed, as well as the total time needed in an eight-hour period for the performance of each type of procedure. In order to simplify the listing, several activities may be included under one heading; for example, planning and evaluation of care may be subsumed under the heading "Conferences." Also list functions that are not presently being performed but that are to be instituted. Provide space on

DAYS	UNIT A			UNIT B			UNIT C			UNIT ___			UNIT ___		
	IN	MO	MI	IN	MO	MI	IN	MO	MI	IN	MO	MI	IN	MO	MI
1 5/1/71	8	8	2	6	11	19	5	11	29						
2 5/3/71	5	6	8	8	8	23	4	10	27						
3 5/5/71	7	7	6	8	9	20	3	6	12						
4 5/7/71	7	5	8	9	11	19	6	12	28						
5 5/9/71	7	4	7	9	9	21	7	12	33						
6 5/11/71	7	6	4	10	7	20	5	11	30						
7 5/13/71	8	9	4	5	9	22	6	9	27						
8 5/15/71	7	5	10	12	6	21	4	12	24						
9 5/17/71	6	7	9	9	8	22	3	11	23						
10 5/19/71	6	6	11	8	7	24	7	8	25						
TOTAL	68	63	69	84	85	211	50	102	258						
AVERAGE	6.8	6.3	6.9	8.4	8.5	21.1	5.0	10.2	25.8						
%	34%	31%	35%	22%	22%	56%	12%	25%	63%						

(On day 3, 5/5/71, Unit C values 3, 6, 12 circled) ← Date on which survey was done

	TOTAL	%
CODE:		
IN = Intensive Care	177	22
MO = Moderate Care	202	26
MI = Minimal Care	413	52

Figure 1. Classification of patients form.

the form for entries to be made on the different tours of duty (day, evening, and night) and for indicating whether the patient requires intensive, moderate, or minimal care. In many hospitals, the admission of patients to units is made categorically on the basis of type of illness, age, or sex. Different forms, listing different activities, may be required for different units.

3. Survey each specialty unit separately. If, however, the hospital is a large one and many of the units have similar types of patients, a representative sample of units may be selected. If the admission of patients to units is made categorically, each such unit should be surveyed separately and data collected on a sufficient number of patients in each unit so that valid

UNIT __C__

PATIENT'S NAME ___Joe Doe___ AGE __58__ ROOM __C-5__ DATE __5-5-71__

CLASSIFICATION: Intensive _X_ Moderate ___ Minimal ___

ACTIVITIES	No./24hrs. D	E	N	Total Time D	E	N	ACTIVITIES	No./24hrs. D	E	N	Total Time D	E	N
A.M. & P.M. Care							Meds/Oral						
Ace Bandage							Meds/PRN						
Admission	1			15			Meds/IM & Subc.	2	2	2	10	10	10
Ambulate/Exercise							Meds/IV	1	1	1	5	5	5
Assessment	1			60			IV's	2	1	1	10	5	5
Assist Doctors	1	1	1	20	20	20	Transfusion						
Baths							Nursing Rounds	1	1	1	2	2	2
Bedmaking							Oxygen Therapy	1	1	1	10	10	10
Bedpans/Urinals	3	3	2	15	15	10	Phisohex Scrubs						
Bladder Irrigations							Post Mortem Care						
Blood Pressure	4	4	4	20	20	20	Psychological Support	1	1	1	15	15	15
Catheterization							Sitz Bath						
Catheter Care							Steam Inhalation						
Change Position	4	4	4	20	20	20	Suctioning	2	2	2	40	40	40
Charting							Teaching Patients	1	1		15	15	
Check Doctors' Orders	1	1	1	5	5	5	Team Conferences	1	1	1	10	10	10
Collect Specimens	2	2	2	10	10	10	TPR	2	2	2	6	6	6
Colostomy Care							Tracheostomy Care	2	2	2	30	30	30
Compresses							Traction Care						
Communication	1	1	1	5	5	5	Transfers/Escorts						
Read CVP							Turn/Cough/Breathe						
Discharge							Urine Reduction						
Dressings							Water Pitchers						
Enemas/Colostomies							Weights	1	1		10	10	
Errands	1	1	1	15	15	15							
Feeding/Nourishments													
IPPB	2	2	2	30	30	30							
Intake/Output	1	1	1	10	10	10							
Isolation Technique													
Levine Tube Irrigation													

Figure 2. Patient data collection form.

averages can be obtained for the different types and classifications of patients.

4. Designate two or three skilled, knowledgeable nurses to collect data on each of the selected units for at least 24 consecutive hours, so that round-the-clock data will be obtained on each patient. Continue for as many days as are necessary to obtain data on a sufficient number of patients on that unit. Having only two or three nurses involved ideally will increase the reliability of the data. These nurses will:

• Survey the card file for medical and nursing orders and interview the head nurse and other nurses caring for the patients to elicit information as to what the individual patient's needs are and what nursing measures ought to be instituted. (The surveyor may suggest additions to or corrections of the nursing care plan.) Record on each patient's *data collection form* (Figure 2) all nursing activities that ought to be performed. Indicate in the appropriate columns the number of times each procedure is to be performed during each tour, including dependent and independent functions and direct and indirect nursing care activities.

• Record on the *indirect activities form* (Figure 3) all those activities that cannot be assigned to a particular patient; at the end of the eight-hour tour of duty, divide the total amount of time for those activities by the total number of patients on the unit to derive an average amount of time spent on indirect activities per patient. This amount is recorded on the *patient data collection form* (Figure 2) of each patient on that unit.

5. Establish the average number of minutes required to accomplish each nursing activity safely and appropriately and record that figure on the *average performance time form* (Figure 4). (The average length of time required to perform certain activities may vary from one patient unit to another and must be determined and taken into account in subsequent calculations.)

6. Specify the amount of time that will be required for new functions that are to be instituted. Time should be included for assessment, planning, teaching, counseling, and evaluation. Record the amount of time on the *average performance time form* (Figure 4).

7. Consider the knowledge and skill required

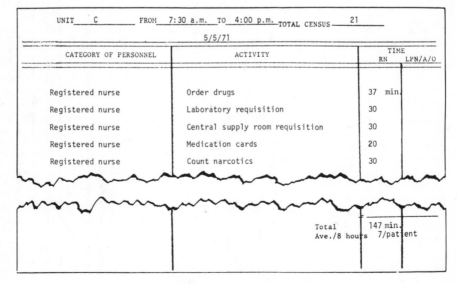

Figure 3. Indirect activities form.

to perform the various nursing activities for patients who are acutely ill and require intensive care, for those who are moderately ill, and for those who are minimally ill. Using the *assignment of nursing activities form* (Figure 5), designate whether each nursing activity should be performed by professional nurses or by auxiliary personnel (LPNs or aides). (This has proved to be the most difficult step in the methodology because of variations in the capabilities of individual members of the nursing staff. It may be helpful, therefore, to focus on defining professional versus nonprofessional activities or on the norm for that particular hospital.)

8. Using the data collected in Step 4 on all of the *patient data collection forms* (Figure 2) and

NURSING ACTIVITY	AVERAGE TIME	NURSING ACTIVITY	AVERAGE TIME
A.M. & P.M. Care	10 min.	IV's	5 min.
Ace Bandage	4	Transfusions	5
Admission	15	Nursing Rounds	2
Ambulate/Exercise	15	Oxygen Therapy	10
Assessment	60	Phisohex Scrubs	10
Assist Physician	20	Post Mortem Care	30
Bath	20	Psychological Support	15
Levine Tube Irrigation	5		
Meds/Oral	3		
Meds/PRN	3		
Meds/IM & Subcu.	5		
Meds/IV	5		

Figure 4. Average performance time form.

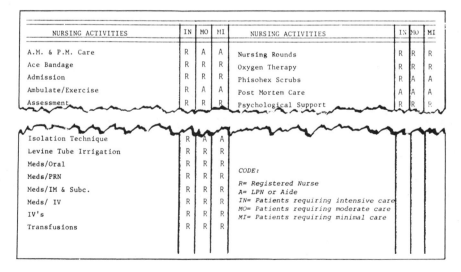

NURSING ACTIVITIES	IN	MO	MI	NURSING ACTIVITIES	IN	MO	MI
A.M. & P.M. Care	R	A	A	Nursing Rounds	R	R	R
Ace Bandage	R	R	R	Oxygen Therapy	R	R	R
Admission	R	R	R	Phisohex Scrubs	R	A	A
Ambulate/Exercise	R	A	A	Post Mortem Care	A	A	A
Assessment	R	R	R	Psychological Support	R	R	R
Isolation Technique	R	A	A				
Levine Tube Irrigation	R	R	R				
Meds/Oral	R	R	R	*CODE:*			
Meds/PRN	R	R	R	R= Registered Nurse			
Meds/IM & Subc.	R	R	R	A= LPN or Aide			
Meds/IV	R	R	R	IN= Patients requiring intensive care			
IV's	R	R	R	MO= Patients requiring moderate care			
Transfusions	R	R	R	MI= Patients requiring minimal care			

Figure 5. Assignment of nursing activities form.

Figure 6. Calculation of nursing unit data form.

UNIT ___C___
DATE ___5/5/71___

	INTENSIVE Total Minutes			MODERATE Total Minutes			MINIMAL Total Minutes			R.N. Total Minutes			LPN/AIDE Total Minutes		
	day	eve	nite	day	eve	nite	day	eve	nite	day	eve	nite	day	eve	nite
Number of Patients	(3)			(6)			(12)								
A.M. & P.M. Care		30			60						30			60	
Ace Bandage															
Admission						15	15	15		15	30				
Ambulate/Exercise	30			15						30			15		
Assessment					60		60	60		60	120				
Assist Physicians					20		20			20	20				
Bath	60			120						60			120		
Bedmaking	30	30	30	60			120						210	30	30
Bedpan/Urinal		15	15	60	60	60							60	75	75
Bladder Irrigation	10	10	10							10	10	10			
Turn/Cough/Breathe	48	48	48							48	48	48			
Urine Reduction							24	24	48	24	24	48			
Water Pitchers				24	24	12	48	48	24				72	72	36
Weights			10		10	10	10	10	60				10	20	80
Other (from Form #3)	21	21	21	42	42	42	84	84	84	147	147	147			
TOTAL	698	610	540	942	916	542	1,331	1,141	877	1,798	1,594	1,187	1,298	1,178	877
	1,848			2,400			3,349			4,579			3,353		
AVE./PATIENT/24 HRS	10.26			6.66			4.65			58% BY RN			42% BY LPN AIDE		

R.N.: day 39% eve 35% nite 26%
LPN/AIDE: day 39% eve 35% nite 26%

Figure 7. Calculation of total staffing form.

UNIT	PROJECTED PATIENT DAYS	PERCENTAGE OF PATIENT DAYS			NUMBER OF PATIENT DAYS			NURSING HOURS/ PATIENT/24 HOURS			TOTAL NURSING HOURS NEEDED ANNUALLY		
		IN	MO	MI	IN	MO	MI	IN	MO	MI	IN	MO	MI
A	6,460	34	31	35	2,196	2,003	2,261						
B	7,373	22	22	56	1,622	1,622	4,129						
C	15,075	12	25	63	1,809	3,769	9,497	10.26	6.66	4.65	18,560	25,101	44,161
												87,822	

PERCENTAGE OF TIME		NURSING HOURS ANNUALLY		PERSONNEL ANNUALLY		PERCENTAGE ON DAYS		PERCENTAGE ON EVENINGS		PERCENTAGE ON NIGHTS		PERSONNEL ON DAYS		PERSONNEL ON EVENINGS		PERSONNEL ON NIGHTS	
RN	LPN/A	RN	LPN/A	RN	LPN/A	RN	LPN/A	RN	LPN/A	RN	LPN/A	RN	LPN/A	RN	LPN/A	RN	LPN/A
58	42	50,937	36,885	27	20	39%	39%	35%	35%	26%	26%	10.5	8	9.5	7	7	5

on the *indirect activities form* (Figure 3), total the data on the *calculation of nursing unit data form* (Figure 6). Calculate for each unit the total amount of time involved in each activity and on each tour of duty, according to patient classification (intensive, moderate, or minimal care). Total each column. Determine the average amount of nursing time required by each patient in each of the three classifications. Allo-

cate the nursing activities to professional or nonprofessional nursing personnel on the basis of decisions made in Step 7. Add the total amount of nursing time in each column. Determine the percentage of time required by each group of patients on each tour of duty. (At this point, it is possible to determine how many staff members are required on duty on a daily basis by multiplying the number of hours of care per

UNIT C FROM Sun. 5/2 TO Sat. 5/15

CATEGORY OF PERSONNEL	ACTIVITY	TIME RN	LPN/AIDE
1 head nurse	Inservice education (1 hr. per mo.)	60 minutes	
27 staff nurses	" "	810	
20 (LPNs (Aides	" "		600
1 head nurse	Staff meetings (1 hr. per mo.)	120	
27 staff nurses	" "	810	
20 (LPNs (Aides	" "		600
Head nurse & team leader	Patient assignments	140	
Head nurse	Time sheets	60	
Head nurse	Evaluation of personnel and counseling	120	
	Assisting faculty and students	420	
	Orientation of new nursing staff	210	
	Orientation of new house staff	140	
	Orientation of new visitors	140	
	Orientation of new managers	140	
	Participation in research projects	60	
	Participation in community activities	240	
	Total	3,470	1,200
	Ave. per day	4.13hrs.	1.4hrs.
	Grand Total	4,670 minutes	
	Ave./Day	5.55 hrs.	

Figure 8. Additional nursing activities form.

patient times the number of patients and dividing that figure by the amount of time an employee works in a day.)

9. Obtain from the business office the number of patient days that are projected for the year on each patient unit. If the business office does not provide such information, a projection may be made from the records of previous years, taking into account any anticipated increases or decreases in patient days.

10. Use the *calculation of total staffing form* (Figure 7) to make the final calculations, using data obtained in Steps 8 and 9. Calculate the total number of nursing hours needed annually for each unit. Then calculate the number that are to be worked by professional and by nonprofessional staff. The number of persons needed depends upon the number of hours each person works in a year, taking into account holidays, vacations, and so forth. Finally, calculate the number of persons required on each tour.

11. After the calculations for staffing for patient care activities have been completed, one additional survey must be conducted, because additional personnel will be required on each unit to permit time for inservice education of personnel; for nursing administration of the unit

(patient assignments, time sheets, evaluation of personnel, counseling, and so forth); for participation in formal educational programs; for orientation of new nursing staff, house staff, and visitors; for participation in community activities; and for participation in research projects. This information may be collected on the *additional nursing activities form* (Figure 8); after the number of requisite staff members is computed, it is added to the numbers needed for each unit.

METHOD IS EASILY ADAPTABLE

The methodology that has been described has been empirically tested in a university hospital over a period of several years and can, I believe, be easily adapted to most, if not all, hospital nursing service departments. The forms referred to have been meticulously designed and numbered so that each step in the methodology moves logically from one form to the next and from one column to the next.

Although nonnursing personnel can perform the calculations, it must be emphasized that the planning of the patient survey, the collection of data, and the analysis of the data in planning for staffing are professional nursing functions and responsibilities and cannot be delegated.

Misconceptions about staffing and patient assignment in primary nursing

KAREN L. CISKE, R.N., M.S.

During the last five years, primary nursing has been the subject of many nursing articles and has been implemented in many nursing departments throughout the country. It has been my privilege to assist in some of these projects.

Reprinted with permission from *Nursing Administration Quarterly*, 1977.

Repeatedly, I am asked questions that illustrate that there is still confusion regarding the practical application of primary nursing. Two major areas are staffing and patient assignment. In this article I will discuss some of the common misconceptions, why they exist and what can be done to reverse them.

STAFFING

"It will cost more to have primary nursing." "You need a higher number of nurse hours per patient." "You need an all RN staff." These are comments often heard from administrators and directors of nursing who associate the increased professionalism expected from primary nursing with increased cost. They also read about pilot units that hire specifically for the project, have more funds for staffing and include research. Some nurse administrators, therefore, dismiss primary nursing as unrealistic for their hospital, "ivory tower-ish," and costly. If the following principles about staffing are understood, then answers to the above statements come forth.

- Assess present staffing to bring it to an acceptable standard of patient care hours.
- Upgrade positions as vacancies occur.
- Utilize all levels of staff more effectively.
- Plan toward future staffing goals.
- Demonstrate what RNs can do as professionals.

The people doing the job

Yes, you may need more nursing hours per patient if your present ratio is inadequate for the acute patient needs and shorter stay in today's complex hospital system. If requests must be made for more and higher quality staff to ensure quality care, then the request is valid, no matter what organization is chosen on the unit. The assessment of staff ratio preceding primary nursing just brings to light a problem that might have been existent for years. But because attempts to increase staffing then follow, it looks like the move to primary nursing required higher staffing.

No, it need not cost any more money if you utilize the present staff more effectively.

Head nurse positions in primary nursing become ones of quality control, management of people, and staff development. She or he must be freed from the management of things, desk work that can be delegated elsewhere, and routine MD rounds. Decentralizing decision making to the bedside requires a unit leader who has assessed the staff's capabilities, provided for their learning, and allowed and trusted them to function as independently as possible. This is no easy process! If the head nurse is available to *share* the clinical expertise that advanced her into the position originally, the staff will develop clinical leadership traits. But if the head nurse previously gained much satisfaction from knowing and being in control of communication about patients or from "running a tight ship," then the adjustment to primary nursing will be difficult and will require defining new satisfactions. Support and education from peers and supervisors will help.

Staff nurses will have intense involvement with a consistent group of primary patients, instead of a superficial knowledge (and consequent superficial involvement) of a whole team. In converting to primary nursing from the team system, two more care givers are gained, the team leaders. This brings a potential for growth of clinical skills, collaboration with other health team members, and satisfaction from direct patient care.

"The part-time RN cannot be a primary nurse" is another misconception regarding staffing. If the RN's work schedule is so sporadic that two or more consecutive days are never worked, then perhaps this person cannot be a primary nurse. However, if the scheduling can be improved, there are short term patients, in for only one to three days, for whom a part-time nurse can be primary nurse. The responsibility would entail admission and care each following day. Continuity, concern, planning, and teaching could occur on a limited basis—if goals were realistic. Another option for the part-timer is being a consistent secondary nurse for short term patients.

Staff LPNs used to perform functional aspects of care for many patients. In primary nursing they perform total care for a few, hopefully with consistent assignments. Considering the various levels of care given by LPNs, can LPNs *be* primary nurses? Many of them want the chance, because they observe the satisfaction and visibility that RNs experience in it. Leaders of primary nursing projects sometimes feel that denying this opportunity establishes LPNs as "second class citizens."

However, the LPN is not prepared or supported legally to be a primary nurse, though it is shocking to admit that some practice bedside nursing at a level comparable with many RNs! We have caused some of this problem ourselves by interchanging LPNs and RNs and assigning LPNs to too much direct patient care—while RNs in some instances have gone farther from the bedside. It should not be surprising to us that the caring skills of LPNs have grown and those of RNs have been stunted.

So, do we take what exists today and assign each qualified, interested LPN as a primary nurse? I don't think so. Fixed accountability for professional nursing belongs only in the RN rank. That is not to say, however, that RNs will not need help! The LPN is prepared to do and plan aspects of nursing care, often using effectively the problem solving process, but that does not make the LPN an RN. What LPNs can provide, which some RNs often do not exhibit, is warmth, concern, and common sense in the approach to patients. If they are older, they also have the life experiences and confidence that most young graduates lack. Accepting responsibility seems more natural to one who has these personal attributes. They can help new RNs grow.

Another reason why the LPN cannot be a primary nurse is that economically RNs would be at a disadvantage in justifying our desire for an upgrading of nursing positions to a higher percentage of RNs. If LPNs and RNs were interchangeable, primary nursing could be performed at a lower cost with more LPNs.

There are hospitals allowing some LPNs to be assistant primary nurses with an RN ultimately responsible for her patients, often the head nurse, usually in situations with long term

employees who have demonstrated excellence in care, judgment, and motivation. There must be good supervision to identify aspects of care beyond their ability, such as dealing with the patient's response to his health problem, initiating actions with planning and interdisciplinary communication, being a change agent and advocate. Effective coordination of what the LPN and RN do takes time and effort—another factor to consider.

Looking to our future, we cannot get boxed into a system that perpetuates no differentiation of nursing role by education. (This also implies a need to study differences in what two-year, three-year and four-year graduates of RN programs provide in primary nursing.) The New York 1985 proposal must also be considered in how we want to utilize LPNs in the future. The principle is to capitalize on the abilities of LPNs within their legal and educational limitations, not expecting that what some *exceptional* ones do in bedside care is applicable to all their colleagues.

Nurse aides are removed from giving much bedside care to doing more cleaning, supply, and errand tasks. Their jobs usually have included these items, which are viewed as less interesting and challenging than patient care. So nobody wants to do them. Nurses sometimes take turns cleaning with the aide! It is true that many aides enjoy and provide well some aspects of patient care, but we cannot perpetuate the practice of allowing the least prepared person the most patient contact. When new aides are hired, it is easier to change the job description to one of supporting the *nurse* to give care by supply, cleaning, transporting functions. New aides will then not expect to be giving care except as asked in assisting the nurse.

If there is a unit whose staffing must include some aides until resignations occur and upgrading is done, there *are* ways to assign aides in primary nursing. An aide is assigned to a nurse, perhaps the same one consistently, and patients—not functions—are assigned within that group with close supervision. Primary nurses enjoy having an assistant, and the aide enjoys having just one "boss."

Insecurities about these job changes will be felt at all levels. LPNs and aides fear for their job security when they see that RNs are increasing their involvement in direct care. They will need reassurance from the nursing administration regarding their jobs and their concern over self-satisfaction. Their contributions are important to recognize and incorporate into the system. However, commitment to the present employee does not prevent restructuring jobs of new employees. Usually there is enough flexibility within a nursing organization to accommodate this action.

RNs might be worried about their nursing care planning and teaching abilities, which will be more visible and, therefore, possibly seen as deficient. Others will be unsure of their satisfaction with more bedside nursing. Communicating directly with the health team can cause insecurities. In all these cases, both education and attention to "people needs" must be provided so that staff can develop into the new role expectations.

The job content

It is appropriate to look at what is done by nurses to see what could be allocated to other departments, what activities are nontherapeutic to patients, or ineffective uses of time. Attention to "who does what" brings up functions that can become battle issues between nursing and other departments unless there is administrative support and departmental cooperation in the project. Transportation of patients is just one of the many examples that we know well. Some hospitals agree to transfer an aide position to other departments to remove concretely some functions that previously were under nursing's broad umbrella.

Routines need to be evaluated, such as bed and bath each day, vital signs at certain frequencies, and the charting of something, no matter how trivial, each shift. We have caused a lot of dry skin with our "cleanliness is next to godliness, and therefore health" ethic! If we had done a good assessment of the patient, we would have known his usual bathing pattern and any changes necessary because of illness. So, if an activity is ritualistic, fulfilling no purpose for the patient or staff, policies should be changed to eliminate this useless time expenditure. We also need better communication with physicians to keep orders up to date as their patients respond. Once written, an order often stands, unchanged, until discharge.

These examples of past misconceptions about staffing and possible solutions illustrate that when principles are followed, there is room for individualization and flexibility.

PATIENT ASSIGNMENT
The method

Some nurses think that there is one *right* way to assign patients. Three patterns have been described in health care literature: geographic, individual, and promotional. Principles to consider in any method are:

1. equal case load depending on staff ability and hours;
2. optimal match between patient need and staff competence made at admission or within 24 hours, and maintained through patient's stay unless:
   a. a patient-nurse personality conflict exists that cannot be resolved,
   b. the nurse is going onto a block of nights or vacation,
   c. the patient condition changes beyond the capability of the primary nurse,
   d. the patient requests a change,
   e. the patient transfers to a room that is inconvenient for the primary nurse;
3. a variety of patient conditions for staff growth, identified and visible to patient, family, nurses, physician, and other staff; and
4. the geographic location of rooms.

There are advantages and disadvantages to each of the three systems as shown in Table 1. There is no perfect system. Considering all your

Table 1. Methods of patient assignment

Advantages	Disadvantages
Geographic	
1. Stable, easy to keep track of.	1. No guarantee of fair case load.
2. Easier to have consistent secondary coverage.	2. Loses patient when transfer to another district.
3. Well-organized.	3. Unclear who is accountable when off duty for long
4. Easier for health team to learn who has what patient.	stretch.
Individual	
1. Case load fair.	1. Much time spent in making original and daily as-
2. Variety of cases.	signment.
3. Can be maintained when readmitted.	2. Wasted steps if patients for any nurse are spread
4. Control by head nurse.	through unit.
Promotional	
1. Screening process, only for best professionals.	1. Large case load.
2. Viewed as more status.	2. Much delegation of direct patient care.
3. Stimulates staff to show competence.	3. Cost of positions.
4. Increased role clarity.	4. Holds back advancement if more nurses are ready
5. Reward of increased pay.	to be promoted than positions available.

unique variables, one or a combination of methods can be chosen, keeping the main principles in mind.

Who are the primary patients?

Is it really true that primary nursing is only for the long term patient and that not every patient needs a primary nurse? The benefit of primary nursing is evident for the patient whose previous care plan, coordination, discharge planning, and continuity were poor. Feedback from satisfaction in the nurse–patient relationship, seeing results in goal accomplishment, and working with other disciplines are easier to experience when the patient's length of admission is more than a week. That is why implementation of primary nursing on medical wards is generally more effective than on surgery, where the average length of stay is shorter. These external rewards are important, and there is just not enough time to accomplish them for the one- to two-day admission.

It is also frustrating to try to establish goals for the healthy, knowledgeable person having minor surgery. Because we deal with extremely serious conditions, we sometimes become immune to the trauma patients experience when admitted for these relatively minor reasons. Still, the minor surgery patient requires a proper evaluation by a primary nurse who will continue to care for the patient the following day and who will instruct the patient concerning the events happening, ensure continuity during other shifts, reduce potential anxiety, and communicate authority and concern. Certainly extensive planning and teaching cannot be done for the short term patient, but if conditions related to planning and teaching are identified as needs, they can be referred to other nurses in the community.

The admitting nurse, when scheduled to work the following days of the patient's expected stay, should be primary nurse for these short term patients. This might not seem like much time to use to implement primary nursing, but it can be a significant period for the patient. Also, this plan allows the part-time RN to be the primary nurse.

Duration of assignment

Some nurses misunderstand the primary nursing assignment to be absolute, never changing. If difficulties occur between the nurse and patient, there is reluctance to discuss a possible change, because the nurse might feel exposure of the situation would reflect inadequacy. This sometimes happens when extremely long term patients clash personalities with their nurse and with patients needing difficult physical or emotional care.

A solution to this is the head nurse's surveillance of all assignments. The head nurse is ultimately responsible for quality of care. Supervision and education can be provided through patient rounds, chart and care plan audits, conferences, etc. When nurses want to change patients, problem solving can help staff see their situations more objectively, learn from them, and possibly stay with the patient rather than requesting reassignment. These conferences could be with the peer group as well. When the patient must be reassigned, it must be decided how it will be done and who will tell the patient. Will patients presume that the first primary nurse does not like them any more? Will they feel guilty for causing the nurse discomfort? Helping the nurse openly and honestly deal with telling the patient should be beneficial. If not, then the head nurse should tell the patient or family so they are aware of the change.

When patients are readmitted, the choice to remain primary nurse with a patient should be left to the nurse. Many times the patient's condition will have deteriorated, as with a cancer patient. It could be stressful for the primary nurse to resume care for such a patient, depending on caseload, emotional reaction to the declining condition, hours, or skills required. When given the option, most choose to remain primary and receive satisfaction in continuing

the relationship, even if the patient is dying. However, most nurses appreciate having an "out" in case they need it.

Temporary relief periods might be necessary for the primary nurse whose patient requires heavy care, physically and/or emotionally. This is possible, if it is limited to a few shifts and the patient is informed. Discussing why relief is needed can help the nurse see the problem more clearly, learn, and be more effective. However, some patients who are hospitalized for several months could request a transfer, but it should be discouraged as much as possible.

Through direct experience as a consultant to hospitals implementing primary nursing, I have learned that there are some common misconceptions in the application of the system. Many of these involve staffing and patient assignment. Only when institutions begin to constructively deal with these misconceptions can a program of primary nursing benefit both staff and patients.

References

1. Anderson, M. "Primary Nursing in Day-by-Day Practice." *American Journal of Nursing* 76:5 (May 1976) p. 802-805.
2. Bowar-Ferres, S. "Loeb Center and Its Philosophy of Nursing." *American Journal of Nursing* 75:5 (May 1975) p. 814.
3. Ciske, K. "Primary Nursing: An Organization that Promotes Professional Practice." *Journal of Nursing Administration* IV:1 (Jan./Feb. 1974) p. 30.
4. Felton, G. et al. "Pathway to Accountability: Implementation of a Quality Assurance Program." *Journal of Nursing Administration* (January 1976) p. 21.
5. Isler, C. "Rx for a Sick Hospital: Primary Nursing Care." *RN* (February 1976) p. 61.
6. Manthey, M. "Primary Nursing is Alive and Well in the Hospital." *American Journal of Nursing* 73:1 (January 1973) p. 85-86.
7. Marram, G. et. al. *Primary Nursing* (St. Louis: The C. V. Mosby Co. 1974) p. 43, 91-93, 137-144.
8. Mundinger, M. "Primary Nurse—Role Evolution." *Nursing Outlook* 21:10 (October 1973) p. 642-645.
9. Page, M. "Primary Nursing: Perceptions of a Head Nurse." *American Journal of Nursing* 74:8 (August 1974) p. 1435-1436.

Chapter 13

POLITICAL INFLUENCES AND NEGOTIATION

A review of collective bargaining and nursing

ARLENE AUSTINSON, R.N., B.S.

Thirty-two years ago, the American Nurses Association adopted an economic security program announcing that one of its important goals was to upgrade the economic position of registered nurses. This stance evolved from years of failure to attain a living wage standard among nurses. While the depression of the 1930's and the inflationary effect of World War II had intensified the problem of substandard wages among nurses, members of labor unions had enjoyed rapid increases in wages. As a result, professionals began to view labor unions as an attractive alternative for upgrading their standard of living (Northrup, 1948). Labor union success pressured the ANA to adopt their economic security program in 1946.

Recognition of the power of group action precipitated a conflict within a variety of professional groups, e.g., teachers, nurses, engineers. The conflict revolved around whether collective bargaining was consistent with "professional ethics" and whether collective bargaining should be controlled by professional societies or by unions (Northrup, 1948).

Now, after years of movement toward an increasingly militant position on the issue of economic security, the majority of the members of the nursing profession have seemed to accept the validity and necessity of collective action to attain economic goals. There

now seems to be less concern for the question of professional ethics and collective bargaining. What continues to remain in conflict is the mechanism and the scope of issues appropriately covered by collective bargaining agreements.

In 1948, there were probably not more than 3,000 to 5,000 registered nurses who were union members (Northrup, 1948). In 1976, a survey indicated that about 25,000 nurses were represented by unions (1975 figures) and that about 84,000 nurses were represented by their professional organization, the American Nurses Association (Godfrey, 1976). While it could be argued that these figures represent a significant change in attitude toward collective bargaining over the years, considering that there are about 495,000 nurses eligible to organize if they so desire (1974 figures, at the time of the Taft-Hartley law revision), it leaves many questions about how nurses are responding to opportunities to organize (Godfrey, 1976). Results of Godfrey's 1976 survey indicated that of the nurses questioned (500 staff and administrative nurses), 28% of the staff nurses were very much in favor of nurses unions; 56% believed that someone should represent nurses, but not unions; and 16% believed that unions were unacceptable for nurses. So while most nurses agree that group action is necessary to attain economic security, there are still some that disagree with that position. In addition, the disagreement among the nurses favoring collective bargaining becomes significant in the areas of (1) inclusion of patient care issues in negotiations and (2) the leadership dilemma of a professional organization functioning as a collective bargaining agent. This article will explore these issues, primarily from the viewpoint of hospital-based nursing, as well as discussing other factors complicating the field of labor relations within nursing.

BACKGROUND OF THE ANA'S COLLECTIVE BARGAINING STANCE

The original impetus for the group action stance by the ANA was economic, in that nurses were among the lowest paid professions, as were hospital employees in general (Northrup, 1948). For years, especially during the 1930's, ANA published employee reference lists and minimum salary schedules and used other tactics to encourage a minimum living standard for nurses. The wartime inflation problem increased pressure on the professional society for stronger economic action. Additionally, the war exacerbated the shortage of nurses and made longer working hours necessary, but without increases in pay to meet increased living costs. As early as 1941, nurses in California were demanding a stronger wage program. Some nurses unionized, some left the profession. When the government initiated a freezing of wages in October 1942, obtaining salary increases became even more difficult. The California State Nurses Association received designation by their members as the sole representative in matters relating to salary and conditions of employment. With this designation the California State Nurses Association went to the War Labor Board and obtained a 15% pay increase for nurses. This successful experience in California aroused members of the ANA to explore the possibility of collective

bargaining activities by other state affiliates. Thus, the eventual adoption in 1946 of the economic security program. Two years later in his article for the *American Journal of Nursing,* Northrup (1949) supported this action with these words:

The professions and the country are certainly suffering from a strange economic malady which permits janitors and truck drivers to earn more than teachers, nurses, and other professionals. Many factors lie at the root of this problem, but surely one of the most important has been the failure of professional groups to press effectively for their just share of the national product. In any society, however realistic its philosophy, competition always exists among individuals and groups who are striving to improve their economic positions. The individual, or group, who fails to press for his rights gets left behind. American professional individuals, except perhaps for doctors and lawyers whose associations are strong and active, have ignored these realities. Postwar inflation has, fortunately, resulted in a general awakening. If the awakening is a permanent phenomenon, it promises to be among the more significant developments of the decade.

At that time, and up until 1966 when California again led the way for change, the ANA program included a no-strike policy. Repeatedly, the literature of those years reiterated the position that strikes were incompatible with nurse's professional responsibilities (Northrup, 1948; St. Sure, 1948; Schutt, 1958; Berlow, 1961). This position changed after the California State Nurses Association (CSNA) endorsed the strike as an acceptable bargaining technique in August of 1966 ("California Nurses Group Endorses Strike as Acceptable Bargaining Technique," 1966). Essentially, this change of position resulted from the action of nurses in the San Francisco Bay area (2,000 nurses in thirty-three hospitals), who submitted their mass resignations over salary demands. CSNA realized they would lose the support of nurses if they did not provide a more effective means of attaining economic goals—thus the change of position on the no-strike issue. The ANA eventually had to follow suit and accept the strike as a legitimate bargaining tool or lose its members to unions.

ATTITUDES OF HOSPITAL ADMINISTRATION TOWARD COLLECTIVE BARGAINING

For the most part, hospital administrations have not been prompt in recognizing the employee's right to organize for collective bargaining purposes. Hospital wages and salaries have been traditionally low over the years. A combination of factors such as the nonprofit status of most hospitals, the ''service'' motive of employees, the lack of legislation to encourage organization of hospitals, and the common belief that quality of patient care would decrease with employee organization have until recently made it possible for most hospitals to avoid collective bargaining with employees.

Hospitals have been a target for union activities, in part because unions needed more members (declining revenues in the industrial sector were an increasing problem), and because health care was becoming big business (Matlack, 1972). In the past, the United States was a goods-oriented society. It has gradually become a service-oriented society, and the hospital sector was, in 1961, already the fourth largest industry in the United States (Berlow, 1961). With a pattern already established of unionization of employees in industry, it was reasonable that both unions and hospital employees were interested in the effects of unionization in the hospital setting (Berlow, 1961).

Despite increased attempts at unionization and employee interest, hospital administrations have preferred not to deal with their employees through unions. In fact, until 1974, hospitals were legally exempt from collective bargaining under the Taft-Hartley Act; most chose to refuse to voluntarily bargain collectively with their employees (McCormick, 1970). The major reasons hospital management gave for this stance were (1) the strike idea, (2) the insubordination idea, (3) the nonprofit status position, (4) the increasing productivity theme, and (5) the social unit idea (McCormick, 1970).

As McCormick (1970) states, hospital administrations believed that the critical nature of their operations could not tolerate the possibility of interference with their mission of caring for the ill and injured as engendered by a strike. Since the ultimate weapon of a union is the strike, it was believed that unionization would increase the likelihood of such action. The strike would prevent a hospital from providing proper care for patients. In addition, hospital management often thought that unionism would lead to insubordination, in that employees might refuse to follow an order and thereby endanger patients' lives. Another position often presented by hospital administration was that nonprofit hospitals have no profits over which to bargain. Since most nonprofit hospitals have some ''surplus'' with which their operations are expanded, replaced, or maintained, this is not a solid position. The ''nonprofit'' term refers to the fact that hospitals are not organized for the purpose of making a profit. For years, hospitals expected their employees to subsidize patients by the acceptance of low levels of compensation, and they justified these substandard salaries with the ''nonprofit'' status theme.

Another aspect of the position of hospitals has been the claim that they could not increase productivity to offset increased costs arising from collective bargaining. Management believed that because of the highly personal nature of patient care, good quality patient care did not lend itself to labor-saving technology. In addition to the questionable nature of such a claim, there are many areas in which hospitals could look to increase productivity, such as better use of existing facilities, alternative or less costly facilities, avoidance of duplication of services, cooperative and centralized operations (shared services), use of computer services, and the like.

The last area of opposition to collective bargaining has come from the claim that hospitals are a social unit, not an economic one. This position is taken due to the nonprofit status of hospitals, the reliance of the community on hospital service, and the requirement of continuity of service (Rice, 1966). The social unit position was effectively nullified by Executive Order #10988, President Kennedy's order giving federal government employees the right to organize; cities and states have followed this example. If various levels of government could operate within a framework of collective bargaining, hospitals also should have been able to do so (McCormick, 1970).

In the 1950's, hospitals were increasingly faced with unionization, especially in the large cities. Nonprofessional workers, whose wages were so low as to be below a living rate, were among the first to unionize. The notion that individuals who worked in hospitals could be paid less than other workers merely because the hospital was doing a good work or were being supported by philanthropy made little sense. The inconsistency between the hospital's commitment to the health and welfare of the community and the failure to recognize the equal responsibility to hospital workers was a situation in need of remedy (Carlson, 1965). Unionization seemed to be the answer for unskilled workers. Nursing professionals also eventually turned to collective bargaining by state nurses associations as an answer to persistently low salaries.

Today, hospital management often still prefers to deal with employees without a union or collective bargaining agreement. Collective bargaining agreements can reduce the flexibility and options open to management and sometimes result in rigid procedures and rules. Some hospitals have avoided unionization through implementation of adequate personnel policies

(Miller, 1971). However, it is difficult to maintain justice and equity within any system, and it is likely that hospitals will continue to feel the pressure of unionization in years to come.

THE DIFFERENCE BETWEEN A PROFESSIONAL ORGANIZATION AND A UNION

Underlying the position of the ANA toward collective bargaining is the conviction that nurses must speak for nursing (Schutt, 1958). This is much more far reaching a concept than the single aspect of economic issues. It is the basis for the difference between a professional organization and a union, and it is the key conflict nursing has with hospital management. Indeed, it is a key conflict among nurses.

Nursing is still struggling to become a profession. Although the public thinks of nursing as a professional service, and the National Labor Relations Board has ruled that nursing is a profession in relation to labor law, that does not make reality out of fiction. A profession controls its own practice. It operates from a unique and identifiable body of knowledge. A professional is responsible for his or her own actions. These characteristics are not represented in all nurses.

The ANA does not represent a majority of nurses (Kelly, 1965). No one does. Economic security is not the primary purpose of the ANA or of nursing practitioners. It is a means to an end (Kelly, 1965). But unless nursing accepts its responsibility to control its own practice, to have nurses speak for nursing, the economic security issue may end up being the end, not just the means. As stated by Pointer and Cannedy (1972), "The association increasingly appears to exhibit quasi-union characteristcis. Further, the Economic Security program seems to be evolving into the raison d'etre of the ANA."

That 1972 statement is in contrast with Dorothy Kelly's (1965) clarification of the real issues of the group action process for nurses.

She describes the key difference between a professional association and a union. Thirteen years later, the situation does not seem to have changed much. She says:

The issue at stake is not just better salaries, pensions, vacations, et cetera. The real issue is who shall control nursing, nursing practice, nursing quality. At the moment, nursing pretty much is setting its own standards of practice but hospitals are dictating the performance of the practice. And the quality? It's a shambles! Nurses have permitted an erosion of both their rights and their responsibilities to result from their employment situation in the modern hospital. This is a failure in public service on the part of nurses at every level: the leaders who stand aloof; the academic nurses who are willing to wait for the next generation; the directors of diploma schools and of hospital nursing service departments who are unwilling to jeapordize their position with management; the rank and file who don't want to be bothered, who can't find any reserves of courage, who won't spend the money, who will not think. Sometimes I believe we are a sorry lot—but most of the time I think we just haven't learned how to loose the bonds of tradition while we maintain what is excellent in that tradition. Each of us hacks away a bit at the fetters but they will not be removed this way. We must think together; we must act together; we must unite in the public interest. Good care for patients and justice and freedom for nurses go hand in hand. Economic Security for nurses is a means to an end. The end, public service, can no longer be attained without this particular means (Kelly, 1965).

The use of collective bargaining to attain better salaries, vacations, pensions, work hours, etc., is an accepted and legally defined arena (Herzog, 1976). Collective bargaining in the area of professional goals is not such an accepted practice. The law does not require employers to bargain over professional issues. Thus, a major conflict between the nursing association and hospital managment exists before anyone ever sits down to negotiate.

There are those who believe that ANA cannot be a professional association and a trade union too (Phillips, 1974). Additionally, as long as legal requirements place the authority, responsibility, and accountability for hospital operations and patient care in the hands of hospital administration, there will be few hospitals willing to allow nursing control of its own quality of care ("Quality Not Negotiable," 1974). Nurses are individually legally accountable for their nursing practice, but as employees of a hospital, management, in the person of the Director or Nursing, is legally responsible for institutional quality. Those issues will not become negotiable until such time as a change in the law occurs, or such time as the nursing profession deals with the issues that so far are not universally understood or accepted—that is, standards for practice, readiness to control practice, and definition of quality (Herzog, 1976).

THE PROFESSIONAL MODEL OF COLLECTIVE BARGAINING

For those who believe that collective bargaining is a means of benefiting professional nursing and its practice, Virginia Cleland has described a professional collective bargaining model (1975). She believes that the labor contract can become the legal instrument through which the profession can implement standards of care. She compares the effect of use of labor contracts to the use of nurse practice acts, which have been the means to gradually upgrade standards for entry into nursing and to legally define the practice of nursing. She believes that labor contracts should include negotiated clauses relating to wages, hours, and conditions of work and that it is "conditions of work" that is of concern to professional collective bargaining.

Cleland states that the combination of the nature of individual licensure as a registered nurse, the legal definition of nursing as a profession by the National Labor Relations Board (NLRB), and the definition of profession are the factors that give nursing an opportunity under collective bargaining to gain control of nursing practice. To achieve that control, she feels the contract should contain certain provisions: (1) shared governance, (2) individual accountability, and (3) collective professional responsibility.

Shared governance would provide for sharing of the rights and responsibility to determine the nature of nursing practice within the institution. Professional policy decisions would be developed jointly by professional staff and professional administration. She suggests that this could take the form of a nursing practice council, with equal representation from nursing service administration and the staff nurse council. The council could develop a feasible nursing practice plan that would avoid the temptation to negotiate staffing patterns into the contract. Cleland believes that clauses relating to staffing requirements inevitably lead to a cessation of innovation and eventually to the promotion of featherbedding.

Individual accountability affects the nature of supervision and the nature of evaluation. A professional model of collective bargaining would look upon supervision as a coordination function rather than the managerial function as described by the NLRB. A strong collective bargaining unit would be desirable in order to maintain leadership and professional commitment. This means that head nurses and supervisors would need to be in the unit in order to help the staff nurse understand and appreciate the institution's many sided problems. It would also help avoid the inevitable schism that would develop between nursing administration and the bargaining unit when weak leadership exists. Poor communication and low morale would lead to rigid contract enforcement and petty grievances. Thus, if a strong bargaining unit is to exist, the definition of the role of a head nurse or supervisor needs to be that of coordinator of efforts of professionally autonomous, legally accountable employees.

The nature of evaluation is affected by individual legal professional accountability within the realm of peer review. A professional model of collective bargaining would provide for peer evaluation of a practitioner's competence. This would be in the nature of reward of meritorious performance.

Unions have traditionally avoided, as being internally destructive, any situation where one worker is judged to be more meritorious than another. To base all salaries on job title, earned degrees, or length of service is an easy escape from a difficult problem, but the simple standardization of such a system can create a haven for the lazy or incompetent. Every employer's resources are finite. If mediocre employees are hired into a lockstep reward system, there will be less money with which to recruit and retain superior employees, and the collegial environment will not be professionally attractive (Cleland, 1974).

Therefore, Cleland recommends a peer review system developed mutually by staff and administration. An effective system would reward staff based on performance and recommend nonrenewal of individual contracts of incompetent staff.

Collective professional accountability is the third type of provision needed in a professional collective bargaining contract. The advantage to nursing for having sets of criteria or standards referenced in the contract would be that standards of patient care would be grievable. Since quality of patient care is now the legal responsibility of hospital administration, it is only through the collective bargaining agreement that nurses would have a chance to protest standards of patient care, and then only if hospital management agrees to negotiate that issue. Cleland's point is that when contracts include a "right to manage" clause (management has the right to determine the number of personnel in the work force, to determine the qualifications of employees, to open or close units, etc.), that there is an obligation too, and that is to perform these acts in the best interests of the public served. "Management is obligated to provide adequate numbers of personnel with appropriate qualifications to serve the public need and, if and where this is not possible, management is obligated to close units of the health facility so that would-be patients may seek health services from other institutions" (1975).

This model requires a high degree of sophistication of nurses prior to its workability. Robert Weatherbee did a study in 1968 (cited in Erickson, 1971) that indicated that staff nurses are not always supportive of professional or patient care issues, and indeed that rank-and-file nurses seem to be primarily motivated by economics. It could be questioned whether staff nurses are ". . . really interested in using collective bargaining to improve patient care, or only to improve their own economic status" (Erickson, 1971).

CURRENT TRENDS

It is projected that by 1980, 70% of the working force in the United States will be employed in service industries (Matlack, 1972). Of these service industries there are more than 7,500 hospitals, with over 2 million employees. The growth of the health care industry will continue to encourage unionization attempts of nonprofessionals and of professionals (Matlack, 1972).

The future of ANA will remain a debatable issue for years to come. One thing seems certain: "In view of the efforts put forth and the successes achieved by the ANA in the field of collective bargaining, we can expect the Association to increasingly assume a trade union posture in the years ahead" (Herzog, 1976). If the ANA truly becomes a labor union, how far can it get with professional issues? A professional model of bargaining would assure the continued professionalism of the organization, but until nurses have agreed upon and accepted sets of standards of practice, the issues of quality and practice will remain controversial. "Who wants to lock into a contract individual or organizational interpretations of quality and practice" (Herzog, 1976)? Collective bargaining by itself will not solve the ques-

tions of standards. Perhaps a profession that trains large numbers of its practitioners at the technical level should expect and provide services at the trade union level.

"If nursing supervisors and administrators continue to be excluded by the NLRB from bargaining units, the ANA stands a good chance of losing an important constituency. It is doubtful that the ANA can effectively represent non-supervisory and non-administrative nurses for the purposes of collective bargaining and also represent the profession on the issues of practice and quality" (Herzog, 1976). Therefore, policies and practices need to be developed that will allow and encourage all nurses, including supervisors and Directors of Nursing, to participate in ANA activities. Otherwise, further division and splintering of the profession will occur. A recent study indicates that Directors of Nursing Services snow no tendency to support the professional organization as a collective bargaining agent and that there is a great deal of ambivalence over collective bargaining activities, which may result in alienation of the Director of Nursing from the ANA (Sargis, 1978).

The current literature seems to reflect the general acceptance, by nurses, of collective bargaining as a legitimate approach to dealing with wage and hour issues. There is some pragmatic information available for supervisors and Directors of Nursing regarding their role in labor negotiations (The Role of the Director in an Organized Nursing Service in Collective Bargaining, 1970; Roscasco, 1974; Fralic, 1977). Also, a disturbing trend is appearing for those who question the ethical right of nurses to strike. Metzger and Pointer (1972) indicate that although professional associations engage in fewer recognitional disputes than unions, they have more instances of work stoppages related to terms of employment. This type of record may reinforce hospital resistance to organization of professional employees. Additionally, an article by David Reece (1977) discussed a decertification effort of a Michigan hospital, in which 175 registered nurses decertified their collective bargaining affiliation with the Michigan State Nurses Association in favor of the hospital's program. The administrative staff of that hospital was able to develop a program to provide a working environment where nurse employees did not feel it necessary to remain aligned with their state nurses association for labor representation. For these staff nurses, economic issues and individual consideration in a compensation and benefit program were the most important gains. Apparently, these nurses did not see collective bargaining as a way to control the practice of nursing. They were either unaware of a "professional model" of collective bargaining, they did not consider it important, or they did not consider it workable.

If recent surveys are representative of nurses thought, then few nurses are ready to understand and implement the "professional model" in their collective bargaining agreements. Additionally, Directors of Nursing will apparently not be a central force in future collective bargaining by registered nurses (Sargis, 1978). Rather, registered nurses will go with whoever will provide them with an adequate economic package and most importantly, job satisfaction (Longest, 1974). Nurses want to be represented by someone (Godfrey, 1976).

References

Berlow, L. Are unions the answer to collective bargaining for nurses? *Hospital Topics,* Vol. 39, No. 5, 1961, 38-42.

California nurses group endorses strike as acceptable bargaining technique. *Hospitals,* Vol. 40, No. 18, September 16, 1966, 201.

Carlson, D. R. Labor union: color it white, black, or red. *The Modern Hospital,* Vol. 105, No. 2, 1965, 107-111; 182.

Cleland, V. S. The supervisor in collective bargaining. *The Journal of Nursing Administration,* Vol, IV, No. 4, 1974, 33-35.

Cleland, V. S. The professional model. *American Journal of Nursing,* Vol. 75, No. 2, 1975, 288-292.

Erickson, E. Collective bargaining; an inappropriate technique for professionals. *Nursing Forum,* Vol. X, No. 3, 1971, 300-310.

Fralic, M. F. The nursing director prepares for labor negotiations. *The Journal of Nursing Administration,* Vol. VII, No. 6, 1976, 4-8.

Godfrey, M. Someone should represent nurses. *Nursing '76,* Vol. 6, No. 6, 1976, 73-85.

Herzog, T. The national labor relations act and the ANA: a dilemma of professionalism. *The Journal of Nursing Administration,* October 1976, 34-36.

Kelly, D. The situation in nursing. *American Journal of Nursing,* Vol. 65, No. 1, 1965, 77-78.

Longest, B. B. Job satisfaction for registered nurses in the hospital setting. *The Journal of Nursing Administration,* Vol. 4, No. 3, 1974, 46-52.

Matlack, D. R. Goals and trends in the unionization of health professionals. *Hospital Progress,* Vol. 53, No. 2, 1972, 40-43.

McCormick, W., Jr. Labor relations in hospitals. *American Journal of Nursing,* Vol. 70, No. 12, 1970, 2606-2609.

Metzger, N., and Pointer, D. D. *Labor Management Relations in the Health Services Industry.* Washington, D.C.: Science and Health Publications, Inc., 1972, 103.

Miller, R. L. The hospital-union relationship, part 2. *Hospitals,* Vol. 45, No. 10, May 16, 1971, 52-56.

Northrup, H. R. Collective bargaining and the professions. *American Journal of Nursing,* Vol. 48, No. 3, 1948, 141-144.

Phillips, D. F. New demands of nurses, part 1. *Hospitals,* Vol. 48, No. 16, August 16, 1974, 31-34.

Pointer, D. D., and Cannedy, L. L. Organizing of professionals. *Hospitals,* Vol. 46, No. 6, March 16, 1972, 70-73.

Quality not negotiable. *Hospitals,* Vol. 48, No. 20, October 16, 1974, 43.

Reece, D. A. Union decertification and the salaried approach: a workable alternative. *The Journal of Nursing Administration,* Vol. VII, No. 6, 1977, 20-24.

Rice, R. G. Analysis of the hospital as an economic organism. *The Modern Hospital,* Vol. 106, No. 4, 1966, 87-91.

The role of the director of an organized nursing service in collective bargaining. *American Journal of Nursing,* Vol. 70, No. 3, 1970, 551-556.

Rosasco, L. C. Collective bargaining: what's a director of nursing to do? *Hospitals,* Vol. 48, No. 18, September 16, 1974, 79-83.

Sargis, N. M. Will nursing directors' attitudes affect future collective bargaining? *The Journal of Nursing Administration,* Vol. VIII, No. 12, 1978, 21-26.

Schutt, B. G. The ANA economic security program . . . what it is and why. *American Journal of Nursing,* Vol. 58, No. 4, 1958, 520-524.

St. Sure, J. P. The meaning of an economic security program. *American Journal of Nursing,* Vol. 48, No. 11, 1948, 692-693.

Nursing ideologies and collective bargaining

NORMA K. GRAND, R.N., Ph.D.

The need to improve the economic and social welfare of nurses has been recognized since the 1930s. Other occupational groups have made notable progress in gaining higher wages and better working conditions by unionizing and using their collective strength to force concessions from their employers. Nurses, on the other hand, have been reluctant to follow the same course of action. The most obvious deterrent to the use of collective action is the tendency of nurses to equate collective action with unprofessional behavior. Many nurses consider collective action in their own behalf irreconcilable with nursing ideology. This is the service ideal, the dedicatory ethic which elevates the ideal of service to others and denigrates material reward as the proper motivation to work.

Since the 1960s, however, an increasing number of nurses have engaged in collective bargaining and have gone on strike. These nurses do not regard themselves as unprofessional or less dedicated to the service ideal. This seeming paradox is explained by a second set of beliefs which has developed in nursing. These beliefs comprise a new ideology, promulgated since the inception of the American Nurses' Association's Economic Security Program, which resolves the apparent irreconcilability of the service ideal and collective action by nurses.

The nature of ideology explains how nurses can believe seemingly contradictory beliefs. An ideology is a body of ideas and sentiments woven together into a fairly consistent pattern. It starts from an ideal and develops into an organized pattern of beliefs which includes both factual and normative elements (the should and

should nots). The normative elements stem from the ideal and in turn direct the selection of facts. The facts selected are not necessarily derived from scientific investigation, but are chosen because they support the "cause" (generally a desire to change or retain the status quo). Since many of the so-called facts may be assumed to be true on the basis of their logicality, an ideology can incorporate both true and false propositions.

Once an ideology has developed, it provides a means whereby an orderly and subjectively meaningful picture of reality can be constructed. It is an arbitrary picture, however, because it does not include social facts in all their complexity, and it may even include what does not exist. Besides being an organized belief system, an ideology is also an organized disbelief system. The faithful are disposed to see only what they have been indoctrinated to see and do what must be done in the light of this vision. Thus ideology defines, explains, and differentiates between what can and what cannot be done.

It has been said that each occupation has its own unique pattern of ideological beliefs. Nursing is not the only occupation with an ideology based on a service ideal (teachers and social workers also have a service ideology), but it has assumed its particular pattern in nursing because of the time in history in which it developed.

When the religious hospitals were founded in England in the twelfth century, the monastic orders took over the care of the sick. The nuns attended the female patients with the help of women of good birth and little training who were devoted to a life of good works. After the Reformation, when no lay orders arose to take the place of the suppressed religious orders, the

Reprinted by permission from *The Journal of Nursing Administration*, March-April 1973.

care of the sick was relegated to women of lower birth with no tradition of devoted service. Nursing came to be viewed as a sordid duty fit only for the lower classes of the community.

In the latter half of the nineteenth century, when the effort was begun to rescue nursing from the bad reputation it had acquired, Florence Nightingale was the popular idol. Her feats in the Crimean War were suggestive of self-sacrifice, heroism, and a passionate belief in the welfare of others. In addition, she was popularly conceptualized as a frail, delicate, and dedicated woman endowed with all the culturally desirable feminine qualities. These characteristics appealed to the romanticism and humanitarianism of the era and presented an ideal symbol for nursing.

The adoption of this idealized conception of Nightingale as a symbol had a decided impact on nursing's social recognition and perceived role. Nightingale's status as a member of England's upper class invested the occupation with the social approval it needed. In addition, the deeds that brought Nightingale wide acclaim brought acclaim to nursing by association. Her representation as a woman of sacrifice enabled nursing reformers to demand sacrifice of nursing recruits; the nurse was to assume the role of nurturant-giving and self-abnegation and to relinquish certain comforts. This meant relinquishing the comforts of home for the work of the hospital and sacrificing themselves to perform tasks that at times were menial and offensive. The role of the nurse was to be a helpmate to the physician, and her dominant interest not in herself but in those committed to her care. There was little money to pay nurses for taking care of the hospital's population—the sick poor—thus nurses were expected to work for little or no pay, and this attitude made irrelevant the question of adequate payment for nurses.

The humanitarianism and ideas of self-sacrifice associated with the popular conception of Nightingale became the prominent values of the occupation. Through the years the idea of sacrifice as originally conceived has come to mean that the primary concern of the nurse is the welfare of the patient and excludes a concern on the part of the nurse with her own economic and social welfare. Inevitably this set of beliefs was named *nightingalism*. Although other factors affect the adoption of collective action by nurses, such as the lack of protective legislation and the negative attitude of their employers toward collective bargaining, this set of beliefs has been the major deterrent.

The economic and social welfare of nurses first became an acute problem when the employment conditions of nurses, which had deteriorated rapidly during the depression, failed to improve in line with the expectations of nurses as the depression lessened. During the 1930s some nurses turned to the labor unions for help and the ANA was confronted with the question of union membership for nurses. Nurses at that time had no organization to represent their economic interests. Even though the ANA had been formed to "promote the usefulness and honor, the financial and other interests of the nursing profession, little had been done about the economic problems of the occupation."[1] The ANA was opposed to union membership for nurses because unions used the strike as a last resort, a sanction felt to be incompatible with the service ideal of nursing. To deter union membership, the ANA urged the state nurses' associations to assume responsibility for nurses' employment conditions. Emphasis was placed on educating the public to the service nurses gave and its importance to the economy. This public relations program met with little success.

California nurses led the way in collective action.

When the California State Nurses' Association (CSNA) developed a basic salary schedule for nurses, which the California hospitals refused to adopt, and the wage freeze went into effect in 1942, the nurses urged the CSNA to act in their behalf. The state association was successful in gaining an increase in salary. Once they had demonstrated the efficacy of collective action, the CSNA became the collective bargaining agent for California nurses.

By 1944 other state associations began asking the ANA if a professional association were obligated to act as the collective bargaining agent for its members. Since the alternative was union representation, the ANA decided that collective bargaining by professional society leadership was preferable to trade union leadership and proposed the Economic Security Program at the biennial convention in 1946. The program was unanimously adopted for, while nurses were reluctant to seem mercenary, they and their families were well aware of the rising cost of living and of the salaries prevalent in other occupations and professions.

One of the major issues for the ANA in developing the Economic Security Program was how to reconcile the service ideal of nursing with the use of collective strength for nurses' economic interests. This issue was resolved by viewing the quality of nursing care as dependent upon nurses' economic status and satisfactory working conditions. When the Economic Security Program was adopted it proclaimed two major objectives: (1) to protect and improve the economic security of nurses and to secure satisfactory working conditions, and (2) to assure the public that professional nursing service of high quality and sufficient quantity would be available.

These objectives are viewed as closely related. It is argued that high quality care is more likely to result when the nurse is provided an environment in which she can work at her best because when employees are dissatisfied with their working environment their work suffers. Sufficient quantity of care depends on attracting recruits to the occupation as well as on retaining those already trained. Hence, the second objective can be achieved only by achieving the first. Making the second objective dependent on the

first places the responsibility directly on the nurse to upgrade her economic status and to improve her working conditions since increased benefits for the nurse should be reflected in better care for the patients.

To appreciate the interdependence of working conditions and quality of care, it is argued that nurses must broaden their concerns about their work beyond face-to-face relationships with patients. Thus it should be a matter of concern to every nurse, e.g., whether or not her work load is too heavy to enable her to give proper care, if she is obliged to perform tasks in a manner incompatible with professional standards or if she continues to perform tasks which can be performed by nonprofessional personnel, because all these factors directly affect her own personal satisfaction, her professional ethics, and the quality of care she gives. Working conditions are also considered to affect the quantity of care available, for unless the occupation offers a well paid and personally satisfying career for future practitioners, nursing will not be successful in the competitive struggle for recruits.

Where the Nightingale ideology stresses the ideal of placing the interests of the patients before the interests of the nurse, this argument stresses the responsibility of the nurse for high quality work, which in turn depends on factors which are in the interests of the nurse: satisfactory working conditions and satisfaction with the quality of her work. Hence, a nurses' strike can be conceived not as a strike against the patient, but as an effort to gain benefits for the nurse that will enable her to provide more and better care for the patients in the long run.

Nursing leaders hope that this rationale will overcome the reluctance of nurses to use collective action since it also is based on concern for the patient. The emphasis has been shifted from the short run to the long run benefits. Because it emphasizes collective action as a professional responsibility, this ideology has been called *professional collectivism.*

There is strong evidence that the professional collectivism ideology was an important influence on the behavior of the nurses in the 1969 Cleveland strike.[2] Both the nurses who went on strike as well as those who did not strike adhered to the Nightingale ideology. The nurses who participated in the strike, however, strongly believed in the professional collectivism ideology whereas those who continued to work did not. In this dispute the new ideology achieved its purpose, for those who accepted it, of overcoming the concern that collective action is unprofessional.

Professional collectivism has an inherent disadvantage, however, because of the assumption upon which it is based. This is the assumption that when working conditions are poor, nurses become restless and unhappy and, as a consequence of their unhappiness, the quality of nursing care deteriorates. Since the low or deteriorating quality of care is the justification for collective action, nurses are impelled to be critical of the nursing care. If they do not use this justification, their employer is free to accuse them of being unprofessional, of having greater concern for themselves than for their patients. The quality of care, on the other hand, is one of the major bases of an employer's public image. To criticize the care is to attack this image, a ploy almost guaranteed to rouse his greatest ire. It may, moreover, increase his resistance to the collective action.

This happened in the Cleveland strike. The nurses aired their concern in the press about the deteriorating quality of nursing care. The hospital administrator immediately took exception to their statement, claiming it was untrue and most upsetting to the physicians, patients, patients' families, and the public. The statement remained an obstacle in the efforts of the nurses and hospital administration to reach a compromise in the dispute. The hospital continued to call for a retraction, and the nurses as adamantly continued to refuse to retract. Thus, it is evident that when nurses use this justification for collective action, they are likely to be placed in the double bind of being damned if they do and damned if they don't criticize nursing care.

Nurses must be under even greater stress when they have difficulty in perceiving the situation as the ideology dictates. The Cleveland data show that although the nurses voiced concern about the quality of care, its importance was minimal as a general issue or as a basis for the strike. The nurses were asked what they felt were the major issues in the dispute. Most of the nurses agreed that job security, communications with administration, and the hospital's hiring and firing policies were the major issues. Significantly, 83 percent did not choose the quality of nursing care as an issue at all. Nor were the nurses who were the most dissatisfied with working conditions at the hospital more likely to view the quality of care as poor. And there was no relation between how the nurses felt about the quality of care and whether or not they went on strike.

These data raise a question about the validity of the assumption that when working conditions are perceived as poor and nurses are unhappy, nursing care will be poor. Although there had been increasing dissatisfaction among the Cleveland nurses for about two years before the strike, 69 percent of the sample felt that the quality of care had remained the same or even improved during their tenure at the hospital.

The ANA does offer other, more pragmatic, justifications for collective action by nurses. One is the argument that women are affected by the same needs and job conditions as men and that the same factors which impel men to try to improve their economic and social welfare exist also for women. Few employers can deny that many nurses work to eat, to pay rent, and to support a family, as do men.

Another argument of the ANA is based on the employee status of most nurses. Employers, on the whole, rarely initiate salary increases and work benefits but pay what their employees will accept; employers of nurses have shown themselves to be no different. Since nurses share this economic reality with other employees, it stands to reason that nurses should also share their method to solve their work problems.

Acceptance of these arguments, however, is weakened by another set of beliefs, namely *employeeism,* the belief that employers of nurses have the best interests of the nurses at heart and will do their best for them. This ideology developed in the years during and following the depression in the 1930s. Many hospitals were forced to close their schools of nursing and few patients could afford the cost of private nurses; many private duty nurses moved into hospital employment. The hospital offered them a livelihood, but under the disadvantageous terms of long and broken hours, little pay, and a home life confined to the hospital nursing residence. Nurses had to depend on the paternalism of their employer at that time; this dependence has continued even though the circumstances have changed. Why this set of beliefs has endured is understandable in the light of the strong hold of nightingalism on the occupation. If nurses are denied the right to be concerned for their own economic and social welfare, it is reassuring to believe that their employers are protecting their interests. Thus one ideology reinforces the other. If a nurse adopts professional collectivism, however, she generally no longer accepts employeeism.

The Nightingale ideology is an integral part of nursing and will probably remain so indefinitely. It still serves as a symbol of status, just as it did at its inception. Until the occupation develops a body of theoretical, scientific knowledge on which to base its practice, the service ideal is nursing's major claim to professional status.

Nightingalism has served and is serving a positive function for the occupation in the eyes of the public because of this equation of altruism with professionalism. At the same time it has actively deterred nursing from taking positive steps to improve its economic position. Lately, this has been viewed as a negative function. It has not been feasible for nursing leaders to justify collective bargaining on a basis which rejects nightingalism because of this professionalizing function. This has necessitated the building of a counter ideology which is compatible with nightingalism in that it is also based on concern for the welfare of the patient, but in terms of the long-range benefits.

The new ideology, professional collectivism, was effective in the Cleveland strike in countering the negative influence of nightingalism on collective action by nurses. It has a built-in disadvantage, however. By making the quality of nursing care the legitimator of the dissatisfaction of nurses with salary and working conditions, professional collectivism impels nurses to be publicly critical of that care. This public criticism is almost certain to rouse or increase the resistance of employers to collective action by nurses.

Unless nurses justify collective action by voicing their concern about the quality of nursing care, they leave themselves open to the charge of selfishness, of being unprofessional. Thus while professional collectivism has helped some nurses loosen the economics fetters of nightingalism, they are now caught in the double bind of being damned if they do and damned if they don't criticize the quality of nursing care.

References

1. *Manual for an Economic Security Program.* 2d ed. New York: American Nurses' Association, 1956, p. 1.
2. Grand, N. K. *Nurs. Forum.* 10(3):289-299, 1972. See also Grand, N. K. The Role of Ideology in the Unionization of Nurses. Case Western Reserve University, 1971. Unpublished dissertation.

Professional employees turn to unions

DENNIS CHAMOT

In March 1975, the nation witnessed a relatively minor, but rather dramatic event. More than 2,000 doctors in New York City went on strike for four days. In the best tradition of more conventional trade unionists, they walked picket lines and demanded improvements in pay, hours, and working conditions. It should be noted that this was an honest-to-goodness labor dispute and not the increasingly common but, in union terms, less significant protest of malpractice insurance problems by established doctors.

This action (and similar, more recent ones in Washington, D.C., Chicago, and Los Angeles) caught many people by surprise. After all, who needs a union less than a doctor? When put in proper perspective, however, these developments are neither strange nor unexpected, and they have important implications far beyond the medical community.

In fact, the men and women who participated in these strikes, and the many more doctors who are currently in unions, are not the highly paid, independent practitioners one usually thinks of. They are, instead, hospital interns and residents, *employees* of large bureaucratic organizations. Thus the similarities between them and other employed professionals are far greater than the more obvious differences.

There are currently almost 3 million members of unions and employee associations who are classified as professional and technical.[1]

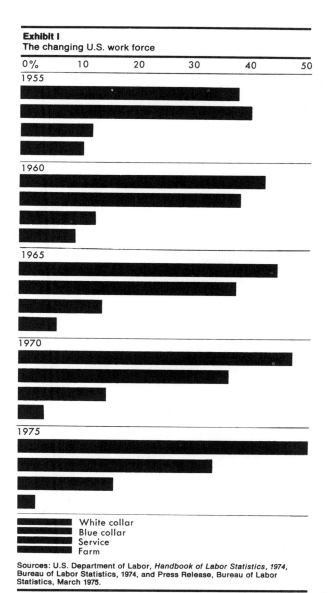

Exhibit I
The changing U.S. work force

White collar
Blue collar
Service
Farm

Sources: U.S. Department of Labor, *Handbook of Labor Statistics, 1974*, Bureau of Labor Statistics, 1974, and Press Release, Bureau of Labor Statistics, March 1975.

Dennis Chamot, "Professional Employees Turn to Unions," *Harvard Business Review,* May-June, 1976. Copyright © 1976 by the President and Fellows of Harvard College; all rights reserved.

[1]U.S. Bureau of Labor Statistics, *Directory of National Unions and Employee Associations 1973* (Washington, D.C.: U.S. Government Printing Office, 1974).

They include public schoolteachers, college professors, musicians, actors, journalists, engineers, nurses, and doctors, among others.

The American work force as a whole is changing. "White collar" now describes one half of all working people, and this figure has been increasing steadily (see *Exhibit I*). The fastest-growing segment, professional and technical employees, currently accounts for one seventh of the total work force, and is expected to increase to one sixth within ten years (see *Exhibit II*). Paralleling these changes has been the upsurge in white-collar union membership, which, in the past decade and a half, increased by over 1 million (to 3.8 million), and now accounts for 17.4% of all union membership; another 2 million employees are in state and professional associations that engage in collective bargaining (see *Exhibit III*).

WHITE-COLLAR UNION GROWTH

Several white-collar unions have experienced spectacular growth over the past few years,

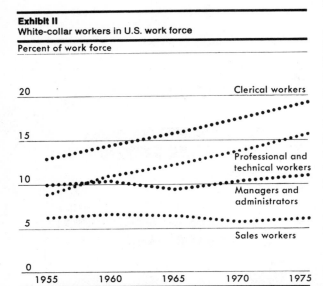

Exhibit II
White-collar workers in U.S. work force
Percent of work force

Source: U.S. Department of Labor, *Handbook of Labor Statistics, 1974,* Bureau of Labor Statistics, 1974.

Exhibit III
Union membership growth (relative to 1963)

Year	AFT	AFSCME	AFGE	CWA	SEIU	UAW	Teamsters	Carpenters
1963	1.00	1.00	1.00	1.00	1.00	1.00	1.00	1.00
1965	1.41	1.07	1.31	1.05	1.09	1.09	1.03	1.03
1967	1.76	1.28	1.88	1.15	1.18	1.31	1.13	1.08
1969	2.33	1.66	2.78	1.28	1.32	1.37	1.20	1.07
1971	2.90	2.02	3.07	1.51	1.48	1.38	1.26	1.11
1973	3.51	2.40	2.76	1.59	1.64	1.30	1.27	1.11
1973 (by thousands)	249	529	293	443	484	1,394	1,855	820

AFT: American Federation of Teachers
AFSCME: American Federation of State, County and Municipal Employees
AFGE: American Federation of Government Employees
CWA: Communications Workers of America
SEIU: Service Employees' International Union
UAW: United Automobile, Aerospace, and Agricultural Implement Workers of America
Teamsters: International Brotherhood of Teamsters, Chauffeurs, Warehousemen, and Helpers of America
Carpenters: United Brotherhood of Carpenters and Joiners of America

with much of the increase occurring in the public sector. For example, by mid-1975, the American Federation of Teachers (AFT) claimed 450,000 members, 4½ times its 1963 membership. Furthermore, 1 in 10 AFT members is on a college faculty. If the professors belonging to other unions are added, it appears that 20% of the American professoriat, on over 420 campuses, have been organized—virtually all within the past decade.

Similarly, the American Federation of State, County, and Municipal Employees (AFSCME) and the American Federation of Government Employees (AFGE) each tripled its membership between 1963 and 1975. It should be noted that many unions represent for collective bargaining purposes more people than are indicated by membership figures, e.g., AFGE has about 325,000 members but represents over 600,000 federal employees.

By contrast, the United Brotherhood of Carpenters and Joiners' membership expanded by only 11% in the decade 1963-1973. Both the Autoworkers (UAW) and Teamsters, mostly blue-collar unions that are trying to increase white-collar membership, did only slightly better (about 30%, although from a larger base).

Growth is not the only measure of success when one is dealing with a finite system. Organization is proceeding slowly in some areas because most eligible workers in these fields are already in unions. This is true, for example, in the performing arts, where union membership is the accepted norm among professional and supporting personnel.

Historically, unions have been most successful among blue-collar workers. Why the rapid and sustained increase in white-collar interest? In the public sector, at least, the situation was helped by changes in the appropriate laws. The Wagner Act, passed in 1935, applied only to workers in the private sector. However, under President Kennedy's Executive Order 10988 in 1962, followed by new laws in state

after state during the 1960s, collective bargaining rights were granted to government employees. Many were quick to use them.

This is only part of the answer, however, since the laws could not have been changed if there had not been a good deal of pressure already for the changes. Furthermore, union interest has increased in the private sector, too, and here the legal framework has been available for decades, permitting, if not mandating, organization.

At the heart of the matter is the nature of modern employment, which is likely to consist of very routine, nonchallenging jobs. Here the problem for nonprofessional white-collar employees is in many ways identical to that of their blue-collar colleagues. It is only natural, then, that they should choose similar means to solve those problems. As the white-collar work force rapidly expands, union successes continue apace.

SPECIAL PROBLEMS OF PROFESSIONALS

The larger number of professional employees presents a more complex situation. Although it is beyond the scope of this article to examine in detail individual professions or industries (which differ from group to group even within the same profession), several important generalizations may be drawn.

It might be useful at this point to note that the word *professional* has two rather different connotations. The first emphasizes the external, economic aspect of the job. A person is a professional because he or she is paid for services rendered. This is one of the differences between Arnold Palmer and a weekend golfer. It is this definition I use in discussing problems with salaries, termination policies, and the like.

The complementary definition involves an internal, psychological view. The professional sees himself as a member of a special group to which admission is gained only after advanced or specialized study. He seeks recognition among his peers and takes great pride in the knowledge he has acquired and the opportunity to use it.

One of the big differences between professional employees and all other nonmanagement workers is that the professional expects that he will have a major role to play in deciding how to perform his job. Unlike a production worker or a secretary, the professional expects to help determine the problems he will work on and the approaches toward their solution. All too often, his expectations fall far short of reality. Dissatisfaction may result from inadequate technical support, insufficient opportunity to pursue interesting ideas, excessive interference by superiors, lack of sufficient input to project assignment decisions, and so on. Whether or not there are overriding economic considerations behind these decisions, the professional employee frequently feels he is not treated with the respect he deserves.

Back in the "good old days," the individual professional enjoyed a one-to-one relationship with his client. He experienced a great deal of autonomy both in making decisions and in determining work assignments and conditions. Further, he had sufficient control to effectively determine adequate compensation.

The professional-client relationship today has been radically altered. Today's professionals are no longer self-employed, independent practitioners, but are instead employees of ever-larger organizations. No matter what the nature of the employing institution—corporation, university, or government agency—few individuals within it feel they have sufficient personal bargaining power to effectively control their careers or their jobs.

The problem is that we are dealing with two very different viewpoints. As Archie Kleingartner of the University of California at Los Angeles put it some years ago in a discussion of industrial engineers, "Management equates professionalism with loyalty to management, and perceives unions as threatening the loyalty of engineers. Any engineer who joins a union is perceived as disloyal, and by extension as behaving unprofessionally. [However,] management opposition to engineer unionism reflects purely managerial interests more than a concern for high professional standards. I would guess that management opposition would be just as strong if professional societies attempted to bargain."[2]

Authority and decision making

Discussion with representatives of several unions that are active in organizing professionals confirms that dissatisfaction with policies relating to authority and decision making is a major issue. For example, at most campuses where faculties have unionized in recent years, the primary concerns were job security and the somewhat related but much broader subject of university governance. Colleges and universities are moving away from the old system of collegiality and are increasingly employing full-time administrators who exercise considerable authority. Attempts to impose business practices (e.g., measurement of faculty "productivity") by people who are perceived, at least, as having insufficient teaching experience, threaten established notions of professional responsibilities, duties, and prerogatives. Unionization is looked on as a way for a faculty to improve its bargaining position with an administration that has grown too powerful in areas that have been traditionally the domain of the educators.

Current union contracts have provisions safeguarding these areas:

- The contract between the Southeastern Massachusetts University Faculty Federation (AFT Local 1895) and the university trustees states: "The faculty shall have the responsibility to determine course content and texts."

---

[2] Archie Kleingartner, "Professionalism and Engineering Unionism," *Industrial Relations,* May 1969, p. 235.

- A recent contract between the faculty union (AFT Local 1600) and trustees of Cook County Community College, District No. 508, has sections limiting class size and teaching loads.
- The Rhode Island College Chapter of the AFT apparently felt that more basic problems existed, because the contract it negotiated in 1972 with the Rhode Island Board of Regents declared: "Each full-time faculty member shall be assigned office space."

In these, and in many other cases, the faculty felt it needed a union to secure rights in areas that are at the heart of its ability to properly perform its professional duties.

Salary and work schedules

Where unions have been active in organizing employees of hospitals and other health care facilities, it has been found that issues involving quality of patient care (e.g., the number of doctors in clinics or emergency rooms, the improvement of nursing and technician staffs, the improvement of X-ray services, the availability of physical therapists, and so on) are of great concern at all professional levels. Salary is the other major issue, although this is far less important at the higher pay levels. Nurses, for example, are much more interested in salary improvement than the better paid pharmacists, but both groups seek greater impact on institutional decision making.

In many cases, concerns overlap: interns demanding shorter schedules will work fewer hours, but they will also provide better care if they get proper sleep; professors fighting enlargement of classes (or elimination of some) are protecting their jobs, but they are also vitally concerned with the effects of proposed changes on the quality of education.

In the federal sector, salary cannot be an issue because the unions are forbidden by law to bargain over congressionally set pay levels. In 1973, NASA engineers at Huntsville, Alabama

joined the International Federation of Professional and Technical Engineers (AFL-CIO). A key issue in the campaign was employee disgruntlement over an extremely complex and rigid organizational structure, which they felt would be changed by a union. One might note that, even before they organized, these engineers were earning an average salary of about $20,000 a year. Engineers in federal, state, and municipal agencies have turned to unions in large part because of a strong desire to have greater impact on managerial decisions.[3]

Although the general concerns noted here seem to be fairly universal, the details of every organizing campaign or bargaining session are different. We are, after all, dealing with groups of *employees,* and, professional or not, they worry about wages, hours, and working conditions.

Furthermore, since professional employees are only human, they do not like to be taken advantage of. For example, they are exempt from the maximum hours provision of the Fair Labor Standards Act. In other words, they are entitled to work overtime for free. As Robert Stedfeld, editor of the magazine *Machine Design,* wrote a few years ago, "Some companies have discovered a new cost-cutting gimmick—force engineers to work overtime without pay. The company saves money. Engineers can be laid off, and the regular work load is imposed on the remaining engineers. The engineers being unfairly exploited are afraid they will lose their jobs if they protest, so they take it."[4]

This situation is still fairly widespread, especially in R&D. Hours are set for the nonexempt clerical and support staff, but the professional employees—scientists, engineers, computer people, and the like—are expected to begin

---

[3] For a more general look at scientists and engineers, see Dennis Chamot, "Scientists and Engineers: The New Reality," *American Federationist,* September 1974, p. 8.

[4] Robert Stedfeld, editorial, *Machine Design,* April 15, 1971, p. 65.

work at least as early as the secretaries and feel a great deal of indirect pressure to stay quite a bit later each day than the official quitting time. The worst offenders are those employers who offer services to others. Here, the pressures can be quite intense as contract proposal or termination deadlines approach.

It should be noted that these pressures are applied to all members of the professional staff, not just to those who are eager to get ahead. Some companies formalize the system by offering compensatory time off, but this is not the norm. Even where this option does exist, it is often abused. For example, one plant has some restrictions on how the compensatory time is taken, limiting it to days approved by the supervisor, and to no more than one day at a time. The rules may be bent a bit, but, in fact, a large part of the overtime put in by those engineers is never paid for in any way.

A recent study of overtime trends by the U.S. Bureau of Labor Statistics shows that nearly a quarter of all professional and technical employees regularly work more than 40 hours a week, but only 18% are paid for overtime.[5] Furthermore, one half of all workers on extended workweeks are white collar, and this number has continually increased, even though overtime for blue-collar workers has fluctuated with changes in general economic conditions.

The reader, especially one in a managerial or executive position, may see nothing wrong with this. The point, though, is that affected employees do. They do not like being required to work overtime routinely. This is particularly true when nonexempt assistants draw premium pay while their professional colleagues get only titles.

Grievance procedures

Another serious problem for the employed nonunion professional is the lack of a realistic grievance procedure. If problems arise, as they invariably do, he is encouraged to complain to his immediate supervisor or perhaps to the personnel department.

Both the supervisor and the personnel people are representatives of the employer; further, their future careers and rewards are in the hands of that same employer. Should the disagreement between the professional and the employer be a serious one that cannot be easily resolved without cost to the company (either in dollars or in "managerial prerogative"), then the employee probably will not get satisfaction through the only channels open to him. His only choice is to accept the unilateral decision of the employer or resign. In neither case is the employee able to demonstrate sufficient professional status to influence the outcome. This can be very discouraging.

It should be emphasized that lists of specific grievances are not as important as are the deficiencies of the system for dealing with them. To be sure, the complaint may be very serious to the individual involved (e.g., dismissal, involuntary transfer, insufficient salary increase, improper job assignment). But, whatever the nature of the specific dispute, a modern organization is not set up to deal directly with individuals. Authority for settling disputes is usually much higher up in the hierarchy than the immediate supervisor or personnel person with whom the complainant tries to bargain.

Frequently, policies are too inflexible in any case, as the following examples show:

A few years ago a physicist at a major corporation was offered a 10% salary increase. He asked if he could have instead an additional week of vacation (which was worth much less in dollar terms). He was refused.

Sometimes a clash may occur over issues of quality of work rather than individual benefits, as in the case of three professional employees of the Bay Area Rapid Transit (BART) in San Francisco. The three, a systems engineer, a programmer analyst, and an electrical engineer, became increasingly concerned

---

[5] Diane M. Westcott, "Trends in Overtime Hours and Pay, 1969-74," *Monthly Labor Review*, February 1975, p. 45.

with defects in the automated train control system being developed by a contractor and with the manner in which the installation and testing of this system was being carried out. When their supervisors continued to disregard their warnings, they complained to the BART board of directors. After a public hearing, the board voted to support management. Shortly thereafter, the three engineers were fired.[6]

Several months later, a BART train overran the station at Fremont, injuring several passengers. Other failures of the automatic system occurred frequently. These three engineers were never rehired by BART and have instituted a court suit.

Whatever the nature of the grievance, if refusal defies common sense, the professional employee in particular feels slighted, impotent, and unsatisfied. Moreover, as the BART engineers found, he may discover that bucking the system invites catastrophe.

Job security

The fear of layoffs among white-collar and professional employees has increased greatly in recent years. There are many contributing factors, but the most important are probably the widespread layoffs of engineers and other white-collar workers that occurred in the early 1970s and the continually poor job market for (and, hence, oversupply of) recent college graduates.

Employees at professional levels used to be encouraged to believe they were a valuable talent pool and a part of the management team. It has come as a shock to them to realize that they are no longer as sheltered from the effects of general economic declines as they once were. They can be fired for any reason (except, ironically, for union activities—these are protected by law). Notice, severance pay, continuation of company-paid health and life insurance after separation, company assistance in locating new employment, all of these benefits are con-

[6] See John T. Edsall, *Scientific Freedom and Responsibility* (Washington, D.C.: American Association for the Advancement of Science, 1975), p. 37.

ferred solely at the discretion of the company. Frequently, policies in these areas are inadequate. And unlike laid-off blue-collar workers, professional employees have virtually no chance of being recalled.

This situation is unfortunate even if the person who is fired is professionally incompetent. But when incompetence is the excuse given for terminations in cases of personality clashes, square pegs in round holes, and economic exigency, then a reasonably sophisticated labor pool can determine for themselves that a colleague is being shafted. It takes only a few clear-cut examples to do a great deal of psychological damage. A union, while it could not prevent a layoff, would eliminate much of the arbitrariness otherwise possible.

A case in point is provided by the American Federation of Musicians, which represents symphony orchestra members, among others. For example, the union at the Detroit Symphony recently won a demand that dismissal proposals be submitted to a committee consisting of 15 musicians elected by the orchestra members. At least 10 must give their approval before management can dismiss a player. Furthermore, a union can negotiate the right of recall, a right that is virtually nonexistent for nonunion professionals.

REASONS FOR RELUCTANCE

There certainly seem to be a lot of reasons for professionals to join unions, and many have. How, then, can we explain the reluctance of some segments (e.g., scientists and engineers) to do so?

A major reason is that unorganized professionals frequently have rather limited knowledge of what unions are and what they can do. They tend to think of unions in terms of not too accurate blue-collar stereotypes: complex and rigid work rules, excessive reliance on seniority, narrow jurisdictional lines, dictatorial power in the hands of union leaders, and so on. They are unaware of the flexibility of collective bargaining and the legal safeguards that exist for protecting their right to influence internal union policies. In short, they need realistic models for professional unions.

No one group's problems are unique, even among professional employees. The questions that are being asked today were asked and answered years ago by other professionals; it is an ongoing, evolutionary process. The renowned educator John Dewey held membership card No. 1 in the American Federation of Teachers, and the highly respected journalist Heywood Broun helped found the Newspaper Guild.

More recently, such professionals as Theodore Bikel, Charlton Heston, Walter Cronkite, and Ed Sullivan have been very active in the affairs of their unions. In the technical world, Albert Einstein spoke in favor of unions for "intellectual workers" 30 years ago. Nobel laureates Linus Pauling and Harold Urey recently wrote in support of unionization among scientists.

Unionization of a particular group may be delayed, but the general outcome is inevitable. There are, after all, inherent differences of interest between employers and those they employ. While they have a common general goal—the success of the business—they often have very different views on specific issues. A prime example should suffice: a major source of income for the employee, his salary, is an expense for the employer. The latter will want to minimize the same flow of dollars that the employee seeks to increase. No matter how enlightened the compensation policy, one is ultimately faced with the basic decision of how to divide limited available dollars between employees and stockholders.

There are only two ways to reconcile the differences, economic and otherwise: either unilateral management decision making or some kind of bilateral, employer-employee system for reaching compromises. (Individual bargaining, philosophically most acceptable to professionals, is totally unrealistic for most employees of large organizations.) It is inevitable that management decisions will not always parallel the personal interests of affected employees. Since employees lack strength as individuals, the logical approach is to join together to support each other.

RESULTS OF UNIONIZATION

Let's take the bad news first. At the very least, and perhaps most important, management flexibility will be reduced. The union will quickly seek to negotiate a contract, and the company is bound by law to bargain with it in good faith. In the course of such negotiations, many areas that were formerly in the exclusive domain of management will become negotiable.

It is probably worthwhile to stress my major caveat—one must not overgeneralize, especially when dealing with unions of professionals. It is fair to say that such unions will be concerned with salaries and fringe benefits. However, in some cases, these may already be at satisfactory levels, so that the main emphasis will be on other areas. In still other instances, the general level of benefits may be satisfactory, but the distribution may be at issue (e.g., a desire for more vacation with very little pressure for major salary increases). In any event, the union's priorities will vary tremendously from place to place, depending almost entirely on local conditions.

The biggest noneconomic change would probably be the establishment of a bilateral grievance system. Quite obviously, this would significantly affect management flexibility. It might require a major overhaul of personnel practices. The union becomes the official representative of that group of employees, and as such, the union, not the individual employee, must be dealt with. Indeed, it could be illegal to make a deal with a particular employee without the knowledge and acquiescence of the union.

Where abuses were rampant in the past, the

union might be interested in having the contract contain sections dealing with overtime (number of hours, as well as extra pay), type of allowable work, relocation policies, and the like.

Uniquely professional concerns will be of interest to the union, too, reflecting the desires of the members. These will vary from one group to another but might include requests for additional technical or supporting staff, tuition refund plans (or improvements thereto), formal peer input to promotion or termination decisions, and the like.

Besides less flexibility in dealing with professional staff, management will probably also face higher costs. In addition, time will have to be spent on contract negotiation and administration. Still, all of the changes can be (and have been) adjusted to.

Unionization need not be all bad for management. A few years ago, the Conference Board surveyed several companies that had recently been involved in successful organizing drives.[7] About 40% saw some advantage to the company as a result of the unionization of their white-collar employees. Some of their comments are indicative:

- ''The presence of the union has made the company much more sensitive in the handling of employee relations matters.''
- ''[It] forced us to formalize and administer properly a merit review program.''
- ''We gained insight into a group of dissatisfied employees. . . .''[8]

Improved worker morale may be the biggest benefit. The union helps employees regain the professional stature and pride that in recent decades were submerged beneath the corporate monolith. The individual union member does not have the freedom enjoyed by members of the learned professions in years past, but, by joining with his peers, he can once again participate meaningfully in decisions that affect his professional life. The results should be more productive, less dissatisfied employees.

CONCLUSIONS

We are dealing here with several rather fundamental assumptions:

1. The fraction of professionals who are employed by others will continue to grow.
2. In spite of similarities in educational background and mores, professional employees and those who employ them have inherently different viewpoints about many aspects of the job situation.
3. White-collar and professional employees will continue to be attracted to unions in ever-growing numbers.

There should be little disagreement with the first two points. As to the third, all trends point to the increasing organization of professionals. The most important factor is the growing size and impersonality of employing organizations. This will make the professional ever more remote from the center of decision making and will inevitably increase his frustrations. It is this professional malaise, rather than strictly monetary considerations, that in the long run will result in a union.

A progressive management will recognize that a unionization attempt at the very least indicates widespread employee discontent with existing conditions and that professional employees in particular desire a stronger voice in solving their problems. The union provides the employees with such a voice.

Should management be less than enlightened, then the union will at least fight to obtain for its members a greater measure of dignity and a larger share of the economic rewards.

---

[7] Edward R. Curtin, *White-Collar Unionization*, Personnel Policy Study No. 220, New York: The National Industrial Conference Board, Inc., 1970.

[8] Edward R. Curtin, *White-Collar Unionization*, p. 66.

Collective action and cooperation in the health professions

WILLIAM B. WERTHER, Jr., Ph.D., and CAROL A. LOCKHART, R.N., M.S.

Most labor-management relationships focus on how to "slice the pie of available benefits." Each side is so concerned about getting a larger slice that the size of the pie is overlooked. Too much effort is expended in a zero/sum arrangement in which benefits accrue to each side only at a cost to the other party. Health care employees obtain higher wages, for example, by forcing their employer to accept smaller profits or net revenues; administrative prerogatives are secured at the expense of less freedom for the health care professional. Efforts aimed at increasing surplus revenues would create more benefits for the health care organization, providers, and clients. This is not to suggest that administrators or employee representatives should allow the other to dictate contract or grievance settlements. However, in evaluating the employment relationship, it becomes obvious that the largest gains for health care professionals, their associations, *and* their employers are down the road of cooperation.

OBSTACLES TO COOPERATION

Unfortunately, mistrust and resentment often exist between employee representatives and administrators. When a state nurses association begins to actively represent its members through collective action, for example, administrators may sense a threat to their ability to manage or a rejection of their past efforts to aid the nurses. These feelings are typically coupled with stereotyped views of employee leaders and

Reprinted with permission from *Journal of Nursing Administration,* July/August, 1977. This article draws heavily from *Labor Relations in the Health Professions* by William B. Werther, Jr., and Carol A. Lockhart, copyrighted by Little, Brown and Company, 1976, and is published with their permission.

demands. Likewise, administrative reactions are seen as a rejection of employee rights and their leader's aspirations. Thus, the stage is set for an escalation of mistrust.

Once they believe a state association is interested in collective action, administrators often adopt an attitude of resistance. Through both subtle and direct remarks, they discourage employees from joining the association. If employee leaders have less formal education or less status than administrators, the latter exploit these differences in an attempt to relegate employee leaders to a subservient role. Attempts by employee representatives to carve out an area of authority within the institution are seen by administrators as an attack on their prerogatives. Rather quickly, it becomes impossible to discern causes from effects as each side acts and reacts.

People do tire of such games, and at some point someone attempts a reconciliation. No matter who initiates it, the other side is suspicious. After months or years of mistrust and open resentment, cooperative gestures are seen as deceptions. The initiator, once rebuffed, reverts to previous approaches. This reinforces the other side's suspicion that the original move was merely a trick. Labor laws and the need to deal with each other act as restraints upon further escalation of the conflict. However, when cooperation is attempted by *both* sides the reaction of each is often, "Why didn't we do this before?"

Admittedly, cooperation will not solve all employee-management problems, nor will it cure problems of ineffective administration. Nevertheless, both parties can benefit in many ways by assisting each other.

The barriers to cooperation are many. This article describes some of the obstacles that each side can put in the way of the other. If employee representatives and administrators can avoid creating these obstacles, mistrust and resentment can be prevented. It may then become possible to implement joint projects that benefit all providers, improve the delivery of health care, and win public support.

PRECAUTIONS FOR MANAGEMENT

Health care administrators who seek the benefits of cooperation often infringe certain labor laws in their zeal to change the labor-management atmosphere. Regardless of good intentions, it is still illegal (an unfair labor practice) for administrators to dominate a state association or labor union through financial or nonfinancial means. One hospital administrator, in an attempt to express her new-found spirit of cooperation, decided to give the organization's vending machines to the machinist union. The machines had depreciated to their residual scrap value and were essentially valueless. Furthermore, she saw no need to provide a food-vending service to employees if the maintenance employees' union would do so. The union agreed, and the hospital signed the machines over to the employee organization. A disgruntled member of a professional association complained to the National Labor Relations Board, and management ended by capitulating to a charge of domination because the act of giving the machines to the union was, technically, a labor law violation. Had the administrator *not* immediately conceded a technical violation of the labor laws, a considerable amount of money might have been spent on legal fees to fight the case—to fight to be cooperative with the union. Therefore, *any* cooperative action by management must be viewed against the backdrop of the labor laws.

Besides the basic laws, there are three concerns that *every* supervisor, *every* middle-level administrator, and *every* top administrator should be made aware of before attempting to cooperate with an employee organization.

1. Survival needs of the union.
2. Political needs of the union.
3. Precedent-setting practices.

Survival needs

Every organization—hospital, nursing home, and especially professional association—has survival needs. These needs can be categorized into those of the organization, its leaders, and its members.

Leaders and members realize that the state association provides them with many satisfactions. It gives members a common identity and it facilitates their professionalism. To the leader it is a source of status, pride, and recognition. Attempts by administrators to undermine the association become a personal threat to its leaders and members. Thus, when administrative actions lead to a loss of professional prerogatives or a rejection of the association's request for automatic dues deductions, reaction is strong. Why would professionals endure a strike for an issue like dues deductions? For much the same reason that administrators sometimes work 80 hours a week during a strike: dedication to their organization. The organization is a major source of satisfaction for employees, professionals, and administrators alike. When the organization is threatened, its members respond. Directors of nursing and other administrators, therefore, should consider decisions in terms of their impact on the employee organization.

The role of employee leaders also tends to be overlooked by administrators. When a change is to be implemented, administrators sometimes fail to advise the appropriate association representatives. The matter may be nothing more complex than a temporary schedule change. But if the association leaders are not consulted, and if members then check with them, resentment of this administrative indifference (that is, lack of consultation) can create problems. To assert leadership (and to obtain the recognition the employee leaders think should be forthcoming), the leader may file a grievance over a contractual technicality. (For example, if the director of nursing changes the schedule, the grievance may state that the director violated the scheduling provisions in the contract.) Administrators, not realizing that the action unintentionally undermined the employee leader's position, cannot understand why the association is so uncooperative. Likewise, the association leader cannot understand why the director is so indifferent to the leadership role of the association officials.

This does not mean that management must seek the association's approval for every action. If the object is cooperation, however, it is not furthered by unilateral decisions. Administrators should reinforce the association leader's position by informing her of planned changes before implementation begins. This allows the association leader to maintain credibility as a leader and makes it less likely that minor actions will be perceived as a threat.

The third survival need is that of the organization's members. This is the one area that most administrators recognize quickly. They know that if a disciplinary action is taken against an association member, the association will respond. The nature of that response can be influenced in several ways. First, any administrative action that is detrimental to union members should be explained, and the explanation should be substantiated with witnesses or documentation. Second, if the supervisors explains the reason for the action to the appropriate employee leader before implementing it, the action will be less threatening to the leader and to other members. Third, if good documentation always precedes administrative actions, the association official is less likely to file a complaint to determine whether the action is justified. Association leaders will sense rather quickly that management can prove its case; otherwise it would not take such actions.

Administrators at all levels must consider the survival needs of the association, its leaders, and its members *before* taking action. Failure to do so breeds mistrust between the association and management.

Political needs

An employee association, even one of professionals, is a political organization. Its leaders are elected officials who retain their position (that is, survive) by winning the support of their constituents. This can lead to a variety of situations that an administrator would label as illogical at first glance. Grievances are filed when it is obvious that management is right, or the association strikes for a minor point in contract negotiations. Underlying political considerations may be the true cause of such acts. Possibly, the association leaders need to demonstrate that they support every member. They may need to use power to assure others they are still in control. Even more simply, employee leaders may be merely reflecting the wishes of their constituents.

The standard administrative response to "irrational" moves is often paranoia: "The association is trying to create trouble again." It is much more probable that the political realities of the association are forcing its leaders into such moves. Generally, even professional associations with union-like goals do not harass management intentionally except in response to an administrative action that is considered ill-advised.

Precedents

For political and survival reasons, the association must represent its members. Much like a good defense attorney, the association tries to win for its clients. Employee leaders will sometimes admit that they knew a member was wrong but feel that each member deserves the best defense possible. Nowhere is this more evident than in a discharge case. When one member is discharged, other members watch the association's response. The leader's credibility is at stake. If the association appears indifferent to the plight of the discharged member, other members may lose faith in the association or in its leaders. Therefore, the association leaders must put on a defense—even if it is obvious that the member was wrong.

What can harm the administrator in such a situation is not the fact that the association goes through the defense motions; instead it is the administrator's past practices. If the violation for which one employee has been discharged led only to a written warning in a previous case involving another employee, the association can argue that the employer has waived the right to fire wrongdoers for that offense. Even if the top administrators do not accept that argument, most arbitrators are impressed by it. It is usually judged unfair to fire one worker for a given offense when others have received lesser penalties for similar infractions.

It is imperative that management develop and follow a uniform personnel policy. When they make exceptions—and they should do so rarely—administrators must emphasize to the association's leaders and members that the case is exceptional and not a waiver of administrative prerogatives.

Cooperation is much more likely to succeed if the employee-management environment is one of fair and consistent treatment. When discipline and other actions by employers appear capricious, the reaction of employee organizations is universally one of hostility and caution, not cooperation.

PRECAUTIONS FOR THE ASSOCIATION

In attempting to cooperate with administrators, some employee leaders lose their positions. If the members think there is a "sweetheart" arrangement between top association and administrative people, the employee leader will be replaced with a "firebrand." It does not matter what the *actual* relationship is. If it *appears* too cozy, members will feel betrayed.

Thus employee leaders must constantly pursue and *appear* to be pursuing the members' objectives.

Aside from this potential problem for the leader, the association has little to lose by cooperation. Success for the health care employer carries with it the implied agreement that all employees will share in the benefits. Any administrator sensitive to the political needs of employee associations will grant association leaders much of the credit for improvements in the work environment. If cooperation is used by administrators merely to further the goals of the facility and not the employees, the resulting harassment from association members will destroy the basis for cooperation. If administrators violate the contract, even with the tacit approval of the association, in order to obtain better performance, the association can always file a grievance. If cooperation improves the facility's financial health, the association may use the negotiation process to obtain its share. It seems, therefore, that state nurses' associations and other employee groups are in a good position to assure themselves the fruits of cooperation. Besides, any management sophisticated enough to overcome years of emotional "hangups" about employee groups is likely to be mindful that a sincere effort at cooperation is the only meaningful alternative to threats of strikes and other disruptions.

Nevertheless, a lack of sensitivity on labor's part to the situation faced by managers can undermine attempts at cooperation. Association leaders and members must be aware of the following:

1. Management's need for efficiency and effectiveness.
2. The image held of collective action by administrators.
3. Precedents set by practice.

Administrative efficiency and effectiveness

Administrators are evaluated, rewarded, and promoted largely on the basis of how well they perform. This means that administrators must be efficient and effective. Efficiency means accomplishing objectives with a minimum of resources and in a timely manner. The desire for efficiency can cause administrators at all levels to react negatively to work rules and jurisdictional standards supported by employee organizations. Administrators are uniformly indifferent to *who does what*. They are more concerned with *what gets done*. In the pursuit of efficiency an administrator may assign a member of the bargaining unit to do some task that should be performed by an employee with a different job description. At times supervisors may themselves do work that should be handled by a member of a specific employee association or union. Employee leaders see such actions as administrative indifference to the labor agreement. However, the supervisor may simply be pursuing goals of efficiency and not intentionally violating the agreement.

If the transgression of the contract is important, a grievance should be filed. If a grievance is being filed merely out of resentment, the employee leader should question the benefits of escalation. Escalation forces both sides into a defensive posture. Attention becomes focused on *how* things are done and not *what* is done, and efficiency suffers. If efficiency declines, there will be a decrease in the pool of resources available to be divided between professionals, workers, and the health care facility. Escalation also results in a strict interpretation of the rules, leaving little room for implicit agreements between administrators and employee leaders. When special circumstances do arise, a strict interpretation of the contract does not permit concessions. Naturally, there is a reduction in the level of enjoyment associated with the work environment.

Effectiveness is more than just being efficient. An administrator may be very quick (efficient) to make decisions, but if he makes the wrong choice, the decision is ineffective. Ineffective decisions are never efficient, because they cause resources to be wasted. If they are forced to follow a literal interpretation of the contract, administrators may also be forced to select less effective solutions to problems— simply because of potential reaction to more effective alternatives. For example, if the most effective order requires a nurse to make an adjustment on a piece of equipment, the head nurse may hesitate to give that order because such work is not the nurse's duty. The less efficient and less effective solution might involve sending a requisition to the maintenance department. The labor agreement is followed to the letter, but organizational effectiveness is reduced. One such incident is irrevelant. When hundreds of minor decisions are made every day, however, and each is slightly suboptimal, efficiency and effectiveness suffer dramatically. This leads to smaller surplus revenues for wage increases, fringe benefits, holidays, and so on.

It is imperative that association officials acknowledge administrators' needs for efficiency and effectiveness without undermining the survival need of the employee organization, its leaders, or its members. Otherwise, the employer *and* the employees ultimately suffer.

Union image

By the time most potential health care administrators graduate from college they have formed an opinion of unions and employee associations. This attitude is often based on incomplete information and reflects the prejudices of parents, peers, and professors. Stories of union violence and corruption are generalized to state professional associations and other employee organizations. Strikes and professional prerogatives increase their negative image of these groups. Even reasonable collective actions are often distorted to substantiate administrative preconceptions. In the minds of administrators, professional associations and unions become merely another obstacle to be tolerated.

If the labor-management relationship is to

grow into one of cooperation, the professional association or union must change its image in the eyes of the administrators. The association must come to be viewed as a contributor to the organization's effectiveness. This is easy to postulate but difficult to implement.

The first step is for the association to evaluate its actions and reactions to administrative initiatives. When grievances are submitted, what is the motivation behind them? Is the association trying to right a wrong or is it merely retaliating against an inconsequential management action? Are association officials allowing political grievances to be formalized—this confirming management's preconceptions? Are terms sometimes put into the contract simply to limit administrative actions? Only association officials can answer these questions accurately. To work cooperatively with management, employee leaders must keep in mind management's goals of efficiency and effectiveness. If the association can further the objectives that labor and management have in common, its image will slowly change.

Second, a professional association or union should offer constructive suggestions for increasing the organization's effectiveness. Employees and employee leaders often see where changes or improvements could be made in the operation of the facility. A common mistake is to inform the supervisor responsible for the area. This may make the supervisor resentful, since suggestions are an implicit form of criticism. A suggestion system established *within* the association allows ideas to be evaluated in terms of how members would be affected. Suggestions that offer a real improvement in efficiency or effectiveness can be presented to top administrators by the employee leaders. Many suggestions may be unworkable for reasons unknown to their originator but those that do hold promise have the advantage of being supported by the employee organization. Thus, the association can help administrators do a better job. This should not be the association's

primary concern, but the establishment of a suggestion committee costs nothing and the employer's gains can be substantial. Astute negotiators will see that some of the savings arising from these suggestions accrue to employees in the form of better contract settlements.

If the benefits of a more enjoyable work environment and improved contracts are to be obtained, the employee association must minimize interruptions to management effectiveness and efficiency. At the same time, the employee organization should make constructive suggestions to the employer. Nothing in the labor laws require such actions, and many union leaders who have unsuccessfully tried to create a cooperative atmosphere would argue that such efforts are a waste of time. Nevertheless, what are the alternatives? Resentment? Open hostility? Who benefits from a belligerent environment?

Precedents

A final word of caution concerns precedents. If administrators are allowed to undertake an action prohibited by the contract, the association may lose the ability to prevent such action in the future. Extracontractual activities by administrators must be scrutinized by employee leaders. Should administrators violate the agreement or past precedents and the association fail to declare a grievance, the employer will have a defense against future grievances on the issue. Arbitrators are very sympathetic to the argument that no complaint was registered when the same action was undertaken previously. For example, suppose the agreement requires that all work schedules be posted a week in advance. One week the secretary fails to post the schedule until four days before it becomes effective. This was an oversight, and in an attempt to be cooperative, the union files no grievance. The following week the director of nursing is away at a convention and the schedule is not posted until three days before it becomes effective. Since this late posting interferes with the plans of several nurses, they tell the director that they will not report to work on Sunday as called for in the new schedule. And, since they did not get a week's notice, these nurses indicate that they can refuse to work a new day according to the contract. The director of nursing disagrees and argues the association waived its rights by not filing a grievance the first time the schedule was posted late. Although the final decision by an arbitrator may be in favor of the nurses, the director's argument will be considered and might control the final decision.

This does not mean that employee leaders should try to interfere with every administrative decision. But when a decision affects contractual rights, employee leaders should complain formally to protect those rights. The complaint may be filed with management and then conceded, as in the case of the secretary's error. However, when a critical issue does arise (for example, the second late posting), the union can show that it has not waived any rights.

There is a delicate balance between protecting rights and filing grievances simply to harass administrators. To avoid destroying cooperation and still maintain contractual rights, when filing the grievance, the union should explain the reason for the formal complaint and point out the need for protecting future rights. If the case at hand has no impact on the employee organization, the union promptly concedes the case. This illustrates to management that the union wishes to cooperate and at the same time puts the employee organization on record as not waiving its rights.

COOPERATION THROUGH CONSULTATION

Cooperation is largely a matter of consultation between the two sides. Most resentment arises because one party has not been informed of the motivations behind the other's actions. In such cases it is only reasonable that motivations will be inferred from past behavior. When the relationship between administrators and professionals is young, inferences are based upon previously held notions, which are too often misconceptions. Even in mature relationships, past experiences often underlie any questions about present actions.

Proactive vs. reactive stance

Each phase of collective action finds one party primarily on the defensive and the other primarily on the offensive. In organizing, the employee association takes the offensive. It is the organizers who decide when to solicit signatures or to request an election. Administrators are forced into a defensive or reactive role; they must react to the collective actions. Contract negotiations follow much the same pattern. The employee organization makes demands, and administrators are forced to defend their positions. In both organizing and negotiations, management can assume the offensive temporarily through careful planning. Well-conceived personnel policies coupled with fair treatment leave the collective action group few areas in which to take the offensive. Likewise, sound counterproposals can take the initiative away from the employee association in contract negotiations. When the association makes demands and management makes a counteroffer, the employee representatives must defend their original demand.

In contract administration the roles are reversed. Normally it is management that is on the offensive and the employee association is on the defensive. Management makes decisions and takes action. The association typically accepts the results or must oppose them by filing a grievance. In rare cases the employee representatives may gain the initiative by submitting positive suggestions. However, since management is responsible for the facility's operation, initiatives by employee representatives are often rejected.

These scenarios are based upon a traditional and reactive model of labor relations: one side acts, the other reacts. If the two parties engage in consultation before carrying out any action, their relationship can become proactive. This leads not only to bilateral commitment to the success of new undertakings, but it also facilitates cooperation, since each party understands the motivations underlying the other's proposed actions.

The proactive approach is applicable primarily to contract administration, although it can be applied to contract negotiations. If employee and employer representatives maintain open communications during the administrative phase of labor relations, they will be familiar with the topics to be negotiated before discussions begin. When each side knows the principal concerns of the other, surprises, which can lead to strikes, are minimized. If the two sides consistently practice consultation in the administration of the contract, they will cooperate more. When they are negotiating, they will be more able to compromise, each side realizing that the other is pursuing positive goals and not merely trying to undermine the other.

Consultation has other direct benefits. Managers find that the implementation of changes is met with employee support, not resistance. If the appropriate employee official is aware of a proposed change and the reasons for it, there is no need for the official to obstruct the project just to assert leadership. Participation modifies the perspective of those involved. When an employee leader can make suggestions that are accepted, a proposal becomes "our" idea and not just "management's." Through the informal organization—the grapevine—the employee leader can work with members on behalf of the change. The motivation to do so comes in large part from the leader's change in perspective. Like most people, employee leaders like to see "their" ideas implemented.

When employee leaders are on the inside of the management decision-making process, they have more information to offer to members. Such information serves to enhance the leaders' power and helps assure their reelection and control over dissident groups within the association, resulting in a more stable employee organization.

Thus, cooperation through consultation benefits the employer, the employee association, its leaders, and its members. It is truly a positive approach to labor relations. Unfortunately, misconceptions and past differences can make it difficult for either side to initiate cooperation.

IMPLEMENTING COOPERATION

Countless factors contribute to the mistrust that commonly exists between employee groups and management officials. To change the employment environment into a cooperative one is a difficult task. If the task is not undertaken, however, employer-employee relations can become an obstacle to the effective delivery of health care. Cooperation can provide new opportunities for giving better care to clients.

There is no one best way to undertake the long journey toward cooperation. Sometimes the first step is made when one side is in a desperate situation and needs a favor. When favors are granted, reciprocation is expected. If they are reciprocated, simple favors and requests for help may slowly create a cooperative relationship. However, one cannot wait for such opportunities, for there is no assurance that they will occur; furthermore, such opportunities do not guarantee a favorable relationship. Positive action is needed.

One technique already mentioned is for the employee association to make constructive suggestions to help administrators. Whether these ideas result from a formal suggestion system within the association or from observations of employee leaders does not matter. It is a positive step.

Another technique for increasing cooperation is labor relations training. Many organizations and employee associations undertake some form of training to inform supervisors and association officials of new changes in the contract. Usually these efforts are carried out independently. In the name of reducing grievances, management might suggest that the training be done jointly at management's expense. Since the nominal purpose is to train employees—both supervisors and workers—in the meaning of the contract, the training can properly be done at management's expense without constituting a labor law violation of domination. The employee association does not lose, since the training allows its officials to be paid while they learn instead of using their free time for instruction. Of course, the trainers include a representative of the employer and of the association; the purpose of the training is training, not indoctrination.

This joint training can provide several benefits. First, misinterpretations of the contract held by either side will not be perpetuated. Ideally the trainers can work out instructional plans together, and resolve misunderstandings before the training sessions start. Second, since association officials and supervisors are given the same presentation at the same time, grievances resulting from misconceptions are likely to be diminished. Third, if supervisors and employee representatives observe higher level association and management officials cooperating in the explanation of the contract, they have a model to follow when they interact.

The training may be nothing more sophisticated than allowing the chief employee representative and the chief management representative (the director of nursing or director of labor relations) to take turns reading and paraphrasing the contract. This permits lower level employee and management representatives to see that there is a single interpretation for each provision of the agreement.

Other joint efforts are possible. Clubs, interest groups, athletic leagues, and charity drives can be sponsored jointly. The primary object of such cooperative efforts is to provide each side with the experience of mutually satisfying interactions—interactions that allow each side to reassess its opinion of the other and build confidence in the possibility of teamwork.

LABOR RELATIONS PHILOSOPHY

Those who provide health services should attempt to develop a reasonable philosophy of labor relations. That philosophy must recognize the needs of all parties—workers, professionals, administrators, and clients. Some components of a labor relations philoslphy are listed below. Other dimensions should be added by each employee to reflect the unique relationship of his or her particular situation.

1. The survival of the employer is the paramount goal. Without the health care facility, the need for an employee organization is nonexistent.
2. Administrators at all levels must recognize the survival needs of the employee association, its leaders, and its members. All management actions should consider the implications of these survival needs.
3. Workers, professionals, and their leaders must respect the employer's need for efficiency and effectiveness.
4. Problem solving should be undertaken jointly with a pragmatic, not an ideological, outlook.
5. Cooperation is the most viable long-term strategy for all parties. It is the only means through which the delivery of health care is improved.

SUMMARY

The success of labor-management relations depends upon cooperation. To achieve cooperation, each side must view the relationship as one in which each can benefit by helping the other. The adversary tradition is strongly reflected in labor laws and in past practices. Overcoming this tradition requires overcoming stereotyped thinking, mistrust, and resentment. Employee leaders must realize that the more effectively management can manage, the greater will be the potential benefits to the employees. Likewise, management must look upon the employee association and its leaders, as allies, not enemies.

Management must not rush into cooperation with such vigor that it dominates the employee association or union. In dealing with the employee organization it is important for administrators to remember that, as an organization, it has *survival needs*. Likewise, its leaders and its members have survival needs, too. Administrative actions that threaten any of these will be met by strong resistance. Furthermore, an employee association is a *political* institution, and its leaders are politicians. Before evaluating actions by the employee organization, administrators should realize that the motivations may be solely political. Administrators should also realize that *precedents* can effectively change the intent of the contract. They should not permit variations from accepted policies without comment.

Employee leaders must be careful not to undermine their credibility with members by appearing too cooperative toward management. They must also be aware of management's desire for effectiveness and efficiency. Many actions that appear to be antiunion or antiassociation moves are simply attempts by the administration to make the facility more effective. Most administrators' image of collective action groups is generally unfavorable. An employee association can overcome this image only through a careful screening of grievances and through contributions to the well-being of the employer. Employee associations must be sensitive to the problem of precedents, too. Failure to protect contract terms may cause those terms to become inoperative.

If professionals, workers, and administrators are to develop a better working relationship, the framework in which they operate will have to evolve from a reactive to a proactive approach. Each side must consult the other before taking action. Unilateral action merely confirms past suspicions and negative images held by the other side.

Affirmative action and nondiscrimination

MELINDA W. GRIER

INTRODUCTION AND BACKGROUND

Affirmative action, equal opportunity, and nondiscrimination are terms heard frequently both in the media and in discussions with managers and administrators. However, the legal requirements to provide affirmative action and equal opportunity are often misunderstood or poorly implemented. Because health care providers today have federal and state obligations to follow nondiscrimination regulations, prudent managers and administrators should be familiar with the concepts and practices needed to fulfill these obligations.

Although our concern with legislation focuses on recent laws and regulations, federal civil rights legislation was initially adopted during the post–Civil War Reconstruction era. However, by the end of the nineteenth century, Supreme Court decisions had nullified much of its potential strength. It was not until the famous *Brown v. Topeka Board of Education* (347 U.S. 483) decision in 1954 that the

Supreme Court reestablished the framework for current civil rights laws. The civil rights movement of the 1950's and early 1960's resulted in the Civil Rights Act of 1964, from which most of the current regulations and obligations regarding nondiscrimination have been written. The initial intent of the Act was to prohibit discrimination on the basis of race, religion, or national origin. Since that time certain prohibitions of discrimination on the basis of sex have been added and new legislation has been passed to deal with discrimination based on age, handicap, and veteran's status.

In addition to federal laws, states, counties and municipalities have passed similar and, in some cases, broader laws prohibiting certain types of discrimination. Although the wording may vary considerably, most of the laws require that practices be utilized which provide equal opportunity for success to persons participating in certain activities without regard to their race, sex, or membership in other protected groups. Except in specific instances, e.g., court-ordered remedial action resulting from past violations or demonstrated state interest, the laws require no preferential treatment but merely proscribe discrimination on certain bases or require action to be taken to increase applicant pools to be more representative of population groups. Nondiscrimination legislation falls into three categories: (1) that which covers virtually all employers (Title VII), (2) that which covers recipients of Federal financial assistance (Title VI; Title IX, Section 504), and (3) that which applies to businesses, agencies, or governmental units having contracts with the federal government (Executive Order 11246, Section 503, Vietnam Veterans Readjustment Act).

Although the wording of these laws may vary, in general they require that practices be utilized which provide equal opportunity for success without regard to various factors (age, sex, race, handicap, etc.) to all persons participating in certain activities. Only in certain specified instances do some of the laws re-

quire, or even allow, actions that could be considered preferential treatment. In fact, the purpose of equal opportunity legislation has been to assure that all people receive equal consideration for employment participation in programs or receipt of services regardless of other factors not related to their qualifications. Because of its history the United States contains many examples of groups whose civil rights have been ignored, and it nas been necessary to pass legislation to enforce what is guaranteed to all by the Constitution.

Both employment and treatment of patients are covered by equal opportunity/nondiscrimination laws. Therefore it is important that everyone who supervises or hires employes or who provides services for patients be familiar with the requirements of these laws.

THE LAWS
Title VII of the Civil Rights Act of 1964

Title VII prohibits discrimination in hiring and/or any other employment practices on the basis of race, color, religion, sex, or national origin by all employers having fifteen or more employees, educational institutions, state and local governments, employment agencies, and labor organizations. The federal government requires that certain employment records be kept and that a biennial report be on file.

Equal Pay Act of 1972

The Equal Pay Act prohibits discrimination on the basis of sex in the payment of wages, including fringe benefits, by all employers.

Executive Order 11246 as amended by 11375, Revised Order #4

All contractors and subcontractors holding contracts of $10,000 or more are prohibited from discrimination on the basis of race, color, religion, sex, or national origin in all phases of employment. All contractors and subcontractors with fifty or more employees or with contracts of $50,000 or more must develop and maintain an affirmative action plan.

Section 503 of the Rehabilitation Act of 1973

All contractors and subcontractors with contracts for $2,500 or more are prohibited from discriminating on the basis of physical or mental handicap in the employment of an otherwise qualified person. All contractors and subcontractors holding contracts of $50,000 or more are required to prepare and maintain an affirmative action plan for handicapped individuals.

Age Discrimination in Employment Act of 1967 with 1978 Amendments

The regulation for enforcement of the act with the 1978 amendments will be issued before January 1979. However, provisions of the bill and testimony during its passage indicate the general requirements of this law. It prohibits discrimination against persons over 45 and prohibits the establishment of mandatory retirement for persons under 70 years of age with a few exceptions (highly paid managerial staff and, until 1982, tenured college and university professors).

Vietnam Veterans Readjustment Assistance Act of 1974

All contractors and subcontractors with contracts of $10,000 or more are prohibited from discriminating against disabled or Vietnam-era veterans. All contractors or subcontractors having contracts of $50,000 or more and fifty or more employees must prepare and maintain an affirmative action program for disabled or Vietnam-era veterans.

Section 504 of the Rehabilitation Act of 1973

Section 504 of the Rehabilitation Act of 1973 prohibits discrimination on the basis of mental or physical handicap against qualified persons in programs receiving federal financial assistance. Because this assistance includes Medicare and Medicaid programs, most medical facilities are covered. In addition to a requirement that employers must make reasonable[1] accommodation to handicapped employes, hospitals are required to provide effective means of communication with hearing-impaired patients in emergency care situations and to provide auxiliary aids necessary to allow prospective patients to benefit from the services.

Other laws

Other federal equal opportunity laws prohibit discrimination in educational programs. Title VI of the 1964 Civil Rights Act prohibits discrimination on the basis of race, color, or national origin in federally assisted educational programs. Because of federal student financial aid, virtually all colleges, universities, and health care training institutions are covered by Title VI.

Title XI of the 1972 Educational Amendments to the Civil Rights Act extends the prohibition to discrimination on the basis of sex. In addition, nursing, medical, and allied health educational institutions that receive assistance under the Public Health Service Act are also prohibited from discrimination on the basis of sex.

State laws and municipal ordinances often prohibit discrimination on various grounds in employment. In addition, many public hospitals or hospitals receiving state financial assistance are required to provide services on a nondiscriminatory basis.

AFFIRMATIVE ACTION TERMS

affirmative action plan An operational plan designed to achieve a work force representa-

---

[1]In determining what is "reasonable" compliance, agencies will evaluate the financial impact of the accommodations on the recipient to assure they do not provide undue hardship on the program.

tive of the diverse characteristics of the available population. An affirmative action plan is required of certain government contractors and if so required must meet the standards of Executive Order 11246, revised 11375, as augmented by Revised Order #4.

affirmative action organizational unit A group of jobs to be considered together for purposes of affirmative action analysis. Examples of an affirmative action unit might be intensive care and cardiology units or emergency care units. Each employer may establish affirmative action units based on organizational similarities and size, so that each unit will be a workable unit and data derived from analysis will be useful in setting goals.

work force analysis A display showing the breakdown of the work force by sex and race for each affirmative action organizational unit and often by salary levels or rank within organizational levels.

availability data The estimated availability of qualified persons for each position by race and sex; shown as the estimated percentage of the total qualified persons available. Availability may be determined from national, regional, state, or local statistics for a given job or profession, if available, or from general census figures of work force. The use of national, regional, state, or local figures should be determined by the scope of the job search for any given position or the majority of positions.

utilization analysis The comparison of the employer's work force by organizational unit, and often levels within the unit, to the work force that would be expected if projected from the availability data. For example, if a unit had 100 employees and the availability data showed that 3% of the available work force were Native American, a representative work force would have three Native Americans in the unit. If, however, there was only one Native American, the utilization analysis would show Native Americans underutilized by two. For most purposes any underutilization greater than .50 is considered significant.

goals and timetables Using the past work force turnover rate, goals and timetables establish hiring goals and the timetables for those goals necessary to eliminate the underutilization of women and minorities. For example, if (1) in a salary range of $18,000 to $25,000 eight blacks would need to be

hired to correct an underutilization, (2) there is, based on past experience, an annual estimated employe turnover of twenty, and (3) blacks represent 10% of the work force, a goal of two positions per year would be expected and could eliminate underutilization in 4 years. The employer may establish higher goals and shorter timetables than could be expected, but the use of unrealistic timetables can lead to a false sense of failure and future compliance problems. In contrast, unrealistically low goals will not eliminate the problem, may lead to a sense of false accomplishment, and may leave the employer open to charges of failure to make a good faith effort.

problem-oriented analysis The analysis of problems that may have caused past and present underutilizations.

action-oriented program Active plans designed to remedy the problems discovered in the program area analysis.

applicant flow data Breakdown by affirmative action classes of all applicants for all positions and subsequent breakdowns at each stage of the hiring process: qualified, not qualified, considered, interviewed, hired.

IMPACT ON PROCEDURES

Affirmative action laws relating to employment do not spell out the types of procedures that must be used. Instead, they are result oriented, establishing rules and using work force composition to evaluate compliance. This provides agencies with a great deal of flexibility to determine what procedures will help them recruit, hire, promote, remunerate, and terminate in a nondiscriminatory manner. However, certain procedures have become common practice or are often recommended for use to help ensure compliance.

Recruitment and hiring

The nature of the recruitment for any position depends on the goals that have been established for that position, the recruitment necessary to locate a person with requisite skills, and, of course, the money available to recruit. Recruitment may be national, regional, statewide, local, or internal. However, if the level of recruitment has been inadequate to meet the affirmative action goal for that position or the unit in which it is included, a more limited recruitment effort than in the past could be viewed as a lack of commitment to achieving one's goals.

Once the level of recruitment is determined, notices should be disseminated in a manner designed to create an applicant pool that would include qualified persons who would help meet affirmative action goals. This might include advertising in minority magazines or newspapers, posting notices at a YWCA, or sending job vacancy announcements to the local organization representing handicapped individuals. In addition, job notices and advertisements should include statements of nondiscrimination and/or equal opportunity/affirmative action policies.

Hiring procedures also should be designed so they are nondiscriminatory. A job description should be developed so that employers and applicants both have a clear idea of the job responsibilities. All applicants should be evaluated on the basis of the skills needed to perform the responsibilities, or bona fide occupational qualifications (BFOQ). It is important that all qualifications be reviewed to assure that they are actually needed to perform the job duties and not that they are merely assumed, or historically considered, to be needed. Frequently those involved in hiring are concerned that the most ''qualified'' person will not be a person who can get along with co-workers or possess certain social traits. If the ability to work with others is necessary to satisfactorily perform the job, it would become a BFOQ. However, if the assumption that the applicant is not able to work with co-workers is based on the person's sex, race, handicap, etc., that is prohibited discrimination and is illegal.

It is important to ensure that all applicants are evaluated equally. Thus the same standards should be used to evaluate all applicants; likewise in interviews, applicants should be given an equal chance to be evaluated. To do this many employers use one set of questions which they pose to all applicants to provide a comparable basis on which to compose responses. Applicants may then be evaluated and the employer may choose the successful applicant based on the hiring criteria.

Promotion, salary, and termination

Equal opportunity laws extend to areas of promotion, salary, and termination. In these areas equal opportunity requirements merely underscore the need to base decisions on performance and to document those decisions. The requirements do not limit the rights of management to determine the criteria for promotion and termination or to establish salary levels. They do require, however, that the criteria be applied equally to male and female, nonwhite and white, nonhandicapped and handicapped, veterans and nonveterans, and people of all ages. In order to accomplish this, many employers have developed written criteria for employment decisions. However, such criteria are not required. It is important that all related employment actions be reviewed in light of performance and to assure that performance is strictly interpreted to mean the activities necessary to perform the job tasks and not other related but commonly associated criteria, for example, the use of accrued sick leave to take care of a sick child, the use of nonwhite idioms, cultural variations in mannerisms.

Grievances arising from promotion, salary, and termination often surround three actions:

1. Promotion of white, able-bodied, young males over other workers with equal or greater seniority or responsibilities. Even in traditionally female professions men often are promoted more quickly than women, because men may be stereotypically considered as more able to assume leadership roles.
2. Jobs that essentially have the same job responsibilities are sometimes given dif-

ferent titles and receive disparate salaries. Housekeepers and custodians are often differentiated merely by title and salary.

3. Similar actions may result in termination for one employee and not for another. For example, two workers repeatedly arrive late to work with hangovers. One worker, a young white male, is teased and receives sympathy for "feeling his oats." A second worker, a middle-aged Native American, is fired because his employer is concerned that he may be becoming an alcoholic. Although an employer may terminate an employee who is often tardy, equal standards must be applied to all employees.

Employee benefits

Health insurance, life insurance, retirement, vacation, leave, and all other employee benefits must be offered nondiscriminatorily. Definitions of nondiscriminatory practices have been the most difficult to define in provision of health care and retirement benefits for men and women.

In a recent case, *Los Angeles Water & Power Dist. et al v. Marie Manhardt et al* (Dkt. No. 76-1810, April 25, 1978), the U.S. Supreme Court ruled that it was discriminatory to require women to make larger contributions to a pension plan in order to receive equal benefits to men.[2] A similar case in which the State of Oregon required equal contribution of men and women employes as members of a retirement fund in which women received lower benefits than men was ended by a consent judgment in Circuit Court subsequent to the *Manhardt* decision. In that case, *Henderson et al v. State*

of Oregon, the state agreed to equalize benefits for all employes.

Another area that has generated considerable controversy and equal confusion is maternity leave and pregnancy benefits. Recent court cases have changed interpretations in this area. In the famous *Gilbert v. General Electric* decision (429 U.S. 125 [1977]), the Supreme Court ruled that employee health insurance policies that do not provide benefits for pregnancy and maternity are not in violation of Title VII.

To overcome this controversial decision, the 1978 Congress passed new legislation[3] establishing that discrimination on the basis of sex included discrimination on the basis of pregnancy, requiring that pregnancy benefits be comparable to benefits for all other temporary disabilities. The bill also prohibits the establishment of arbitrary time limits within which pregnant women must be considered disabled.

In subsequent opinions the Supreme Court has ruled that women granted maternity leave must regain their seniority when they return to work under Title VII if men also regain seniority after leaves for temporary disabilities. Institutions covered by Title IX are required to provide benefits for pregnancy equal to those for other temporary disabilities under that Regulation. The Regulation specifically states that pregnancy and related conditions shall be treated as other temporary disabilities. If health insurance coverage and leave are available for other temporary disabilities they must also be available for pregnancy and related conditions. In addition in the State of Oregon a 1977 law required that all public employers provide such benefits to their employees.

AFFIRMATIVE ACTION—A MANAGEMENT PERSPECTIVE

Affirmative action puts additional requirements on management. However, if one looks at these requirements, most are procedures al-

[2]The Court found that although women as a group lived longer than men, the use of such a group constituted discrimination because individual women were discriminated against who did not fit the average description used. That is, any individual woman who does not live longer than the average life expectancy for women has been discriminated against solely on the basis that she is a woman.

[3]1978 Amendments to the 1964 Civil Rights Act.

ready used by competent managers. Certainly a thorough search to provide candidates most able to perform the job without consideration of other non–job-related information is in the employer's best interest. The clear documentation of employment records and the establishment of employment policies assist in other personnel activities. Affirmative action regulations leave the decisions regarding job qualifications and standards for comparison of employee performance to the employer. That is not to say that certain affirmative action requirements do not increase the level of accountability of managers to government, especially in two areas: record-keeping and grievance management.

Record-keeping. Aside from the affirmative action requirements of managers, increased record-keeping is one of the burdens of modern managers. It is a sound business practice to adopt other personnel procedures so that affirmative action requirements (hiring records, job descriptions, work force and utilization analysis) can be incorporated into other personnel data requirements. Record-keeping requirements are not specific, but adequate data should be kept to evaluate the nondiscriminatory nature of an employer's practices. In general, these records should include applicant flow data, salary and general personnel data, personnel evaluations, and documentation of decisions regarding hiring, promotion, and terminations. The length of time that records should be kept is under revision; 3 years from the last action is the generally accepted standard. Thus, if a decision to terminate took place on January 1978, but due to a grievance action regarding the termination the final action on the grievance did not take place until June 1978, related records should be kept through June 1981.

Grievance management. Employers of union-organized employees are usually familiar with the administrative requirements of grievance management. Where union contracts provide a mechanism for grievance resolution that may be employed for nondiscrimination griev-ances, some contracts may require the utilization of the negotiated grievance procedure for all grievances. Whether or not a preexisting grievance procedure exists, managers need to approach grievances in the proper manner with the intent of making grievances a useful personnel tool. The following are essentials of grievance management:

1. Quick informal resolution of grievances should be sought where possible. Timely resolution is less costly and reduces the tendency for polarization of positions.

2. Approach grievances from a problem-solving perspective. Although it is very natural to defend one's own behavior or the behavior of one's employees, a grievance points up a difference of values or a lack of communication that is hindering the effective operation of the agency or business. Defensiveness only increases the resolve of the grievant and tends to push grievants and respondents into adversary positions.

3. Ask the grievant what she or he would consider an adequate resolution to the complaint. Establishment of a proposed solution provides a basis for compromise and perhaps an immediate resolution. It is often surprising to a respondent how reasonable an acceptable resolution is.

4. Keep the grievance procedure as simple as possible. There is no one perfect system. A grievance procedure must be designed to complement the organization and the people implementing it. Stay away from the Perry Mason type courtroom setting. Even if each party has a trial lawyer to represent them, this style is far too complex and time consuming to be used effectively.

5. In all but informal cases keep records. If the grievance is not adequately resolved, it may become a court case.

Obtaining assistance

As in other areas of management, proliferation of regulations and theory has made it difficult for a manager or responsible employee to thoroughly know all the requirements of non-discrimination and affirmative action regulations. However, at many levels help is available. Within the organization personnel officers and affirmative action officers are often well versed in procedures and requirements. On the local level, city and county governments may have affirmative action or human rights' specialists who work to assist employers and employees with questions. Most states have trained specialists. Federal assistance should not be overlooked. The Departments of Labor and Health, Education, and Welfare have staff in their enforcement agencies who are often willing to provide assistance. A request for information and advice to a federal enforcing agency is not, as many people fear, considered an automatic signal to investigate the agency. Federal agencies understand the regulations they enforce can be complex and ambiguous. It should be kept in mind that requests for advice and interpretations are merely that and thus are not legally binding.

Consequences of noncompliance

Even the most diligent institution can be found in noncompliance due to oversight or the incorrect interpretation of a requirement. The willful attempt to circumvent the rules or the failure to be informed about requirements is far more serious. Although in determining whether a practice or policy is discriminatory, enforcing agencies and courts look at the impact or result rather than the intent; in determining the penalties for noncompliance, intent becomes an important factor. Frequently the institution's good faith efforts to follow both the spirit and the language of the laws or the lack of such effort affects the penalties assessed.

An institution can face serious penalties for violations of civil rights laws. Fines may be assessed against the institution. If the institution receives federal funds, those funds may be cut off or, more seriously, a federal contractor may

be debarred, preventing it from applying for future federal contracts as well. Institutions that are successfully sued by individuals or classes of individuals claiming their civil rights have been violated face substantial costs to cover back pay, cost of lost benefits, and punitive damages.

In addition to institutional cost liabilities, responsible individuals may be fined, found criminally responsible, or held liable. The U.S. Supreme Court has held that a school official could not be held liable

so long as they could not reasonably have known that their action violated . . . clearly established . . . rights, and provided that they did not act with malicious intent to cause injury.[4]

Implicit in this decision is the possibility that a person might be considered liable for a purposeful violation or one in which the person should have reasonably known that the law existed.

Other management considerations reinforce arguments for avoiding unnecessary violations that come about willfully or through ignorance: legal costs, time costs, employee morale. Health institutions are already experiencing unprecedented increases in their need for legal counsel. The costs of litigation and legal assistance for civil rights violations are often expenses that can be avoided by the use of adequate procedures or receipt of competent advice before a complaint is filed. Civil rights disputes also tend to be time consuming. Many violations have occurred because institutions failed to spend a few hours to learn compliance requirements, only to spend hundreds of person-hours over 2 or 3 years in resolving a complaint.

Finally, the effect of inadequate policies and

---

[4]*Imbler v. Pachtman,* 424 U.S. 409 (1974). The finding here is consistent with the early finding, *Wood v. Strickland,* 420 U.S. 308 (1975) which also deals with a violation by a school official.

procedures on employee morale can be disastrous. Good management procedures and fairness contribute more to an institution than a lack of compliance complaints. The development of procedures to assure that each employee is evaluated on the basis of her or his ability to successfully perform the duties of their position will benefit all aspects of the institution by placing the most qualified person in each position and rewarding him or her accordingly.

CONCLUSION

We are faced with a complexity of legal requirements, among which are those aimed at establishing fair and equitable employment and provision of services. Rather than to view non-discrimination compliance requirements as obstacles to be feared or ignored, with the help of qualified assistance compliance requirements can be used by good administrators as tools to achieve effective management.

Affirmative action program: its realities and challenges

GOPAL C. PATI[1] and PATRICK E. FAHEY

With the advent of governmentally-imposed affirmative action plans, it is hoped that minorities will receive a greater share of the national economy. However, companies operating under such plans face never-before-encountered problems in accomplishing their duties. Where does one find qualified minority employees? Must incompetents be hired to satisfy the specified goals? What is the cause of the hostility and resentment some recruiters receive when contacting potential minority employees? Add these questions to the simmering internal discontent of the company's own middle line supervisors and the end result can approach panic—a lost federal contract is an economic blow. The authors examine the situation faced by modern business in complying with federal minority hiring goals.

Managers in many business organizations are increasingly feeling the impact of public policy in many functional areas of management.[2] This has created an unusual fermentation of mixed feelings of hope and frustrations. It has been further compounded by the complexities and ineptness of the technological society which has demanded an unprecedented emphasis on

human resource utilization and development.[3] As a matter of fact, in the last several years it has been the area of manpower planning and development in general, and equal employment opportunities in particular, where the role of government has been increasingly observed.[4] Many government-initiated and supported programs to ameliorate poverty, unemployment and wastage of human resources have generated numerous kinds of anxieties, debate and bewilderment among educators and practitioners. The affirmative action program is that part of the public policy which has induced many organizations to undertake a more vigorous approach to reach out for members of the minority groups, who have been traditionally left out as a consequence of socio-economic deprivation. More specifically the objective here has been to provide them with training, jobs and an opportunity to share the fruits of our economic system, thereby enabling them to assimilate themselves better in the greater participating democracy.

The experience of the last several years in the area of affirmative action program has been characterized by learning, relearning, and ad-

Reprinted from *Labor Law Journal*, June 1973, *24*(6), 351-361, by permission of the publisher and the authors.

justing to things unheard of before, and clearly indicates the ineptness of many approaches to meet the great challenge. This has also required tremendous change in internal organization, values, climate and many organizational adjustments that were not thought of before. Consequently, the objective of this paper is not only to point out these changes and challenges, but also to point out the bumpy roads and detours that have been encountered by managers within the last several years. The issues to be examined will not only have implications for traditional personnel functions and practices but also for an unprecedented philosophical change that a corporation will have to undertake in order to keep up its commitment to the government and society.

LEGAL REQUIREMENTS IN PERSPECTIVE

On July 2, 1965, Title VII of the Civil Rights Act of 1964 became effective. Title VII "Equal Employment Opportunity" covers companies, labor organizations, and employment agencies. It *prohibits* discrimination because of race, color, religion, sex or national origin. During the 1971 Fiscal Year, the Equal Employment Opportunity Commission (EEOC), established by Title VII as the primary federal enforcement agency for the Civil Rights Acts, received 22,920 new charges. This was a substantial increase over the 14,129 charges received during the previous fiscal year.[5]

Under the 1964 law, the EEOC was limited to "informal methods of conference, conciliation and persuasion" unless the Department of Justice concluded that a person or practice of resistance to Title VII was involved. If the employers refused to accept the conciliation conditions, it was the individual victim of discrimination who carried the burden of obtaining an enforceable court order.

Under the recently signed "Equal Employment Act of 1972," the EEOC, if unable to secure an acceptable agreement within thirty (30) days, may bring action in a U.S. District Court. In addition to the above, other provisions of the "Equal Employment Act of 1972" include: coverage of stat and local government agencies, coverage of educational institutions, coverage of employers of fifteen (15) or more persons and labor unions with fifteen (15) or more members. The latter coverage is effective March 24, 1973.

The changes enacted by the "Equal Employment Act of 1972" will make increasingly stringent demands on employers in the future.

The other federal agency with jurisdiction in the field of employment discrimination is the Office of Federal Contract Compliance (OFCC). The authority of the OFCC is derived from Presidential Orders 11246 and 11375. These orders resulted from the government's decision to use its immense purchasing and regulatory powers to enforce equal employment opportunity.

A federal contractor, which term includes virtually every employer with a contractual, financial, or regulatory relationship with the federal government, is required to go beyond the prohibition to discriminate under the Civil Rights Act. The contractor must take "affirmative action," that is, results-oriented activities, not mere passive compliance.

The Office of Federal Contract Compliance has shifted the burden of proof from the government to the contractor and made eligibility for government contracts, services, financing, etc., dependent on compliance with OFCC guidelines.

Previously "Order #4" and currently "Order #14" set forth the components of an acceptable written affirmative action program, the basis for the compliance review.

An acceptable affirmative action program must include an analysis of minority and female participation in all levels of the organization to determine if minorities or women are being underutilized. Underutilization is defined as "having fewer minorities or women in a particular job category than would be reasonably expected by their availability."[6] Once the deficiencies are identified, the contractor must set goals and time-tables to which good-faith efforts will be directed to increase the utilization of minorities and women at all levels where deficiencies exist.

Despite the confusion caused by President Nixon's declaration against quotas in his renomination speech on August 24, 1972, it is improbable that the current method of goal setting will be abandoned. Though the difference between goal and quota might be subtle, it is generally accepted that a goal is a reasonable objective based on the availability of qualified people and a quota would restrict employment opportunities to members of a specific group without regard to qualification.

Emerging trend

The above material provides a framework and perspective for understanding the role of government in the personnel decisions and suggests the kind of direction a manager will have to take in reexamining his own values and then reconciling these with those of corporate philosophy and posture in the area of manpower planning and development. Furthermore, it definitely indicates the emergence of more stringent rules and regulations as an answer to the partial failure of many organizations in achieving the result-oriented goals of the affirmative action program. The spirit and the realities of the regulations require that it is not just the personnel manager or department that has to carry the burden, but line and operating managers will also have to do their share to achieve the company objectives. In other words, it does affect the whole organization.

More specifically, this means that the operating manager will have to do things that he has never done before and yet his organization is

demanding that he: (1) modify his recruitment, selection and testing policies; (2) vigorously and systematically reassess his training needs and criteria; (3) rechannel his training and developmental facilities and faculty; (4) become involved in better manpower inventory, manpower audit and control. He is further responsible for doing these things within the limitation of budget, without duplicating effort and coordinating better with the federal and state program without annihilating organizational climate. This requires not only broadening the knowledge base of individual managers, but also a serious effort in defrosting old ideas, relearning new developments and refreezing this newly learned knowledge to be useful in organizational growth. Thus, this challenge can only be met by more aggressive consolidation of managerial expertise supplemented by a strong corporate commitment.

RECRUITMENT

The immediate impact of AAP and the EEOC regulations has necessitated broadening the base of manpower supply. The basic objective of a traditional recruitment and selection policy has been to get the most qualified people at the least cost from those traditional sources which would be consistent with the organizational way of life in meeting the needs of the available job openings. The frequently used external sources have been (1) employee referrals, (2) private employment agencies, (3) walk-in recruiting, (4) newspaper ads, (5) major senior colleges and universities, (6) (to a lesser extent) vocational and correspondence schools. The traditional internal sources have been (1) transfer, (2) promotion, (3) job upgrading, without giving much attention to the potential of minority manpower within the organization.

Indeed, these sources once served their purpose in the past and still are doing so; however, in light of the developments in the area of reaching new elements of manpower these traditional sources may not be adequate. Consequently, the following sources are emerging as the kind of places that the employers are increasingly contacting to find people as required by the law:

1) Urban league offices,
2) Individual ministers and local religious organizations,
3) Minority-oriented media,
4) Senior and junior colleges with large minority populations,
5) Schools in the inner cities,
6) Local Spanish-American organizations,
7) Trade schools (more vigorously used now),
8) Women's organizations,[7]
9) Agencies dealing with correctional manpower.

As a consequence of this enlargement of the recruitment base, companies are definitely seeing more people to meet legal requirements as well as corporate ethic.

However, the rejection rate is usually high which can lead to many uneasy moments during a compliance review.

One company provided the following information which illustrates the difficulties that might arise as organizations appeal to minority-oriented agencies to fulfill their affirmative action commitments. During the effective period of an affirmative action program, the rejection rate for black female hourly applicants was 80 per cent while the rejection rate for white female hourly applicants was 68 per cent.

Though it certainly does not account for the entire disparity in rejection rates between black and white applicants, one statistic does give some insight into the depth of the problem employers are currently facing. In job categories for which a typing test meets the OFCC requirements for testing, the average black female applicants ($N = 70$) typed 30 WPM—approximately 25 per cent below the average typing speed of the remainder of the applicant population.

Furthermore, many agencies do refer people without any skills who miserably fail to meet even the minimum requirements of the company. When qualified individuals are available, frequent lack of transportation to a suburban plant location may prevent them from even appearing for an interview. In addition, many agencies are often speculative about their knowledge of job availability and send applicants to plants without any job openings, creating frustration for many individuals. Needless to say, there is a steep competition among the companies themselves to attract the best qualified personnel available. Consequently, some companies in the area are facing difficulty even in gaining entrance to an organization or institution which might have qualified minority manpower.

Confrontation with the new types of manpower and the sources has also caused reconsideration of the qualification of company recruiters. Today, a recruiter has to be a person who understands the minority culture; if not, at least make an attempt to understand and be sensitive to the needs of divergent groups. Several examples will clarify this point. In one instance a company representative went to a Spanish-American organization meeting to recruit. Ironically, no one spoke English and the entire meeting was conducted in Spanish. The recruiter could not communicate with the prospects and he returned to his office, of course, without recruiting anyone. The second example is of the case of a recruiter who went to a prominent black educational institution only to be asked "what the hell are you doing here?"[8] In another instance at a female dominated institution, a recruiter was asked about the real intention of the company for recruiting females. More specifically, a question such as, "Why, Honey, suddenly are you interested in us?" baffled the recruiter.

The implications of these examples are crucial. There exists a tremendous amount of mistrust about the real intent of the corporation in hiring minority groups. They are not sure about their future in these organizations where organizational posture of active recruitment is being considered as the ultimate consequence of severe government prodding and pressure rather than a genuine attempt by the organizations to hire them on an equal basis in any real sense. Accordingly, it is imperative that a recruiter know the sensitiveness of the issue, understand the dilemma, and is prepared to represent the corporation and carry on its objectives in spite of the realities of complex attitudinal crisis.

EMPLOYMENT TESTING

One employment procedure that has come under close scrutiny since the 1966 EEOC published guidelines is employment testing.

The field of industrial testing has grown substantially since World War II. Far too often, testing programs have been incorporated in the selection process based only on the "professional judgment" of personnel executives with little or no expertise, or on the recommendation of consultants motivated more by their fee than by the service they provide to industry.

Though the professionals in the field have for decades been recommending validation of personnel tests for their intended purpose, the widespread failure to establish criterion-related validity has resulted not only in the denial of employment to minorities but also in a waste of money. Contrary to generally accepted business practices, top corporate executives have been approving expenditures for testing programs that screen out people who would be productive employees and select people who will be marginal employees at best. Funds are allocated to production, advertising, research, etc., only if a reasonable return is anticipated but this requirement is lacking in the allocation of funds to personnel department testing programs in most cases.

In the U.S. Supreme Court decision *Griggs v. Duke Power Company*,[9] the Court adopted the interpretative guidelines of the EEOC that

tests must fairly measure the knowledge or skills required in a job in order not to unfairly discriminate against minorities.

Nothing in the Act precludes the use of testing or measuring procedures; obviously they are useful. What Congress has forbidden is giving these devices and mechanisms controlling force unless they are demonstrably a reasonable measure of job performance.[10]

The supreme Court decision in upholding the EEOC guidelines settled much of the confusion centered around test usage. A test can be used only if professionally developed and validated against job performance in accordance with the standards found in *Standards for Educational and Psychological Tests and Manuals*[11] and the burden of proof is placed on the employer in the area of business necessity.

Government contractors subject to the Rules and Regulations of Order #14 are required to provide an analysis of testing practices used in the past six months to determine if equal employment opportunity is being offered in all job categories. This will include the number of men and women acceptable on the test, the number of men and women not acceptable on the test, the same information for Negroes and Spanish-surnamed Americans, American Indians, Orientals and others when the group constitutes 2 per cent or more of the labor market or recruiting area for non-minority men and women. If there is a disparate rejection rate the test must be validated in accordance with the OFCC Testing Order (except for language arising from different legal authority, this order is the same as the EEOC guidelines).

Test validation will not bring about equal employment opportunity but will allow the employer to determine the relationship between the test and job performance and determine the significance of the test as a predictor of job performance for racial, sex or national origin groups. A test that has been validated against job performance, used with other selection or assessment tools, can significantly aid in the development and maintenance of an efficient work force. Such a test does not violate the civil rights law nor is it forbidden by the executive orders.

At this point it seems appropriate to discuss the validation study recently completed by one industrial organization.

A test battery was administered to 165 applicants over a four-month period. Though the battery included five, short, professionally-developed tests and the tests were chosen only after a thorough job analysis by an individual with a graduate degree and experience in both job analysis and testing, only one of the battery met the requirements for test usage.

The job is an inspection job that requires a background in electrical circuitry. The applicants selected for employment are enrolled in a company training school program for eleven days prior to actually starting on the job. During this period each employee is paid approximately $300.00. The selection tools used prior to the test validation study were considered unsatisfactory and the company considered it necessary to find additional tools to reduce the failures in the training school and the turnover on the job. (It should be noted that the training school evaluation was also validated against subsequent job performance by the Pearson product moment coefficient method with a coefficient of .4965.) The sample size was sixty-seven and the coefficient .4965 is significant at the 1 per cent level and satisfies the requirents of both the EEOC and OFCC.

The test was one of the Purdue Vocational Tests with two forms. In the study, Form B was used and Form A would be available for retesting purposes. Though the test carries a twenty-five minute time limit, this was disregarded and it was considered a work limit test.

The above clearly indicates that the classes protected by Title VII are adversely affected, that is, 48 per cent of Caucasians tested were subsequently enrolled in the training program

Number tested	Mean score	Race	Enrolled in training school
108	38.75	Caucasian	52
41	24.92	Negro	13
1	—	Oriental	1
1	—	American Indian	0
14	29.53	Spanish-American	5

but only 32 per cent of Negroes and 36 per cent of Spanish-Americans. As there is a disparate rejection rate, the test must be validated. The related criteria considered were (1) training school evaluation and (2) job performance criteria.

The training school evaluation consists of four paper and pencil tests on the subject matter taught during the eleven-day program. As noted previously the correlation coefficient between Training School Evaluation and job performance criteria is .4965.

I. Validity—test correlated to training school evaluation

$N = 67$
Mean $= 39.7$
Standard Deviation $= 10.2$
Correlation Coefficient $= .4877$

The Pearson product moment method results in a .4877 coefficient which is significant at the 1 per cent level and satisfies the testing requirements.

II. Validity—test correlated with job performance criteria

In this case the performance criteria consisted of a thirteen-week average percentage of a standard set by the Time-study Department.

$N = 38$
Mean $= 41.2$
Standard Deviation $= 10.05$
Correlation Coefficient $= .3788$ which is significant at the 5 per cent level and satisfies the requirements of the order and the guideline.

Therefore it is considered that the above meets the requirements set by the OFCC and EEOC. The authors are aware of the issues not considered above, that is, differential validity, etc. These were part of the study but not noted here.

III. Reliability

The method chosen was the split half estimate. The number in the sample was 158, none of which were retests. The scores of the odd number items were correlated against the even number items by the Pearson product moment correlation coefficient. The resultant correlation coefficient .857 was corrected by the Spearmen Brown formula to correct the reliability coefficient for the full length test to .9229, certainly in the acceptable area for continued test usage.

The test was validated in a period of economic downturn as clearly indicated by the number who successfully completed the training school (59) and the number included in the efficiency study (38). Nineteen employees were transferred out of the inspection group prior to the time meaningful proficiency data was available.

In view of the above, expectancy charts were constructed but a cutoff score was not determined until a later date and was based on "need" for inspectors as well as test score.

Though a complete explanation of the statistical data is not included here, it is obvious that the efforts generated to validate the test will not only reduce costs of failure and turnover, it will also be a more objective evaluation of prospective employees which is expected to increase the chances of minority group members to be selected.

There was not a disparate rejection rate for female applicants and the test validity study did not report validity correlation coefficients by sex.

PROMOTION

Promotional opportunities for minorities and women have been thus far a neglected subject primarily because of the initial emphasis on economic opportunities and its delivery system rather than vertical mobility within the organizational structure. Since some progress has been made in the employment opportunity area, the promotional aspect becomes the next logical step. This is a recent phenomenon and has been effectively dramatized in those organizations with a large population of female employees. An example of this was the recent EEOC charge against the Bell system for lack of females in management level jobs.[12] As a result of this charge and consequent negotiations, Illinois Bell has agreed to promote 2,500 women employees by 1974. On the national level, the AT&T system has agreed to promote 50,000 women into higher paying jobs, including 10 per cent into management posts. Furthermore, 6,600 members of the minority groups will be promoted into higher paying jobs, 12 per cent of them into management. Before specifying the regulations for government contractors in this section, one must pause to consider the significance of the AT&T agreement. If it took eight long months for AT&T to conclude an agreement such as this, other organizations traditionally less committed to equal employment opportunity must now recognize that they cannot ignore this enormous responsibility they are charged with.

The emerging government regulations require government contractors to insure that minority and female employees are given equal opportunity for promotion. Suggestions for achieving this result include (1) post or announce promotional opportunities, (2) take inventory of current minority and female employees to determine academic skill and experience level of individual employees, (3) initiate remedial training and work study programs, (4) develop and implement formal employee evaluation programs, when apparently qualified minority or female employees are passed over for upgrading and require supervisory personnel to submit written justification, (5) establish formal counseling programs and hold supervision responsible for having qualified and promotable minority or female employees in their organization.

The question of promotional opportunity is a twofold question.

One, minorities have been historically hired in the least desirable jobs, if hired at all. It appears that recruiting minorities for supervisory, technical and clerical jobs is a step in the right direction. It will only be after qualified minorities are on the payroll that the question of promotion will occur. Promotions of minorities must be made on the basis of qualification and potential, not on how well they measure up to some undefined profile that has no proven relationship to job performance. The problem in this area is also related to the structural condition of the economy and the labor market in particular. During recent years there has been little turnover in managerial jobs and new jobs have not been created as anticipated. This has been further compounded by the lack of manpower planning and developmental efforts within organizations and the lack of consideration for people with potential within the organizational reservoir, particularly women and minorities.

Two, qualified women have always been hired but often not on jobs that truly utilize their abilities. To alleviate this problem organizations must open up their training program for females with management potential. Failure to open the facilities to women or minorities will invite stringent rules and regulations imposed by governmental authorities. This means that the burden of proof will not only affect personnel people but other line personnel who will be required to spend a great deal of time in manpower inventory and audit. This will be an additional burden to the line organizational personnel who will have to spend more time and energy in developing human resources, a task for which they are seldom trained.

SUPERVISORY AND CORPORATE ATTITUDE

Perhaps it is the preoccupation with our own frustrations that emotionally isolates us from one another. This is particularly true for many supervisors and foremen who are frustrated because they feel that they are being "left-out" from some of the action of the great society. Affirmative action programs are a traumatic experience for them. To them government pressure signals the practice of dual standard; company commitment appears phony in view of his usual assumption of the role of responsibility without accompanied authority. His own values and his inability to understand the motivation of youth, women and black employees; his own changing neighborhood, his own employer's emphasis upon his reeducation for organizational mobility or survival; increasing economic demand on him to make any significant headway in the inflationary economy—all these baffle him and place him in a very defensive mood. Thus, when the personnel department tries to select people *in,* the foreman seems to select them *out.* The supervisory groups just do not believe that "equal employment opportunity" is really happening and do not believe that the company is serious.

An unprecedented amount of attitudinal modification on the part of the top as well as supervisory groups is necessary if this program has to succeed. A strong support system within the organization is a necessity if any significant progress is intended to be made. And that support system can be developed if,

1) A vigorous organizational renewal program is pursued (at least partially),
2) an organizational development effort is seriously launched,
3) company reassurance of supervisory job security is strengthened,
4) 100 per cent company commitment is demonstrated, and
5) reward is given to the supervisory and

various support personnel for their co-operation in an effort to create a better organizational climate.

If the above-mentioned is not being done (and in most cases we studied it is not), then we should not be surprised about the dubious impact of the action-oriented affirmative action program. First line supervisors in most instances do not know what it takes to make a good worker and performer out of an individual. Under this condition it is very unlikely that a person without training and previous work experience will survive in an organization once hired.

IMPLICATIONS

One, increasingly stringent goals and time-tables as well as increased pressure from municipal Human Relations Commissions will emerge in the future. Only with specific goals derived from factual analysis will a company be able to carry the burden of proof against the OFCC and sell the program internally to non-persuaded upper management.

Two, the proposed regulations to require federal contractors to keep records of employees' religious and ethnic background will eventually be adopted in spite of protests from groups that consider such regulations an invasion of privacy.

Three, federal contractors will find it necessary to appoint a full-time Compliance Officer. An effective affirmative action program requires a strong results-oriented executive, not the average impotent personnel executive nor the unqualified token minority, too often administering programs at present.

Four, a considerable amount of money has been spent in recent years to fund neighborhood agencies to train and assist minority group members to secure employment. Many of these organizations have failed miserably. In the future, business organizations must take an interest both financially and with their training

expertise, to ensure that qualified applicants are available from the sources an affirmative action program requires companies to contact.

Five, this indeed is a very sensitive area and will continue to be a serious problem for those organizations who are passive. A strong corporate commitment supplemented by an internal support system will have to be undertaken to live up to the real spirit of the equal employment practices.

Six, in light of our experience in the Midwest it is very clear that recruiting a few warm bodies to meet the legal requirements is not enough. The real spirit of the law requires reevaluation of corporate philosophy, changes in traditional personnel practices, modification of attitude of the operating managers and a type of complete involvement which will help minorities to retain a job and grow within the organization. Otherwise, more interesting laws will be forthcoming.

And finally, with regard to continued progress by minorities in all job categories, comparative data for about 31 million employees covered by 1970 EEO-1 employment reports indicate that since 1966, Negro employment as a proportion of total employment is up 1.9 per cent in total employment, 1.0 per cent among officials and managers, 1.2 per cent in professional category, 2.1 per cent among technicians, 1.9 per cent among sales workers and 3.7 per cent in office and clerical category. Spanish-surnamed Americans and women also showed increases in each of these job categories. While it can be assumed that the percentage gains would have been higher in a more dynamic economy, that is, minorities remain in a great many cases "last in," "first out," our conclusion is that minorities remain grossly underrepresented in the more desirable jobs in industry in spite of law and moral suasion. Furthermore, if we are to use our human resources to their potential, organizations must make total commitments to expend time, money, energy and expertise at least to the extent imparted to the other factors of production, for example, finance, plant acquisitions, technology, etc. If this is not done, the chances of living up to the real spirit of the burgeoning laws is very slim.

Notes

1. Gopal C. Pati was a senior assistant professor of industrial relations and management at Indiana University Northwest at the time of publication of this article. Patrick E. Fahey was manager of manpower planning and compensation with the Stewart-Warner Corporation.

2. Leon C. Megginson, *Personnel; A Behavior Approach to Administration,* Homewood, Illinois, Richard D. Irwin, Inc., 1972, pp. 244-245.

3. Elmer H. Burack and Gopal C. Pati, "Technology and Managerial Obsolescence," *MSU Business Topics,* Spring, 1970, Vol. 18, pp. 49-56.

4. Robert A. Gordon, *Toward a Manpower Policy,* New York, John Wiley and Sons,Inc., 1967, also see Garth, L. Mangum, *The Emergence of Manpower Policy,* New York, Holt, Rinehart and Winston, Inc., 1968, Elmer H. Burack, *Strategies for Manpower Planning and Programming,* New Jersey, General Learning Press, 1972.

5. Equal Employment Opportunity Commission, *6th Annual Report,* CCH, Chicago, June, 1972, p. 25.

6. *Federal Register,* Section 60-2.11, Vol. 36, No. 234, October 4, 1971.

7. For example, National Organization for Women, Professional Women's Caucus, Talent Bank from Business and Professional Women.

8. Descriptive adjectives have been omitted in the interest of scholarship.

9. *"Griggs v. Duke Power Company,"* Labor Law Reports, Commerce Clearing House, Inc., p. 15, 1971. (39 U.S.L.W., 4317)

10. Ibid.

11. *Standards for Education and Psychological Tests and Manuals,* Washington, D.C., American Psychological Association, 1966.

12. Chicago Sun-Times, Thursday, September 21, 1972.

Unit three □ STUDY GUIDE

1. Have a peer group member interview the Director of Nursing Service. What process is used to involve nurse management personnel in budget preparation? How is accountability delegated? What budget training is needed? What time frame is incorporated in fiscal preparation? Is a historical data base or zero-base approach used?

2. Interview the person who prepares the budget for your clinical unit. How do they go about it? What preparation did they have before doing it for the first time? What advice would they have for someone else preparing to do it? Are computer read-out sheets utilized on a regular basis? What satisfactions or frustrations are experienced related to budget preparation?

3. In conference, discuss what the major revenues and expenses are for several different types of units. Determine how the patient occupancy rates and lengths of stay affect revenues. Identify the major items of capital equipment.

4. How much are patients charged for the supplies you order and use? Make a price list of the supplies regularly used on your unit. Use the list in a staff conference as a means of identifying ways of eliminating unnecessary waste. Post the list in a strategic place after the conference.

5. Examine carefully the staffing of one or more units in an agency and determine:
   a. What is the agency philosophy regarding staffing and nursing care hours per patient?
   b. Who is responsible for staffing and how does this relate to staff salaries?
   c. Are the personnel satisfied with the staffing policies?
   d. Is the staffing ratio for clients adequate for quality care?
   e. Is continuity of care provided for? How does this affect the salary budget?

6. a. Survey a sample of professional nurses in an agency; collect data and analyze the prevailing attitudes related to collective bargaining.
   b. Find out from the top administrative persons of the agency what the management philosophy is concerning collective bargaining.

7. Survey a sample of physicians, residents, interns, and other health professionals in your agency. Collect data and analyze the prevailing attitudes of these persons related to unionism and collective bargaining.

8. If you had a grievance against an employment policy or an administrative action, what active steps could you take to change the policy or reverse the action?

9. Discuss the current status of nursing with someone active in the political aspect of nursing in your community (lobbyist, nursing association representative, grievance committee member, etc.). What changes have occurred in your community in the last few years as a result of increasing political activity of nurses nationally? Is this seen as a positive or negative influence in your community?

10. Have a member of your clinical group in-

terview the affirmative action officer or the person responsible for that program in your agency. What are the goals of the program? When was it implemented? How do the specifics of the program affect nurse-managers?

11. Randomly interview some staff nurse personnel. Determine their knowledge of and appraisal of the agency's affirmative action program.

INDEX